Kidney MRI: Preclinical Applications

Kidney MRI: Preclinical Applications

Edited by Sarah Brown

STATES
ACADEMIC PRESS
www.statesacademicpress.com

States Academic Press,
109 South 5th Street,
Brooklyn, NY 11249, USA

Visit us on the World Wide Web at:
www.statesacademicpress.com

ISBN: 978-1-63989-317-1

Cataloging-in-Publication Data

Kidney MRI : preclinical applications / edited by Sarah Brown.
p. cm.
Includes bibliographical references and index.
ISBN 978-1-63989-317-1
1. Kidneys--Magnetic resonance imaging. 2. Kidneys--Diseases--Diagnosis.
3. Imaging systems in medicine. I. Brown, Sarah.
RC904.5.I42 K53 2022
616.610 757--dc23

Table of Contents

Preface

In my initial years as a student, I used to run to the library at every possible instance to grab a book and learn something new. Books were my primary source of knowledge and I would not have come such a long way without all that I learnt from them. Thus, when I was approached to edit this book; I became understandably nostalgic. It was an absolute honor to be considered worthy of guiding the current generation as well as those to come. I put all my knowledge and hard work into making this book most beneficial for its readers.

Magnetic resonance is a medical imaging technique which is used for taking detailed pictures of the soft tissues and organs of the body through radio waves and magnets. Unlike X-rays and CT scans, it does not make use of ionizing radiation. Therefore it can be used in cases where exposure to radiation is dangerous. The soft tissues as well as masses, cystic structures, lymph nodes and blood vessels can be seen in detail. The MRI functions by directing radio waves at the molecules of water inside the body, exciting and relaxing the protons in them. This energy from the water molecules is read and a 3-D image is produced which shows the different types of tissue. It can be used for the detection of acute renal failure and chronic kidney disease. It also helps in finding out changes in kidney function which could indicate inflammation or obstruction. The book aims to shed light on some of the unexplored aspects of magnetic resonance imaging and its clinical and experimental applications. It is an upcoming technique in the field of medical science that has undergone rapid development over the past few decades. Researchers and students in this field will be assisted by this book.

I wish to thank my publisher for supporting me at every step. I would also like to thank all the authors who have contributed their researches in this book. I hope this book will be a valuable contribution to the progress of the field.

Editor

1

Fluorine (^{19}F) MRI for Assessing Inflammatory Cells in the Kidney: Experimental Protocol

Min-Chi Ku, Adrian Schreiber, Paula Ramos Delgado, Philipp Boehm-Sturm, Ralph Kettritz, Thoralf Niendorf, Andreas Pohlmann, and Sonia Waiczies

Abstract

Inflammation is one underlying contributing factor in the pathology of acute and chronic kidney disorders. Phagocytes such as monocytes, neutrophils and dendritic cells are considered to play a deleterious role in the progression of kidney disease but may also contribute to organ homeostasis. The kidney is a target of life-threatening autoimmune disorders such as the antineutrophil cytoplasmic antibody (ANCA)-associated vasculitides (AAV). Neutrophils and monocytes express ANCA antigens and play an important role in the pathogenesis of AAV. Noninvasive in vivo methods that can quantify the distribution of inflammatory cells in the kidney as well as other organs in vivo would be vital to identify the causality and significance of inflammation during disease progression. Here we describe an noninvasive technique to study renal inflammation in rodents in vivo using fluorine (^{19}F) MRI. In this protocol we chose a murine ANCA-AAV model of renal inflammation and made use of nanoparticles prepared from perfluoro-5-crown-15-ether (PFCE) for renal ^{19}F MRI.

This chapter is based upon work from the COST Action PARENCHIMA, a community-driven network funded by the European Cooperation in Science and Technology (COST) program of the European Union, which aims to improve the reproducibility and standardization of renal MRI biomarkers. This experimental protocol chapter is complemented by two separate chapters describing the basic concept and data analysis.

Key words Magnetic resonance imaging (MRI), Fluorine (^{19}F), Nanoparticles (NPs), Inflammation, Kidney, Mice

1 Introduction

Inflammation is one underlying contributing factor in the pathology of acute and chronic kidney disorders [1]. Studies also suggest that systemic inflammation can cause ischemic injury in a vital organ, such as the kidney, which could then result in repercussions in another distant organ downstream of the ischemic event, such as the heart [2–4]. Early inflammatory events governed by cells of the innate immune system, such as macrophages, probably promote

Andreas Pohlmann and Thoralf Niendorf (eds.), *Preclinical MRI of the Kidney: Methods and Protocols*, Methods in Molecular Biology, vol. 2216, https://doi.org/10.1007/978-1-0716-0978-1_30, © The Author(s) 2021

renal tissue injury but may also support repair [5–8]. Phagocytes such as dendritic cells (DC) and macrophages are considered to play a deleterious role in the inflammatory outcome of chronic kidney disease but may also contribute to organ homeostasis [9].

The kidney is often a target of systemic autoimmune disorders that are compounded by complex inflammatory processes [10]. Examples of life-threatening autoimmune disorders that affect the kidneys are the antineutrophil cytoplasmic antibody (ANCA)-associated vasculitides (AAV) manifesting as rapidly progressive necrotizing crescentic glomerulonephritis (NCGN) [11]. Neutrophils and monocytes express ANCA antigens and ANCA induces neutrophil extracellular traps that cause RIPK1-dependent endothelial cell (EC) damage via activation of the alternative complement pathway [12]. While the central role of neutrophil activation in ANCA-associated vasculitis and NCGN is clear, the role of monocytes/macrophages was only recently uncovered in a renal ANCA-associated vasculitis model [13].

Noninvasive in vivo methods that can quantify the level of inflammation in the kidney as well as other organs in system autoimmune disorders such as ANCA-associated vasculitides would be vital to identify the causality and significance of inflammation during the course of disease. One method to visualize inflammation by MRI makes use of MR contrast agents that modulate T_2^* and that are easily taken up by phagocytic inflammatory cells [14, 15]. Iron oxide particles including ultrasmall iron oxide agents (USPIO) have been used as susceptibility (T_2^*) MR contrast agents to target inflammatory cell populations. These particles are engulfed by phagocytic cells in the blood. Drawbacks of USPIO-based T_2^* studies include MR signal quantification and difficulty to distinguish contrast created by labeled cells from other intrinsic tissue contrasts [14].

Here we describe an alternative noninvasive technique to study inflammation in rodents in vivo using fluorine (^{19}F) MRI. ^{19}F MRI is performed in association with intravenous injections of perfluorocarbon (PFC) nanoparticles (NPs). These NPs are taken up by cells of the immune system traveling through the circulation into the inflammatory regions. Thus ^{19}F MRI is ideal for studying distribution of inflammatory cell in vivo. In this protocol we chose a murine AAV model of renal inflammation that has been described in greater depth elsewhere [16] and made use of nanoparticles prepared from perfluoro-5-crown-15-ether (PFCE).

This experimental protocol chapter is complemented by two separate chapters describing the basic concept (please *see* the chapter by Waiczies S et al. “Functional Imaging Using Fluorine (^{19}F) MR Methods: Basic Concepts”) and data analysis (please *see* the chapter by Starke L et al. “Data Preparation Protocol for Low Signal-to-Noise Ratio Fluorine-19 MRI”), which are both part of this book.

This chapter is part of the book Pohlmann A, Niendorf T (eds) (2020) Preclinical MRI of the Kidney—Methods and Protocols. Springer, New York.

2 Materials

2.1 Animals

This experimental protocol is tailored for mice with a body mass of 20-30 g (e.g., wild type C57BL/6 mice or a disease model of renal inflammation). Here we describe briefly how to generate the AAV animal model. More thorough detail on the immunization, bone marrow transplantation as well purification of mouse MPO is given in the study establishing the MPO-AAV animal model [16]. Wild-type (WT) C57BL/6J mice (B6) (Jackson Laboratories, Bar Harbor, ME) and myeloperoxidase-deficient ($MPO^{-/-}$) mice (generated by Aratani et al. [17]) were used in this protocol. $MPO^{-/-}$ mice were immunized with murine MPO at the age of 8–10 weeks, subjected to lethal irradiation, and then transplanted with MPO-expressing bone marrow cells. Animal experiments should be approved by animal welfare authorities and guidelines to minimize discomfort to animals (86/609/EEC).

2.1.1 Lab Equipment

1. NP preparation: Ultrasonic device with ultrasonic power (400 W) and frequency (24 kHz) for stand-mounted operation such as UP400S (Hielscher, Teltow, Germany) to prepare PFCE nanoparticles.
2. NP preparation: Titanium sonotrode for emulsifying samples from 5 to 200 ml (e.g., H3 from Hielscher, Teltow, Germany).
3. NP characterization: Dynamic light scattering instrument such as Zetasizer Nano (Malvern Instruments, Malvern, Worcestershire, UK) to characterize particle size (Z-average) and polydispersity index (PDI) of the PFCE nanoparticles.
4. NP application: Mouse restrainer for intravenous administering the PFCE nanoparticles.
5. Anesthesia: Isoflurane inhalation system which can adjust different levels of isoflurane such as Isoflurane Vapor 19.1 (Draeger, Draegerwerk, Luebeck, Germany). The range of isoflurane level that is used for anesthesia in mice is 0.5–1.5%. Please refer to the chapter by Kaucsar T et al. “Preparation and Monitoring of Small Animals in Renal MRI” for an in-depth description and discussion of the anesthesia.
6. Anesthesia: Mouse chamber connected to isoflurane inhalation system and gas-mixing system to anesthetize mice by inhalation narcosis prior to transfer to the MR scanner.
7. Gases: O_2, and compressed air, as well as a gas-mixing system such as FMI (Föhr Medical Instruments GmbH, Seeheim-Ober Beerbach, Germany) to achieve the required physiological O_2/air mixture in combination with the isoflurane gas.

2.2 MRI Hardware

The general hardware requirements for renal ^{1}H MRI on mice and rats are described in the chapter by Ramos Delgado P et al. "Hardware Considerations for Preclinical Magnetic Resonance of the Kidney." The technique described in this chapter was tailored for a 9.4 T MR system (Biospec 94/20, Bruker Biospin, Ettlingen, Germany) but advice for adaptation to other field strengths is given where necessary.

1. $^{1}H/^{19}F$ dual-tunable volume RF coil (35 mm inner diameter, 50 mm length; Rapid Biomed, Würzburg, Germany).
2. $^{1}H/^{19}F$ dual-tunable volume RF coil (18 mm inner diameter, 39 mm length) for ex vivo imaging [18].
3. ^{19}F cryogenic quadrature RF surface probe (^{19}F-CRP) operated at ~28 K (*see* **Note 1**).
4. A physiological monitoring system that can track respiration and temperature during the MR procedure such as the Monitoring & Gating System and PC-sam software from SA Instruments (SAII, Stony Brook, NY, USA).
5. Mouse sled with a breathing mask connected to the isoflurane system.

2.3 MRI Techniques

Typically, ^{19}F MR studies applying PFC compounds such as PFCE to study inflammation in vivo employ the turbo spin echo (SE) rapid acquisition using relaxation enhancement (RARE) sequence [18–22]. This method reduces acquisition time by accumulating multiple echoes within a single repetition time [23]. Typically T_1 of these ^{19}F compounds is in the range of 0.5–3 s, depending on the compound and also magnetic field strength (B_0). However, if employing paramagnetic macrocyclic PFC compounds complexed to lanthanides, T_1 values can be reduced to the order of 1–15 ms and T_2* values correspondingly reduced to 0.4–12 ms and a radial zero echo time (ZTE) sequence might be better suited [24].

1. *^{1}H MR sequence*: 2D and 3D FLASH protocols are standard sequences on Bruker MRI systems, where they are called "FLASH_2D", "FLASH_3D" or "1_Localizer_multi_slice" (*see* **Note 2**).
2. *^{19}F spectroscopy sequence*: Block pulse for nonlocalized (global) is a standard sequence on Bruker MRI systems, where it is called "SINGLEPULSE" (*see* **Note 3**).
3. *^{19}F MR sequence*: 3D RARE protocol for measurements. This is a standard sequence on Bruker MRI systems, where it is called "TurboRARE_3D" in Paravision 5, "T2_TurboRARE_3D" in Paravision 6 (*see* **Note 4**).

3 Methods

3.1 MR Protocol Setup

3.1.1 ^{19}F MR Imaging

Typically T_1 of PFC compounds is in the range of 0.5–3 s, depending on the compound and also magnetic field strength (B_0). When working with a standard diamagnetic PFC such as PFCE that is documented in the literature, it is recommended that the T_1 and T_2 of the compound be studied at 37 °C before starting with the first in vivo experiments to study inflammation. According to the measured relaxation times (T_1/T_2), the optimal settings for RARE, namely echo train lengths (ETL) and repetition time (TR) should be calculated to improve sensitivity thresholds.

1. *Repetition time (TR)*: for RARE, TR will be limited by ETL and the number of slices. A short TR is desirable for SNR efficiency (0.8–1.5 s depending on T_1) keeping in mind that T_1 will change with changes in oxygenation status (*see* **Note 5**).
2. *Flip angle (FA)*: for the block pulse and RARE sequence, the FA for the excitation pulse should be at 90°. Additionally the RARE sequence has a refocusing pulse with a FA of 180°. To maximize the SNR and contrast, the flip angle has to be separately calculated for FLASH considering the Ernst angle: $\alpha_E = \cos^{-1}\left(e^{-TR/T_1}\right)$ which relates FA, T_1 and TR (*see* **Note 6**).
3. *Echo train length (ETL)*: in RARE, use a value as high as possible to reduce scan time. In the TurboRARE sequence on Bruker MRI systems, ETL is referred to as "rare factor".
4. *Echo time (TE)*: use the shortest effective TE and echo spacing (ΔTE) possible. Especially for very high ETL, TE can become very long. Centric encoding can be used to reduce the effective TE, generally at the cost of introducing minor image artifacts.
5. *Acquisition bandwidth (BW)*: long enough to shorten the ΔTE without compromising the SNR, which decreases with increasing BW as a result of increased noise level.
6. *Geometry*: Adapt so that whole abdomen fits into FOV in L-R direction (approx. 25 mm for mice) and use frequency encoding in H-F- direction. Choose a 3D volume suited to cover the whole body width and as much of the length of the mouse that the RF coil can afford as possible. With a typical mouse body resonator as the one used in this protocol one could use a FOV of 60 × 30 × 30 mm and matrix size of 400 × 200 × 200 (for ^{1}H) and 128 × 64 × 64 (for ^{19}F).
7. *Resolution/acceleration*: Use the highest in-plane resolution that the SNR allows, typically around 100–150 μm for ^{1}H MR scans and 250–500 μm for ^{19}F MR scans. Zero-filling in phase encoding direction can be helpful to speed up acquisition while increasing the number of averages to improve SNR

especially for ^{19}F MR scans. One may use half Fourier in read direction (asymmetric echo) to further shorten the first TE. Reducing the excitation pulse length to below 1 ms would then also help to shorten TE.

8. For an example of parameters used in this chapter, please *see* **Notes 7** and **13**.

3.2 ^{19}F Nanoparticle Preparation, Characterization, and Application

1. *NP preparation*: Emulsify 1.2 M PFCE (Fluorochem, Derbyshire, UK) in Pluronic F-68 (Sigma-Aldrich, Germany) for 10 min using a cell disrupting titanium sonotrode connected to an ultrasonic device and employing a continuous pulse program for 60 s. Use ear protection while sonicating the mixture to avoid hearing damage and loss.
2. *NP characterization*: Measure mean particle size (in nm), polydispersity index (PdI), and zetapotential (mV) by using a dynamic light scattering machine such as the one listed above. Use the *z*-average diameter for particle size since it gives an intensity-weighted harmonic diameter and is ideal for comparing different analyses. The nanoparticles should have a PdI < 0.3 indicating a relatively low polydispersity and narrow size distribution (*see* **Note 8**).
3. *NP application*: Administer ^{19}F nanoparticles via tail vein at a dose of 5–80 μmol of PFCE molecules, depending on the frequency of the bolus injections. Start administering ^{19}F nanoparticles at relevant time-points of your inflammatory model, for example, in MPO immunized $MPO^{-/-}$ mice subjected to lethal irradiation we started intravenous application of PFCE nanoparticles 4–8 weeks following transplantation of MPO-expressing bone marrow cells (*see* **Note 9**).

3.3 Preparation Prior to ^{19}F/^{1}H MRI Scans

Four to 18 h following the last intravenous administration of ^{19}F nanoparticles prepare the mice for ^{19}F/^{1}H MRI:

1. First anesthetize the mice by inhalation narcosis using a mouse chamber connected to a isoflurane inhalation system and gas-mixing system (*see* **Note 10**).
2. Adjust the flow rate for air and O_2 at 0.2 and 0.1 l/min respectively and 3% isoflurane (adjusted from a vaporizer) for about 2 min until the required level of anesthesia is reached (no response following toe pinch).
3. Transfer mice to the MR scanner. Should a quantification of inflammation be required, a reference tube with a known concentration of ^{19}F nanoparticles should be placed in proximity to the region of interest. For quantification of signal please refer to the chapter by Starke L et al. "Data Preparation Protocol for Low Signal-to-Noise Ratio Fluorine-19 MRI."

4. While keeping the flow rate for air and O_2 constant, adjust the isoflurane vaporizer to 0.8–1.5% until an optimal breathing pattern is reached.
5. Set up the temperature monitoring (rectal probe) and respiratory monitoring (balloon on chest) unit. A respiratory rate of 70–90 breaths per minute is recommended. Keep the body temperature at 36–37 °C during the experiment by employing a warm water (or alternatively warm air) circulation system.
6. Tune the RF coil to both the ^{1}H resonance frequency (e.g., 400.1 MHz for 9.4 T) and to the ^{19}F resonance frequency (e.g., 376.3 MHz for 9.4 T) and match the characteristic impedance of the coil to 50 Ω using the tuning monitor of the animal MR scanner.
7. Perform anatomical imaging as described in the chapter by Pohlmann A et al. "Essential Practical Steps for MRI of the Kidney in Experimental Research." Set up a 2D FLASH protocol for the acquisition of anatomical kidney ^{1}H scans (*see* **Note 7**).
8. Perform localized shimming on the kidney imaging as described in the chapter by Pohlmann A et al. "Essential Practical Steps for MRI of the Kidney in Experimental Research" (*see* **Note 11**).
9. Save the parameters of all adjustments (such as iterative shimming calculations and reference power values) performed during the first ^{1}H scans for application into the ^{19}F scans.

3.4 ^{19}F/^{1}H MRI of the Kidney

Following acquisition of the anatomical ^{1}H kidney scans, in vivo ^{19}F MR images of the kidney can be acquired and later overlaid onto the ^{1}H MR images. An example of an in vivo ^{1}H/^{19}F MRI is shown in Fig. 1.

3.4.1 In Vivo ^{19}F/^{1}H MRI Using a Room Temperature Mouse Body Volume ^{19}F/^{1}H RF Resonator

1. Load the SINGLEPULSE FID-sequence with a TR of at least 1000 ms.
2. Set nucleus to ^{19}F (e.g., in "Open Edit Scan" in Bruker's Paravision 5.1 or "System" tab in Bruker's Paravision 6). Since the ^{19}F MR signal is too low for automatic adjustments, apply the same settings used for the ^{1}H anatomical scans (*see* **Note 12**).
3. Deselect the automatic reference gain (RG) and set on maximum (e.g., in Edit Method in Bruker's Paravision 5.1 or using the "Instruction" tab (GOP) and "Setup" tab in Paravision 6).
4. Start the SINGLEPULSE sequence using setup mode. If the ^{19}F spectral signal within the acquisition-window is too low, add more averages until a signal is clearly visible. Adjust the basic frequency in order to center the ^{19}F spectral peak at 0 Hz in the acquisition window. Apply this basic frequency, press Stop and apply.

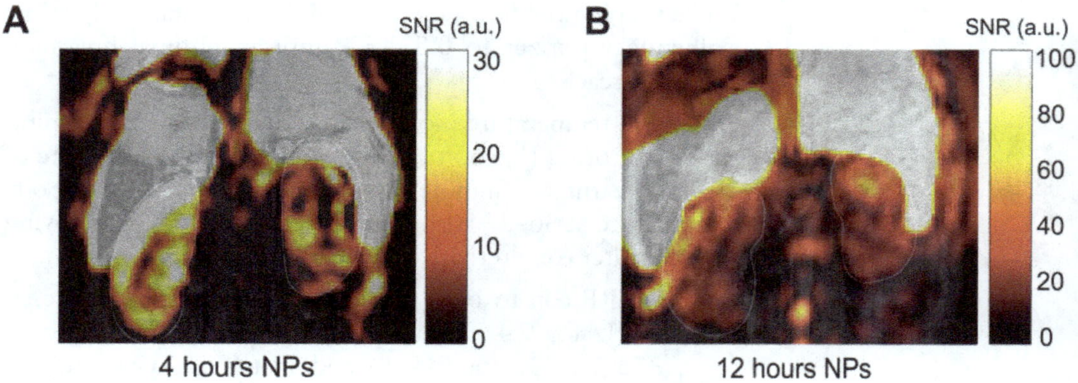

Fig. 1 In vivo $^{19}F/^{1}H$ MRI of a murine ANCA-AAV model of renal inflammation using the $^{1}H/^{19}F$ dual-tunable volume RF coil (35 mm inner diameter). Eight weeks following transplantation of bone marrow cells, MPO-AAV mice were administered one bolus of PFCE nanoparticles (NPs) intravenously (80 μmol in 100 μl) and $^{19}F/^{1}H$ MRI was performed 4 h (**a**) and 12 h (**b**) thereafter. (1) ^{1}H 2D FLASH protocol: TR = 579.4 ms, TE = 5 ms, FA = 75, matrix = 256 × 128. (2) ^{19}F 3D RARE protocol: TR = 800 ms, TE = 6.16 ms, Matrix = 256 × 128 × 128, RARE Factor = 32

5. Setup a TurboRARE 3D protocol for the ^{19}F scans.
6. Use the same geometry used for anatomical ^{1}H imaging but reduce the matrix size for increased SNR and use a rare factor of at least 32. Set nucleus to ^{19}F. Deselect automatic adjustments (as above). For an example of parameters, please *see* **Note 7**.
7. When the scans are finished retract the mouse-holder from the MR scanner. Disconnect the mouse carefully from the holder. If the mouse is not sacrificed for ex vivo analysis (e.g., high resolution ^{19}F MRI of the kidney, see below) following the MR scans, closely monitor until it has completely recovered from anesthesia. Body temperature regulation might still be affected after the anesthesia, so during the recovery process, put the mouse in a separate cage that is placed on a warm temperature regulated pad. Once the mouse has completely recovered from anesthesia, you may return it to its holding cage and to the animal room.

3.4.2 High Spatial Resolution ^{19}F MRI of Ex Vivo Kidney Using a ^{19}F CryoProbe

Kidney inflammation can also be studied with high spatial resolution ex vivo ^{19}F MRI, for example, by using a transceive ^{19}F CryoProbe, which we previously used to study brain inflammation in a model of CNS autoimmunity [25]. An example of a high resolved ex vivo $^{1}H/^{19}F$ MRI of the kidney is shown in Fig. 2.

1. At the end of the in vivo experiment, anesthetize mice with a terminal dose of ketamine and xylazine. Ensure the required level of anesthesia is reached (no response following toe pinch).
2. Transcardially perfuse mouse with 20 ml PBS followed by 20 ml 4% paraformaldehyde.

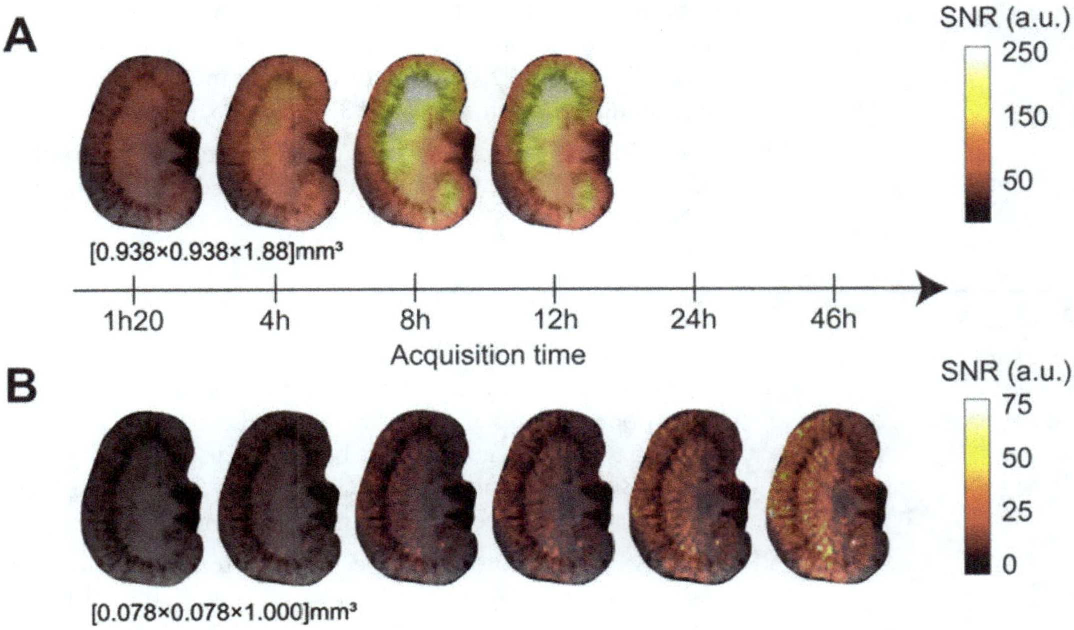

Fig. 2 Ex vivo $^{19}F/^{1}H$ MRI of an inflamed kidney from the ANCA-AAV model. (**a**) Low spatial resolution images acquired using the $^{1}H/^{19}F$ dual-tunable volume RF coil (18 mm inner diameter). At this resolution [0.938 × 0.938]mm^2, a high ^{19}F signal can be achieved already after 1 h acquisition time. However, anatomical detail is lacking in the ^{19}F MR images. (**b**) High spatial resolution images acquired with the ^{19}F cryogenic quadrature RF surface probe (^{19}F-CRP). The gain in SNR achieved by the ^{19}F-CRP was used to increase the in plane spatial resolution [0.078 × 0.078]mm^2

3. Harvest relevant organs (e.g., kidney, liver, and spleen).
4. Transfer organs to a container filled with 4% PFA and store at 4 °C.
5. Prior to the high resolution ^{19}F MRI of the kidney, embed the kidney in 1% low melting agarose in a 1.5 ml Eppendorf tube.
6. ^{19}F-CRP adjustments: since the ^{19}F signal is too low for automatic adjustments, use a ^{19}F calibration phantom (fill highly fluorinated substance such as trifluoroethanol with water in a 1.5 ml Eppendorf tube. Place the ^{19}F calibration tube under the ^{19}F-CRP and repeat steps 13–16 to calculate the working frequency. Load and run a 1_Localizer_multi_slice sequence (see above). Adjust the reference power using the adjustments platform: select a coronal slice of 2 mm thickness and place it close to the RF coil's surface. Select an initial power two orders of magnitude smaller than what is usually expected and press start. Run the rest of the adjustments using the same sequence. Save the shim settings.
7. ^{19}F-CRP imaging: place the ex vivo kidney embedded in a 1.5 ml Eppendorf tube under the ^{19}F-CRP surface. Run the working frequency adjustments as per 13–16, load the shim

calculations, and adjust the reference power as described above. Set the RG to maximum. Load a 2D FLASH protocol and set it up for ^{19}F imaging. Examples for high and medium resolution ^{19}F imaging are given in **Note 13**.

8. Set up a 2D FLASH protocol for the acquisition of anatomical kidney ^{1}H scans. Use the same geometry used for ^{19}F imaging (*see* **Note 13**).

4 Notes

1. The transceive ^{19}F cryogenic quadrature RF surface probe (^{19}F CryoProbe) operates at ~28 K with a dual cooled preamplifier at the base running at ~77 K. It has a similar geometry to the existing Bruker ^{1}H quadrature CryoProbes. More details on the ^{19}F CryoProbe are available in our previous study [25].
2. The FLASH_3D protocol is especially adapted for whole-body imaging of mice (the gradient-system and the volume-resonator need to have a linear region of about 8 cm).
3. The block pulse program (SINGLEPULSE) contains the necessary elements for a simple transmit/receive experiment, sending a pulse and acquiring an FID afterward.
4. A 2D version of this sequence is also available, which allows thicker slices for a general overview but suffers from low SNR for most in vivo applications.
5. Special attention should be given when studying inflammation in models where tissue oxygen levels are likely to change, for example, following ischemic events. In these cases, T_1 weighting needs to be reduced at cost of SNR efficiency by increasing $TR \gg T_1$ (typically $TR = 3–5 \times T_1$).
6. When using transmit-receive surface coils a B_1 correction should be considered in order to compensate for the intrinsic spatial gradient in coil sensitivity (B_1^-) and excitation field (B_1^+ inhomogeneity), which results is signification variation in the excitation FA, decreasing with increasing distance from the RF coil surface. This severely reduces image homogeneity and hampers the acquisition of the absolute signal intensity values for ^{19}F quantification techniques.
7. Example for a 30 g mouse at 9.4 T and FOV of $50 \times 25 \times 25$ mm, (1) ^{1}H 2D FLASH protocol: TR = 579.4 ms, TE = 5 ms, FA = 75, matrix = 256×128. (2) ^{19}F 3D RARE protocol: TR = 800 ms, TE = 6.16 ms, Matrix = $256 \times 128 \times 128$, RARE Factor = 32–64.

8. The polydispersity index (PdI) is extrapolated from the DLS function and quantitatively describes the particle size distribution best. PdI ranges from 0.01 for monodispersed particles to 0.7 for particles that have a very broad size distribution. The *z*-average diameter gives the mean diameter based on intensity of scattered light and sensitive to presence of large particles, peak diameter, peak width, and PdI.
9. In MPO-AAV mice we administered one bolus of PFCE nanoparticles intravenously (80 μmol in 100 μl) 8 weeks following transplantation of bone marrow cells.
10. Mice can be alternatively anesthetized with an intraperitoneal injection of ketamine and xylazine.
11. Shimming is particularly important, since macroscopic magnetic field inhomogeneities affect the exact resonance frequency of the PFCE compounds and might affect quantification of the ^{19}F MR signal. Shimming should be performed on a voxel enclosing both kidneys using either the default iterative shimming method or the Mapshim technique (recommended). However, the Mapshim technique is not available for X-nuclei-only RF coils. An alternative in this case is to use a highly fluorinated sample to calculate the shims.
12. Since the NMR properties of ^{19}F and ^{1}H are similar, the same MR setup and MR parameter settings can be used for both nuclei.
13. Example for ex vivo *high-resolved* ^{19}*F MRI* at 9.4 T using the ^{19}F-CRP and a 2D FLASH: TR = 11 ms, TE = 2.7 ms, FA = 30, Avg = 2250, Repetitions = 35, FOV = 20 × 20, matrix = 256 × 256, 1 mm slice thickness. Example for ex vivo *low-resolved* ^{19}*F MRI* at 9.4 T using the ^{1}H/^{19}F dual-tunable volume RF coil (18 mm inner diameter) and a 3D RARE method: TR = 800 ms, TE = 5 ms, Avg = 256, Repetitions = 13, FOV = 60 × 30 × 30, matrix = 64 × 32 × 16. ^{1}H 2D FLASH protocol: TR = 18.7 ms, TE = 5.5 ms, FA = 25, matrix = 171 × 256, 1 mm slice thickness.

Acknowledgments

This work was funded, in part (Adrian Schreiber, Ralph Kettritz, Thoralf Niendorf, Sonia Waiczies, and Andreas Pohlmann), by the German Research Foundation (Gefoerdert durch die Deutsche Forschungsgemeinschaft (DFG), Projektnummer 394046635, SFB 1365, RENOPROTECTION. Funded by the Deutsche Forschungsgemeinschaft (DFG, German Research Foundation), Project number 394046635, SFB 1365, RENOPROTECTION).

Also, our research is funded by the Deutsche Forschungsgemeinschaft to SW (DFG WA2804), AP (DFG PO1869), and AS (DFG SCHR7718).

This chapter is based upon work from COST Action PARENCH IMA, supported by European Cooperation in Science and Technology (COST). COST (www.cost.eu) is a funding agency for research and innovation networks. COST Actions help connect research initiatives across Europe and enable scientists to enrich their ideas by sharing them with their peers. This boosts their research, career, and innovation.

PARENCHIMA (renalmri.org) is a community-driven Action in the COST program of the European Union, which unites more than 200 experts in renal MRI from 30 countries with the aim to improve the reproducibility and standardization of renal MRI biomarkers.

References

1. Chawla LS, Eggers PW, Star RA, Kimmel PL (2014) Acute kidney injury and chronic kidney disease as interconnected syndromes. N Engl J Med 371(1):58–66. https://doi.org/10.1056/NEJMra1214243
2. Levy EM, Viscoli CM, Horwitz RI (1996) The effect of acute renal failure on mortality. a cohort analysis. JAMA 275(19):1489–1494
3. Jorres A, Gahl GM, Dobis C, Polenakovic MH, Cakalaroski K, Rutkowski B, Kisielnicka E, Krieter DH, Rumpf KW, Guenther C, Gaus W, Hoegel J (1999) Haemodialysis-membrane biocompatibility and mortality of patients with dialysis-dependent acute renal failure: a prospective randomised multicentre trial. International Multicentre Study Group. Lancet 354(9187):1337–1341
4. Brouns R, De Deyn PP (2004) Neurological complications in renal failure: a review. Clin Neurol Neurosurg 107(1):1–16. https://doi.org/10.1016/j.clineuro.2004.07.012
5. Chawla LS, Bellomo R, Bihorac A, Goldstein SL, Siew ED, Bagshaw SM, Bittleman D, Cruz D, Endre Z, Fitzgerald RL, Forni L, Kane-Gill SL, Hoste E, Koyner J, Liu KD, Macedo E, Mehta R, Murray P, Nadim M, Ostermann M, Palevsky PM, Pannu N, Rosner M, Wald R, Zarbock A, Ronco C, Kellum JA (2017) Acute kidney disease and renal recovery: consensus report of the Acute Disease Quality Initiative (ADQI) 16 Workgroup. Nat Rev Nephrol 13(4):241–257
6. Humphreys BD, Cantaluppi V, Portilla D, Singbartl K, Yang L, Rosner MH, Kellum JA, Ronco C (2016) Targeting endogenous repair pathways after AKI. J Am Soc Nephrol 27 (4):990–998
7. Kurts C, Panzer U, Anders H-J, Rees AJ (2013) The immune system and kidney disease: basic concepts and clinical implications. Nat Rev Immunol 13:738. https://doi.org/10.1038/nri3523. https://www.nature.com/articles/nri3523-supplementary-information
8. Bellomo R, Kellum JA, Ronco C, Wald R, Martensson J, Maiden M, Bagshaw SM, Glassford NJ, Lankadeva Y, Vaara ST, Schneider A (2017) Acute kidney injury in sepsis. Intensive Care Med 43(6):816–828
9. Weisheit CK, Engel DR, Kurts C (2015) Dendritic cells and macrophages: sentinels in the kidney. Clin J Am Soc Nephrol 10 (10):1841–1851. https://doi.org/10.2215/cjn.07100714
10. Kurts C, Panzer U, Anders H-J, Rees AJ (2013) The immune system and kidney disease: basic concepts and clinical implications. Nat Rev Immunol 13:738. https://doi.org/10.1038/nri3523. https://www.nature.com/articles/nri3523-supplementary-information
11. Furuta S, Jayne DRW (2013) Antineutrophil cytoplasm antibody–associated vasculitis: recent developments. Kidney Int 84 (2):244–249. https://doi.org/10.1038/ki.2013.24
12. Schreiber A, Rousselle A, Becker JU, von Mässenhausen A, Linkermann A, Kettritz R (2017) Necroptosis controls NET generation and mediates complement activation, endothelial damage, and autoimmune vasculitis. Proc Natl Acad Sci 114(45):E9618–E9625. https://doi.org/10.1073/pnas.1708247114

13. Rousselle A, Kettritz R, Schreiber A (2017) Monocytes promote crescent formation in anti-myeloperoxidase antibody–induced glomerulonephritis. Am J Pathol 187 (9):1908–1915. https://doi.org/10.1016/j.ajpath.2017.05.003
14. Grenier N, Merville P, Combe C (2016) Radiologic imaging of the renal parenchyma structure and function. Nat Rev Nephrol 12 (6):348–359
15. Hueper K, Gutberlet M, Bräsen JH, Jang M-S, Thorenz A, Chen R, Hertel B, Barrmeyer A, Schmidbauer M, Meier M, von Vietinghoff S, Khalifa A, Hartung D, Haller H, Wacker F, Rong S, Gueler F (2016) Multiparametric functional MRI: non-invasive imaging of inflammation and edema formation after kidney transplantation in mice. PLoS One 11(9): e0162705. https://doi.org/10.1371/journal.pone.0162705
16. Schreiber A, Xiao H, Falk RJ, Jennette JC (2006) Bone marrow-derived cells are sufficient and necessary targets to mediate glomerulonephritis and vasculitis induced by anti-myeloperoxidase antibodies. J Am Soc Nephrol 17(12):3355–3364. https://doi.org/10.1681/asn.2006070718
17. Aratani Y, Koyama H, Nyui S, Suzuki K, Kura F, Maeda N (1999) Severe impairment in early host defense against *Candida albicans* in mice deficient in myeloperoxidase. Infect Immun 67(4):1828–1836
18. Waiczies H, Lepore S, Drechsler S, Qadri F, Purfurst B, Sydow K, Dathe M, Kuhne A, Lindel T, Hoffmann W, Pohlmann A, Niendorf T, Waiczies S (2013) Visualizing brain inflammation with a shingled-leg radiofrequency head probe for 19F/1H MRI. Sci Rep 3:1280. https://doi.org/10.1038/srep01280
19. Srinivas M, Morel PA, Ernst LA, Laidlaw DH, Ahrens ET (2007) Fluorine-19 MRI for visualization and quantification of cell migration in a diabetes model. Magn Reson Med 58 (4):725–734. https://doi.org/10.1002/mrm.21352
20. Flögel U, Ding Z, Hardung H, Jander S, Reichmann G, Jacoby C, Schubert R, Schrader J (2008) In vivo monitoring of inflammation after cardiac and cerebral ischemia by fluorine magnetic resonance imaging. Circulation 118 (2):140–148
21. Jacoby C, Temme S, Mayenfels F, Benoit N, Krafft MP, Schubert R, Schrader J, Flögel U (2014) Probing different perfluorocarbons for in vivo inflammation imaging by 19F MRI: image reconstruction, biological half-lives and sensitivity. NMR Biomed 27(3):261–271. https://doi.org/10.1002/nbm.3059
22. Flögel U, Burghoff S, van Lent PL, Temme S, Galbarz L, Ding Z, El-Tayeb A, Huels S, Bonner F, Borg N, Jacoby C, Muller CE, van den Berg WB, Schrader J (2012) Selective activation of adenosine A2A receptors on immune cells by a CD73-dependent prodrug suppresses joint inflammation in experimental rheumatoid arthritis. Sci Transl Med 4(146):146ra108. https://doi.org/10.1126/scitranslmed.3003717
23. Hennig J, Nauerth A, Friedburg H (1986) RARE imaging: a fast imaging method for clinical MR. Magn Reson Med 3:823–833. https://doi.org/10.1002/mrm.1910030602
24. Schmid F, Höltke C, Parker D, Faber C (2013) Boosting 19F MRI—SNR efficient detection of paramagnetic contrast agents using ultrafast sequences. Magn Reson Med 69 (4):1056–1062. https://doi.org/10.1002/mrm.24341
25. Waiczies S, Millward JM, Starke L, Delgado PR, Huelnhagen T, Prinz C, Marek D, Wecker D, Wissmann R, Koch SP, Boehm-Sturm P, Waiczies H, Niendorf T, Pohlmann A (2017) Enhanced fluorine-19 MRI sensitivity using a cryogenic radiofrequency probe: technical developments and ex vivo demonstration in a mouse model of neuroinflammation. Sci Rep 7(1):9808. https://doi.org/10.1038/s41598-017-09622-2

2

Functional Imaging Using Fluorine (^{19}F) MR Methods: Basic Concepts

Sonia Waiczies, Christian Prinz, Ludger Starke, Jason M. Millward, Paula Ramos Delgado, Jens Rosenberg, Marc Nazaré, Helmar Waiczies, Andreas Pohlmann, and Thoralf Niendorf

Abstract

Kidney-associated pathologies would greatly benefit from noninvasive and robust methods that can objectively quantify changes in renal function. In the past years there has been a growing incentive to develop new applications for fluorine (^{19}F) MRI in biomedical research to study functional changes during disease states. ^{19}F MRI represents an instrumental tool for the quantification of exogenous ^{19}F substances in vivo. One of the major benefits of ^{19}F MRI is that fluorine in its organic form is absent in eukaryotic cells. Therefore, the introduction of exogenous ^{19}F signals in vivo will yield background-free images, thus providing highly selective detection with absolute specificity in vivo. Here we introduce the concept of ^{19}F MRI, describe existing challenges, especially those pertaining to signal sensitivity, and give an overview of preclinical applications to illustrate the utility and applicability of this technique for measuring renal function in animal models.

This chapter is based upon work from the COST Action PARENCHIMA, a community-driven network funded by the European Cooperation in Science and Technology (COST) program of the European Union, which aims to improve the reproducibility and standardization of renal MRI biomarkers. This introduction chapter is complemented by two separate chapters describing the experimental procedure and data analysis.

Key words Magnetic resonance imaging (MRI), Fluorine (^{19}F), Kidney, Inflammation, Tissue oxygenation

1 Introduction

The need for methods to assess renal function that are both robust and noninvasive is increasingly becoming recognized. One approach is to use MRI in combination with contrast agents that are responsive to physiological changes [1]. The most common type of MR contrast agents are paramagnetic agents that enhance contrast on MR images. These contrast agents act by modulating proton (^1H) relaxation, either during recovery (T_1 component) or

Andreas Pohlmann and Thoralf Niendorf (eds.), *Preclinical MRI of the Kidney: Methods and Protocols*, Methods in Molecular Biology, vol. 2216, https://doi.org/10.1007/978-1-0716-0978-1_17,

decay (T_2 component) of the MR signal. In order for a contrast agent to be useful to identify changes in a specific physiological phenomenon, its sensitivity to detect and quantify physiological changes on MRI and its pharmacokinetic properties must be balanced [2].

From a technical point of view, paramagnetic contrast agents have a concomitant effect on all components of MR relaxation; the interplay between T_1 and T_2 relaxation depends on the dose and location of the contrast agent as well as the MR imaging sequence used [3]. This complexity is exacerbated by intrinsic factors such as deoxygenated blood or air cavities that may confound the signal being investigated [4]. A case in point is when imaging cells labeled with contrast agent: changes in contrast created by such intrinsic tissue factors could render the labeled cells indistinguishable from the surrounding tissue. This drawback is heightened by the signal sensitivity constraints due to the low concentrations of contrast agent (<μM range). As a result, any quantification of the physiological observation is hampered, and in some cases, no definitive conclusions can be made.

The use of fluorinated agents in combination with fluorine (^{19}F) MRI overcomes the hurdle of signal ambiguity because the ^{19}F MR signal is specific to the administered ^{19}F agent. While the ^{19}F nucleus has similar MR sensitivity and resonance frequency as ^{1}H, unlike ^{1}H, it is practically absent in vivo, that is, there are no endogenous ^{19}F organic forms in vivo. Therefore, any exogenous fluorinated compounds introduced in vivo can be detected with high selectivity and absolute specificity. This has been exploited to noninvasively track cells in vivo using ^{19}F MRI after labeling them with ^{19}F compounds, typically in the form of nanoparticles (NP). Interestingly, the chemical shift range for ^{19}F is much larger than that of ^{1}H. Organofluorine compounds span a chemical shift range of over 350 ppm [5]. Thus multiple ^{19}F nuclei resonances for organofluorine compounds can be easily separated, even under rather inhomogeneous conditions [6]. The unique properties of ^{19}F nuclei as well as ^{19}F compounds have been the driving force behind the increasing interest in ^{19}F MRI. However, the application of ^{19}F MRI to a wide range of biomedical research fields has been restricted by the low abundance of ^{19}F nuclei in vivo following exogenous administration. This constraint is compounded by the fact that the signal sensitivity of current MR hardware remains limited, making the detection of ^{19}F compounds present at low concentrations extremely challenging. Therefore, one strategy in ^{19}F MRI to circumvent this is to boost the signal-to-noise ratio (SNR) as a function of time, that is, the SNR efficiency to enhance signal sensitivity and improve detection limits.

From a biological perspective, several key components must be considered when using contrast agents to study renal function. Among other physicochemical properties, size will determine the pharmacokinetic properties of the contrast agent as well as its uptake by cells in vivo. For example, low-molecular-weight-gadolinium-based contrast agents (GBCAs) are filtered through the glomerulus and are not reabsorbed by the renal tubule. Conversely, larger contrast agents such as paramagnetic iron oxide particles or ^{19}F nanoparticles commonly follow a one-compartment pharmacokinetic model within the blood [7]. These nanoparticles are too large to be filtered by the glomerulus and are eventually taken up by phagocytic blood cells. Such nanoparticles including the iron replacement therapy ferumoxytol have a long intravascular half-life (>14 h) and are therefore useful for vascular and perfusion-weighted MRI [8]. Unless inflammatory processes are ongoing, these particles will localize primarily in the liver and will eventually undergo elimination via hepatic clearance. The clearance of nanoparticles via liver or kidney is dependent on their size and surface properties [9] but also on the health status of these organs, such that clearance should be critically studied [10] especially prior to patient studies.

This introduction chapter is complemented by two separate chapters describing the experimental procedure and data analysis, which are part of this book.

This chapter is part of the book Pohlmann A, Niendorf T (eds) (2020) Preclinical MRI of the Kidney—Methods and Protocols. Springer, New York.

2 Overview of Applications

Quantitative measurements of renal function are necessary to detect changes already during the early stages of kidney disease, to support disease staging and to screen emerging therapeutic strategies. Non-invasive and rapid MR methods are needed to quantify disease components such as inflammation, hypoxia and tissue damage. While commonly available MR contrast agents act by modulating ^{1}H relaxation, contrast agents containing ^{19}F have also been developed to investigate disease components such as inflammation and to quantify pathological changes in the tissue microenvironment (e.g., changes in tissue oxygenation (pO_2) or pH) using ^{19}F MRI.

2.1 ^{19}F MRI to Study Environmental Changes in the Kidney In Vivo

There is an abundant repertoire of exogenous MRI contrast agents that act by modulating ^{1}H relaxation and which are triggered by changes in pO_2, pH or temperature as well as changes in protein, metabolite or metal ion concentrations (reviewed elsewhere [1]). Here we focus on the application of ^{19}F probes that elicit a desired MR signal following changes in pO_2 and pH and hold promise as tools for screening kidney disease.

2.1.1 Renal Tissue Oxygenation

Healthy kidneys operate under relatively low O_2 conditions, requiring extensive extraction of O_2 from flowing blood. While several regulatory mechanisms act to maintain oxygenation within homeostatic limits, the kidneys are nonetheless particularly susceptible to hypoxic injury [11]. While O_2 consumption determines perfusion in most nonrenal tissue such as the brain, perfusion determines O_2 consumption in the kidney [12]. Therefore, a sudden temporary impairment of the blood flow to the kidney results in acute kidney injury (AKI) as a result of impaired O_2 delivery. Approaches for identifying and treating AKI as early as possible should aim at detecting and restoring imbalances the homeostasis between renal oxygenation and factors such as nitric oxide that control the renal microcirculation [13].

Noninvasive methods to measure kidney function in vivo, specifically tissue pO_2 and blood perfusion, are crucial. Arterial spin labeling MRI determines intrarenal perfusion without the need of exogenous contrast agents, and will be reviewed in a separate chapter of this book. MRI techniques that utilize the native ^1H contrast from blood—blood-oxygenation-level-dependent (BOLD) MRI—have been proposed [14]. The level of renal oxygenation within each voxel is quantified by mapping the shortening of ^1H T_2^* induced by deoxyhemoglobin—deoxyHb [15]. However, the relation of T_2^* to tissue pO_2 may be confounded by factors such as hematocrit, oxyHb dissociation curve, and the vascular volume fraction. This underscores the need for careful scrutiny of this relation in order to make quantitative interpretations [16].

Perfluorocarbon (PFC) emulsions offer an alternative to quantify changes in tissue pO_2 during vascular pathology [17, 18]. More recently PFC NPs were also employed as a theranostic strategy for studying perfusion and treating AKI [19]. Primarily PFC NPs have been used to assess perfusion in the renal microvasculature following AKI [20]. ^{19}F MRI sensitively detected decreased RBV and pO2 in the cortical–medullary (CM) junction 24 h following unilateral (left) renal ischemia–reperfusion [20], where increased T_2^* was also observed by ^1H BOLD MRI (Fig. 1a). The T_2^*, ^{19}F signal, and pO_2 in the renal cortex of injured kidneys were all comparable to the contralateral control kidney, suggesting recovery of perfusion and oxygenation in this region. In the inner medulla, however, vascular leakage and hemorrhage-induced extravascular retention of PFC NPs (Fig. 1b, c) resulted in a false readout of reduced ^1H T_2^*, increased ^{19}F signal intensity, and unchanged pO2.

PFCs and oxygen exhibit similarly low cohesive energy densities, such that both require little energy for mutual solubility [21]. The high oxygen-dissolving capacity of PFC emulsions makes them ideal as O_2 carriers. PFCs were, in fact, considered as artificial blood substitutes [22]. Fluosol-DA—a mixture of perfluorodecalin (PFD) and perfluorotributylamine—was the first PFC emulsion studied in humans in a trial of Japanese patients [23]. It was soon recalled due to its rather low oxygen transport capacity compared to that of red blood cells [24]. PFCs ultimately failed as blood substitutes (even as next generation products

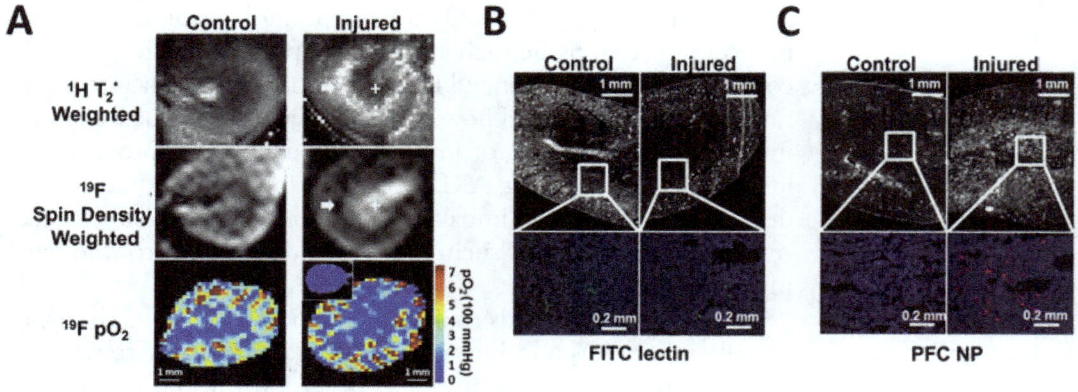

Fig. 1 Assessing perfusion in the renal microvasculature following acute kidney injury using PFCs. (**a**) Composite Representative ^{1}H T2*-weighted image (top row), ^{19}F spin density weighted image (middle row), and p0$_2$ map (bottom row) in the left control and right injured kidneys of the same mouse. (**b**) Fluorescence images showing FITC-lectin labeled perfused blood vessels in control and injured kidneys (top row) and zoom-in view of FITC-lectin (green) labeled perfused vessels in the CM junction (bottom row). (**c**) Fluorescence images showing rhodamine labeled PFC NPs in injured and control kidneys (top row) and zoom-in view showing PFC NPs (red) in the renal medulla (bottom row). Adapted from Hu L. et al. (2013) [20] with permission from John Wiley & Sons Inc.

appeared in the clinic). Although O_2-deprived tissues easily extract O_2 in PFCs, the oxygen dissociation curve of PFC emulsions is linear and monotonic, in contrast to the sigmoidal hemoglobin dissociation curve. Therefore, most of the O_2 dissolved in PFCs is released at high O_2 partial pressure in the arteries, with little O_2 being available for the capillaries where O_2 partial pressure is low but needed the most [22]. Interestingly Fluosol-DA (the first PFC that was used in patients [23]) was also used to acquire the first ^{19}F MR images in vivo, showing its accumulation in the rat liver [25]. The PFC in this emulsion gives complex MR spectra and has since been replaced by other PFCs with better imaging properties [26].

The longitudinal relaxation rate ($1/T_1$) of ^{19}F in PFCs was shown to depend linearly on O_2 partial pressure [27]. This led to the first noninvasive in vivo tissue O_2 assessments in tumor tissue and liver [28] and later in myocardial tissue [29]. The latter study provided the first proof of concept study for rapid, noninvasive measurements of O_2 oxygen tension changes in response to ischemia and reperfusion [29]. It is claimed that the size of PFC nanoparticles (>100 nm) confers upon them a good safety profile without renal toxicity, since they are not expected to be cleared through glomerular filtration. Therefore, unlike other imaging agents that undergo renal clearance (e.g., iodinated CT compounds, gadolinium MRI chelates), PFC emulsions do not increase the workload of the kidney and are not immediately considered as nephrotoxic [10].

2.1.2 Acid–Base Homeostasis in the Kidney and pH Sensors

The kidney plays a major role in acid–base homeostasis; this balance depends on its capacity to reabsorb filtered bicarbonate, mainly from the proximal tubule, and to excrete an equivalent amount of protons at the distal tubule [30]. CEST MRI was originally developed to measure pH with exogenous pH-responsive MRI contrast agents [31]. The pH in the kidney following AKI gradually increased from 6.7 to 7.2 as measured with CEST-MRI pH-responsive probes [32]. A major drawback of paramagnetic probes is that signal intensity is not only proportional to the pH but also to contrast agent concentration. Particularly in tumors, in vivo pH mapping assumes a constant contrast agent concentration across tissue notwithstanding poor perfusion where acidolysis occurs [33].

Approaches such as ratiometric $^{19}F/^{1}H$ probes have been developed to overcome the issue of quantification; the signal is normalized to the concentration of the contrast agent by means of a concentration reporting (^{19}F) moiety [34]. Another advantage of ^{19}F MR probes is the larger range in chemical shifts in ^{19}F (compared to ^{1}H). These chemical shifts are highly sensitive to the immediate surroundings, such that small chemical changes can lead to dramatic changes in chemical shift [6]. The first ^{19}F MR probe identified as a candidate to probe cellular pH was the vitamin B6 analog 6-fluoropyridoxol (6-FPOL) reported to have a pK_a in the physiological range and large chemical shift response [35]. Subsequently the feasibility of using 6-FPOL to probe cellular pH was demonstrated in whole blood [36]. The concept of employing ^{19}F MR probes for in vivo imaging was introduced when a series of fluorinated vitamin B6 analogs with a chemical shift sensitivity in the range 7.4–12 ppm were synthesized as pH indicators [37]. The sensitivity of ^{19}F MRS probes can be further improved by incorporating paramagnetic metal ions that further amplify the chemical shift between protonated and deprotonated forms by the presence of covalent and dipolar contributions [38, 39]. Iron (II) complexes were also explored to exploit the pH-dependent spin-state population change; the ^{19}F NMR chemical shift was in a sensitivity range of 13.9 ppm per pH unit at 37 °C [40]. More recently fluorinated nickel (II) complexes with diamagnetic and paramagnetic properties were designed for ratiometric pH mapping by ^{19}F MRI [41]. Supramolecular nanostructures formed by fluorinated peptide amphiphiles transitioning from cylindrical to ribbon-like shape as pH increases from 4.5 to 8.0 resulting in enhanced MR signals. These nanostructures represent a good strategy to design stimulus-responsive ^{19}F MRI contrast agents for responses to pH changes in vivo [42].

2.2 ^{19}F MRI to Study Renal Inflammation In Vivo

Together with renal tissue hypoxia and tubular injury, inflammation is one underlying component in the pathology of AKI [43]. Studies suggest that systemic inflammation causes ischemic injury in one organ and that repercussions follow in distant organs downstream

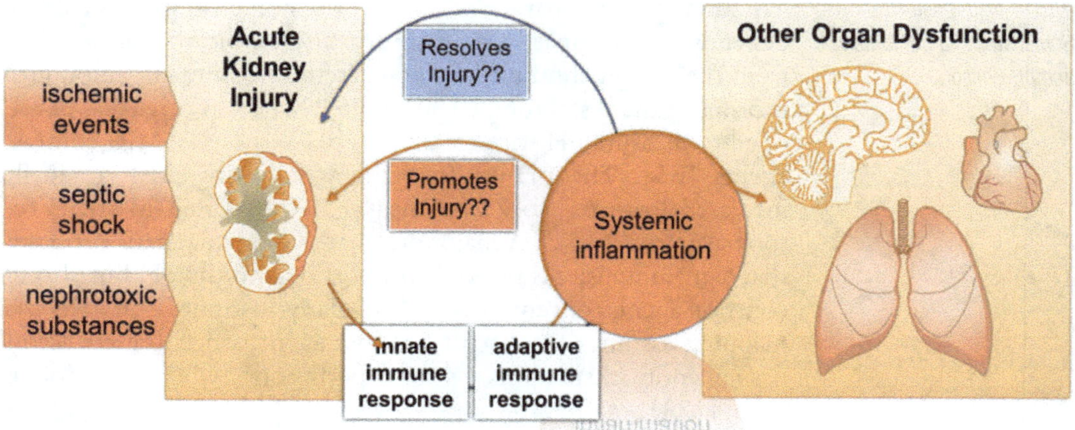

Fig. 2 Inflammation as one underlying factor in the pathology of AKI. AKI can be triggered by a variety of clinical disorders ranging from renal ischemic events to sepsis and exposure to nephrotoxic substances. The kidney is tightly connected with the interior milieu of the body such that even the slightest of changes will be rapidly detected and communicated between the kidney and the rest of the body

of the ischemic event [44–46] (Fig. 2). Therefore, methods that can non-invasively quantify the level of inflammation in different organs would be crucial to identify the causality and significance of inflammation during both systemic and kidney-specific disease.

^{19}F MRI is commonly used in association with an intravenous administration of PFC emulsions to study the distribution of inflammatory cells in vivo [26, 47–51]. ^{19}F MRI is performed after an in vivo labeling of inflammatory cells with a ^{19}F compound—typically in nanoparticle (NP) form. The ^{19}F-NPs are administered intravenously in order for them to be taken up by inflammatory cells that are migrating through the systemic circulation into inflamed organs. Typically, PFCs such as perfluoro-15-crown-5 ether (PFCE) are used to prepare NPs for cell labeling. PFCE is biologically stable and provides a high payload of ^{19}F nuclei since it contains 20 chemically equivalent ^{19}F spins.

In a rat model of orthotopic kidney transplantation, ^{19}F MRI was used to study inflammation in the kidney undergoing rejection [48]. Three days following transplantation, PFCE NPs were administered intravenously and ^{1}H/^{19}F images acquired 2 and 24 h following NP infusion (Fig. 3a). At the earlier time point, the ^{19}F signal was mainly found in the circulation but also in small but roughly equal amounts in both the native and transplanted kidneys (Fig. 3a). By day 4 posttransplantation (i.e., 24 h following PFCE NP), the transplanted kidney underwent moderate (Grade 2) rejection and showed an intense signal in the allograft kidney and in liver and spleen, but the ^{19}F signal was virtually undetectable above the level of image noise in the native kidney (Fig. 3a). T_2*-weighted

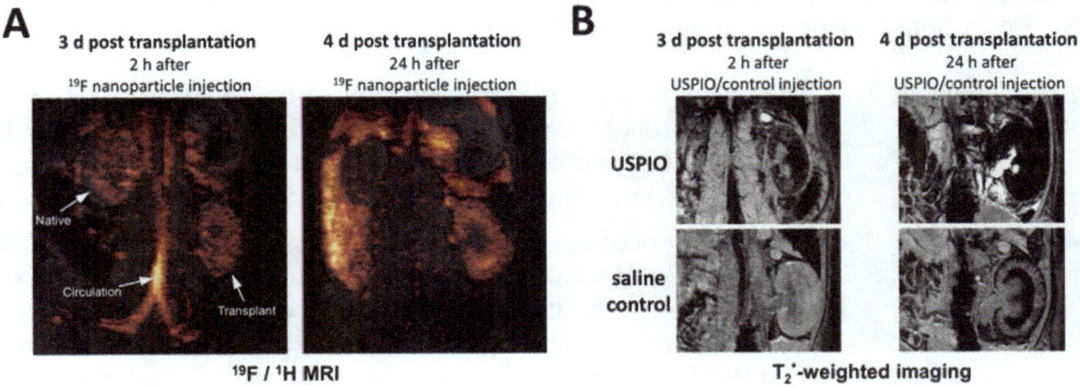

Fig. 3 Inflammation in the kidney in a rat model of orthotopic kidney transplantation experiencing rejection. (**a**) Composite $^{1}H/^{19}F$ images of an orthotopic kidney transplant recipient ~2 h post–PCE injection on POD 3 with ^{19}F signal found in the vasculature and equally in both the native (upper) and graft (lower) kidneys (left) and ~24 h post–PCE injection with ^{19}F signal in the allograft kidney, as well as other organs (right). (**b**) Allograft kidney on POD 4 following an injection (left) of 6 mg/kg BW USPIO (upper row) or following an injection of saline (lower row) and 24 h later (right). Adapted from Hitchens T.K. et al. (2011) [48] with permission from John Wiley & Sons Inc.

imaging reveals hemorrhaging in the medulla on day 4 post-kidney transplantation, which can be detected both in animals administered ultrasmall superparamagnetic iron oxide (USPIO) NPs but also in transplants without USPIO (saline control) (Fig. 3b). This can confound the detection of USPIO-labeled macrophages and exhibits one of the advantages of ^{19}F MRI over iron oxide-based NPs.

Apart from labeling inflammatory cells in vivo, NPs have been used to label specific immune cell types such as dendritic cells (DCs) ex vivo, prior to their administration in vivo [52–54]. This kind of labeling is particularly useful to label cellular therapies that will be administered in patients as part of a treatment strategy [55]. In addition to cancer patients, kidney transplantation patients would also benefit from cell-based therapies, specifically the types of cells inducing tolerance [56]. Monocyte-derived suppressor cell products are currently being investigated alongside immunosuppressive therapies in kidney transplant recipients with promising results [57]. These candidate therapies would benefit from a labeling strategy that will enable them to be tracked in vivo over time with ^{19}F MRI. The possibility of quantifying the ^{19}F MR signal would allow an objective assessment of the spatial and temporal cellular distribution within the same individual. This kind of labeling and ^{19}F MRI would result in absolute cell quantification, since the ^{19}F MR signal is generated from the cells alone, by direct detection of the ^{19}F spins in the cells labeled with ^{19}F NPs, without any confounding background MR signal. However, several biological and technical considerations need to be made, in order to achieve a truly absolute MR signal quantification: not all cell types can be labeled with the ^{19}F NPs currently available (Subheading 3.1.1).

3 Basic Concepts of ^{19}F MRI

3.1 ^{19}F imaging Probes

The design and synthesis of novel fluorine-rich molecular labels and imaging probes is an important domain for ^{19}F MRI. For several years, a wide range of fluorine probes has been available for experimental and even clinical applications [58, 59].

3.1.1 ^{19}F Probes for Cellular Uptake

Current procedures used to label cells with nanoparticles take advantage of the intrinsic nature of cells to engulf foreign bodies, a cellular property known as phagocytosis. Dendritic cells are intrinsically phagocytic and therefore ideal candidates for tracking with ^{19}F MRI [52, 53, 55, 60–62]. Cells labeled with clinical grade ^{19}F nanoparticles have been administered as immunotherapies in cancer patients [55]. This tracking method could support several other cell therapy studies, including those dealing with kidney transplantation [63].

Enhancing cellular uptake is desirable, even for cells that are intrinsically phagocytic. Several studies have investigated the incorporation of phosphatidylserine (PS) in nanoparticle-based therapeutics to enhance their uptake [64]. After renal ischemia–reperfusion, the signal from PS-containing microbubbles was two-fold higher than that for standard lipid microbubbles [65]. Phospholipids such as PS and phosphatidylethanolamine (PE) are important components of biological cell membranes and are important components for endocytosis in phagocytic cells such as DCs [66]. We previously reported that enrichment of ^{19}F nanoparticles with 1,2-dipalmitoyl-sn-glycero-3-PE (DPPE) resulted in a striking increase (at least one order of magnitude) in cytoplasmic uptake in DCs [62]. Interestingly, membrane lipid-raft processes have been proposed as trafficking mechanisms for transporting therapeutic cargo such as siRNA [67] or targeting ligands [68] into the cytoplasm, circumventing the usual endosomal uptake pathway.

Labeling cells with low intrinsic phagocytic properties (such as T cells) will prove more difficult using the above strategy, even if the nanoparticle size is lower than 180 nm [69]. Some research groups claim to have labeled T cells using the same above principles [70]. T cells are not able to internalize nanoparticles, even small iron oxide nanoparticles (core diameter = 12.5 nm), as has been clearly shown by transmission electron microscopy (TEM), considered to be a definitive method, and also by confocal microscopy [71]. For the latter method nanoparticles with fluorescent tags were used to corroborate the in vivo ^{19}F signals with ex vivo fluorescence microscopy signals, but the authors also included a cell membrane stain [71]. This is a necessary control to distinguish membrane association from intracellular distribution, in light of the point spread function contribution [72]. Another key point is that the fluorescent tag dissociates from the fluorine label over time, both in vitro and in vivo [73]. This has a critical impact on the interpretation of long-term experiments validated by standard fluorescent techniques.

Before taking the next steps toward administering cells in vivo, it is essential to understand how nanoparticles are recognized, internalized, trafficked, and distributed within the specific host cell [74]. This is critical when contemplating labeling of cells that may ultimately be applied in vivo to patients in a therapeutic context. Cells that are not intrinsically phagocytic will not readily internalize NPs but might still exhibit a ^{19}F MR signal ex vivo, due to reasons such as transitional binding of NPs to the cell membrane or incomplete clearing of noninternalized NPs from the cell culture medium. The ^{19}F MR signals following administration of ineffectively labeled cells with contaminating NPs would be misrepresentative of the actual distribution of the cells in vivo. Therefore, we need to ask the right questions regarding the specific cell type to be labeled, and the methods used prior to transfer of the cells into living organisms [75].

3.1.2 ^{19}F Probes with Increased Signal Sensitivity

Fluorinated probes are commonly designed with the goal of improving signal strength by increasing the number of fluorine atoms per molecule [59]. Linear ^{19}F polymers such as perfluoropolyethers (PFPEs) are the simplest choice to achieve increased fluorine content but the NPs produced with these polymers are polydisperse and the presence of multiple chemical shifts presents several peaks in the ^{19}F spectra [76]. Superfluorinated branched ^{19}F probes such as ^{19}FIT [77] and PERFECTA [78] promise several advantages, specifically a very high fluorine nuclei density with a single ^{19}F spectral peak. These probes therefore afford enhanced sensitivity and better imaging performance than linear perfluoropolymers. Unlike PERFECTA [78], the bispherical fluorocarbon ^{19}FIT is water soluble [77] and therefore possesses low organ retention, but it cannot be emulsified into nanoparticles for cell labeling strategies. Increasing the density of ^{19}F nuclei can only go so far in terms of increased sensitivity of ^{19}F probes. Ultimately, a limit to this density will be reached.

Another strategy to promote ^{19}F MR signal is to manipulate the MR properties of the ^{19}F probes in order to favor ideal conditions for MR signal acquisition. One approach is to decrease the T_1 of the ^{19}F nuclei, which is typically in the range of 0.5–3 s for diamagnetic compounds. Paramagnetic metal ions such as lanthanides(III) or iron(II) reduce the T_1 of ^{19}F compounds [38]. Paramagnetic centers affect the relaxation of ^{19}F nuclei (paramagnetic relaxation enhancement or PRE effect) via a number of mechanisms, most notably electron–nucleus dipole–dipole interaction and Curie relaxation [39], both of which are influenced by the effective magnetic moment (μ_{eff}) of the paramagnetic metal [79]. Other than the μ_{eff} of the metal ion, the PRE effect is also influenced by the distance separating the ^{19}F nuclei and the paramagnetic metal ion [39]. While long distances will severely diminish PRE, short distances will substantially shorten the spin–spin relaxation time T_2. Thus T_1 reduction by molecular design should be dealt with carefully since it could also lead to a reduction in the T_2 and thereby line broadening of the resonance, which ultimately affects sensitivity [80]. The most sensitive metal-based probes are, in fact, not those whose metal ions have the highest μ_{eff}, but rather those who have the ideal distance separating ^{19}F from the paramagnetic metal ion (4.5–7.5 Å) thus resulting in higher T_2/T_1 ratios [81]. Nonetheless even at larger ^{19}F–M distances (>10 Å), the PRE effect can still be notable as is the case for a DOTA-based ^{19}F chelator [82]. In paramagnetic PFC nanoparticles, the ^{19}F MR relaxation enhancement has also been explained by diffusion mechanisms attributed to the changes in Brownian motion of PFC molecules inside the NP in conjunction with their ability to permeate into the lipid surfactant coating [83].

Introduction of paramagnetic metals in the design of ^{19}F probes not only results in a decrease T_1 of ^{19}F nuclei but also leads to paramagnetic induced chemical shifts. The CEST signal generated by paramagnetic involvement (PARACEST) will also be modulated by pH (Subheading 2.1.2). A macrocyclic Fe (II) complex bearing both exchangeable ^{1}H and ^{19}F was shown to behave as a ratiometric pH-responsive MRI contrast agent, whereby the CEST, but not the ^{19}F MR signal was pH-dependent [84]. This enables accurate pH mapping without the use of multiple probes. More recently a DOTA macrocyclic structure complexed with Ni(II) metal was shown to exhibit larger separations between the ^{1}H CEST signal and water [85]. Though the in vivo application of ^{19}F PARACEST probes remains to be investigated, the available complexes will likely provide valuable information in the near future when probing pH changes in vivo.

3.2 MR Data Acquisition

3.2.1 Pulse Sequence Optimization

One way of improving signal sensitivity is to avoid signal losses such as those occurring during spin relaxation. Most fluorinated compounds generally have long T_1 relaxation times, which effectively increases the acquisition time. Together with the fact that there is a large range of relaxation times for ^{19}F MR, this motivates more reliable optimization of pulse sequences that is informed by the MR properties of the ^{19}F compounds under investigation. Sequence performance is largely dependent on the relaxation times of the addressed spin system but also on the conditions the nuclei are in, such as tissue oxygenation level [17].

The choice of the best pulse sequence and acquisition method is dictated by the MR properties, particularly the relaxation times, of the nuclei being measured. The acquisition protocol for each sequence should be optimized by tailoring detection schemes to the properties of the nucleus—also in relation to its environment—using relationships empirically drawn from simulations [86]. Relaxation times determine the time frames of signal losses, so the time orchestration for data acquisition should be assigned correctly. Other parameters, such as acquisition bandwidths, should also be properly planned to avoid recording unnecessary noise and to achieve the highest possible SNR [87].

A number of ^{19}F MR studies using different pulse sequences have aimed to optimize the acquisition method to promote SNR efficiency and signal sensitivity [17, 87–90]. A large proportion of ^{19}F MR studies, especially those applying perfluorocarbons (PFCs) in vivo, have employed the turbo spin echo (SE) rapid acquisition using relaxation enhancement (RARE) sequence [26, 47, 50, 51, 91]. This method reduces acquisition time by accumulating multiple echoes (dictated by the turbo factor) within a single repetition time [92]. Optimal settings for echo train lengths and repetition time (TR) according to measured relaxation times (T_1/T_2 combinations) were calculated for RARE to improve sensitivity thresholds [90].

Although RARE is commonly been for studying PFCs in vivo, other sequences will be better suited for ^{19}F compounds that unlike typical PFCs have short T_2 relaxation times. In such cases signal detection might be technically challenging and will demand acquisition strategies properly adapted for the compound and its environment. Gradient echo (GE) sequences were used to maximize SNR efficiency for imaging paramagnetic macrocyclic ^{19}F molecules complexed to lanthanides [87]. These molecules exhibit T_1 values in the order of 1–15 ms and T_2* values in the order of 0.4–12 ms [88]. In the latter study a radial zero echo time (ZTE) sequence yielded a sensitivity gain of 27-fold when compared to nonparamagnetic molecules, while the GE sequence yielded a gain of 11-fold [88]. Additionally, the highest SNR efficiency gain was achieved when T_2/T_1 were close to 1, particularly for the ZTE pulse sequence, and when T_1 was in the range of 1–5 ms [88]. Even ^{19}F molecules with unique spectral properties will require a more individualized adjustment of the MR parameters; such molecules might benefit from sequences such as ultrashort echo time (UTE) that acquire signal before the spins dephase, taking into consideration destructive phase interference [93]. An efficient k-space sampling strategy will be necessary to achieve maximal SNR and artifact-free MR images [94]. To image perfluorooctyl bromide (PFOB) that has a rich spectrum with large chemical shifts, a radial UTE with a balanced steady-state free precession (bSSFP) pulse sequence showed superiority above other sequences, such as SE, GE, or bSSFP with Cartesian sampling [89]. However, radial sampling might not always be viable since k space sampling pattern effects need to be considered, which might altogether result in reduced SNR efficiency [86]. Another way to speed up data acquisition is synchronous multinuclear imaging. For this, the MR system needs to have the architecture suited to acquire images from more than one nucleus in a single pulse sequence [95]. Simultaneous proton and ^{19}F MRI was performed in a preclinical model using a clinical MR scanner at 3 T [95].

3.3 Hardware Considerations

The similarity between ^{19}F and ^{1}H MR properties with respect to sensitivity and resonance frequency is an advantage, from an engineering perspective since similar pulse power settings can be used, and dual-tuned radio frequency (RF) coils for ^{19}F and ^{1}H MRI are more convenient to design [50, 96]. One way of improving the ^{19}F MR signal in vivo is to increase SNR by improving the sensitivity of the measuring instrument. Two hardware strategies to improve sensitivity for ^{19}F MR are to increase the strength of the static magnetic field (B_0), and to increase the sensitivity of the RF coil by cryogenic cooling.

3.3.1 Cryogenic Cooling

The sensitivity of the RF coil is an important factor limiting SNR and thereby the level of spatial and temporal resolution that is targeted for ^{19}F MRI [97]. Even when employing an RF coil with a homogeneous transmit field (B_1^+) distribution and dedicated for brain ^{19}F and ^{1}H MRI, the spatial resolution of in vivo ^{19}F MRI was limited to approximately 600 μm [50]. This level of spatial resolution prohibits a detailed understanding of inflammation dynamics. To overcome the sensitivity constraints in ^{19}F MR and improve detail of inflammatory cell location, we applied the concept of cryogenically cooling RF coil hardware to improve SNR by reducing thermal noise [98–100]. The cryogenically cooled RF coil (CryoProbe™) technology is commercially available for small animal MRI of ^{1}H and X-nuclei such as carbon (^{13}C) and phosphorous (^{31}P). For these X-nuclei this technology is expected to be particularly useful for increasing SNR. A gain in SNR of 3.0- to 3.5-fold was reported for the ^{13}C CryoProbe [101]. We recently compared a ^{19}F CryoProbe with a room temperature ^{19}F RF coil of similar size and reported on a maximal SNR gain of 15-fold and were able to study inflammation at an isotropic resolution of 150 μm [100].

Surface RF coils provide a very high SNR close to the region where they are applied. However, a decrease in signal amplitude with increasing distance from their surface is inherent to the geometry of their design. Inhomogeneities in the transmit (B_1^+) field cause a spatially varying flip angle (FA) and as a result signal quantification is hampered. Likewise, the receive (B_1^-) field of surface RF coils is position-dependent [102]. In the particular case of the ^{19}F CryoProbe, we observed a strong FA decrease with increasing distance from the surface of the coil [100]. Using a receive-only surface RF coil in combination with a volume resonator used for transmission would overcome B_1^+ inhomogeneities. With this configuration the transmitted FAs will be homogeneous, thus enabling quantification [103]. This option is not available when using CryoProbes, since they are typically built in the form of transceive (transmit–receive) RF coils with no active decoupling.

Particularly for quantitative ^{19}F MRI, a correction of the B_1^+ inhomogeneity will be necessary when comparing concentrations of PFC in vivo with an external standard of known ^{19}F concentration. Differences in the B_1^+ field between the region of interest in vivo and the external standard will result in errors when quantifying in vivo ^{19}F signals. Several approaches have been implemented to correct B_1^+ inhomogeneities retrospectively, even for ^{19}F MRI [104, 105]. These approaches typically include RF pulse sequences for which an analytical knowledge of the signal intensity dependency on the FA exists.

3.3.2 Magnetic Field Strengths

Increasing the strength of the static magnetic field (B_0) will increase SNR of the measured signal [106], a strategy which is actively being pursued for clinical application [107]. Intrinsic SNR is expected to grow at least linearly with increasing B_0 strengths [97, 108, 109]. The principle of reciprocity can be used at low field strengths to calculate the receive field (B_1) sensitivity of a single channel RF coil in terms of the transmit field (B_1^+) that can be easily measured [110]. In studies performed at frequency (f) <1 MHz the maximum sensitivity was calculated to be proportional to the f: sensitivity $\propto f1.75$ [97, 108]. When going to higher magnetic field strengths, the increasing f and the influence of wave propagation need to be considered [106]. The homogeneity of the B_1^+ field is expected to decline with increasing B_0, thereby influencing the overall SNR gain. An experimental study investigating SNR dependency on B_0 in the human brain revealed that SNR $\propto B_0 1.65$ in the range of 3.0–9.4 T [109]. A recent simulation study also showed that SNR grows superlinearly with frequency, particularly in deeper regions of the sample; in less deep regions the SNR versus B_0 trend approached linearity [111].

An increase in magnetic field strength is particularly beneficial for X-nuclei imaging. An increase in B_0 from 9.4 to 21.1 T results in an SNR gain of ~3 compared to a gain of ~2 for ^{1}H MR [112]. We recently studied the influence of increasing B_0 on improving ^{19}F MR signal sensitivity [113]. Prior to the practical experiments, we estimated the expected SNR gain when moving from 9.4 to 21.1 T to be 2.7 [113]. We estimated SNR gain using the principle of reciprocity [110] and ignoring all flip angle, sequence and relaxation-dependent effects. The estimated SNR gain represents a baseline expectation, based on the information available for the specific hardware of each system. When introducing the relationship of the reference power for both MR systems, we estimated an SNR gain of ~3.8. In our practical experiments the ratio in SNR efficiency (SNR/$\sqrt{t}$ ratio) was estimated to be 7.29, when comparing the best possible conditions for both 21.1 and 9.4 T, and when including T_1 relaxation effects [113]. Differences between the actual SNR gains determined experimentally and those expected from simulations are conceivable, due to minor inaccuracies in the assumptions made for the EMF simulations.

All research efforts ranging from new ^{19}F probe design, through optimization of ^{19}F MR data acquisition methods up to hardware developments hinge on the need for promoting ^{19}F MR signal in vivo, in order to answer crucial questions during pathology including kidney disease. Most of the efforts devoted to discovery and proof-of-principle research will benefit from an integration of all available tools and technologies, in order to reach the maximum potential for practical applications for patient health care.

Acknowledgments

This work was funded in part (Thoralf Niendorf, Sonia Waiczies, Andreas Pohlmann) by the German Research Foundation (Gefoerdert durch die Deutsche Forschungsgemeinschaft (DFG), Projektnummer 394046635, SFB 1365, RENOPROTECTION. Funded by the Deutsche Forschungsgemeinschaft (DFG, German Research Foundation), Project number 394046635, SFB 1365, RENOPROTECTION).

Also, our research is funded by the Deutsche Forschungsgemeinschaft to S.W. (DFG WA2804) and A.P. (DFG PO1869), by the European Research Council, ERC to T.N. (ThermalMR, EU project 743077), by the State of Florida and National Science Foundation Cooperative Agreement No. DMR-1157490 and DMR-1644779 to J.R. and the Visiting Scientist Program of the NHMFL to S.W. and H.W. (227000-110, Project 12643). We thank Professor Samuel Wickline from the University of South Florida for valuable feedback on the manuscript.

This publication is based upon work from COST Action PARENCHIMA, supported by European Cooperation in Science and Technology (COST). COST (www.cost.eu) is a funding agency for research and innovation networks. COST Actions help connect research initiatives across Europe and enable scientists to enrich their ideas by sharing them with their peers. This boosts their research, career, and innovation.

PARENCHIMA (renalmri.org) is a community-driven Action in the COST program of the European Union, which unites more than 200 experts in renal MRI from 30 countries with the aim to improve the reproducibility and standardization of renal MRI biomarkers.

References

1. Hingorani DV, Bernstein AS, Pagel MD (2015) A review of responsive MRI contrast agents: 2005–2014. Contrast Media Mol Imaging 10(4):245–265. https://doi.org/10.1002/cmmi.1629
2. Grenier N, Merville P, Combe C (2016) Radiologic imaging of the renal parenchyma structure and function. Nat Rev Nephrol 12 (6):348–359

3. Martinez GV, Zhang X, García-Martín ML, Morse DL, Woods M, Sherry AD, Gillies RJ (2011) Imaging the extracellular pH of tumors by MRI after injection of a single cocktail of T1 and T2 contrast agents. NMR Biomed 24(10):1380–1391. https://doi.org/10.1002/nbm.1701
4. Brooks RA, Brunetti A, Alger JR, Di Chiro G (1989) On the origin of paramagnetic inhomogeneity effects in blood. Magn Reson Med 12(2):241–248
5. Günther H (2013) NMR spectroscopy: basic principles, concepts and applications in chemistry. John Wiley & Sons, Hoboken, NJ
6. Dolbier WR (2009) Guide to fluorine NMR for organic chemists. John Wiley & Sons, Hoboken, NJ
7. Arami H, Khandhar A, Liggitt D, Krishnan KM (2015) In vivo delivery, pharmacokinetics, biodistribution and toxicity of iron oxide nanoparticles. Chem Soc Rev 44 (23):8576–8607. https://doi.org/10.1039/c5cs00541h
8. Toth GB, Varallyay CG, Horvath A, Bashir MR, Choyke PL, Daldrup-Link HE, Dosa E, Finn JP, Gahramanov S, Harisinghani M, Macdougall I, Neuwelt A, Vasanawala SS, Ambady P, Barajas R, Cetas JS, Ciporen J, DeLoughery TJ, Doolittle ND, Fu R, Grinstead J, Guimaraes AR, Hamilton BE, Li X, McConnell HL, Muldoon LL, Nesbit G, Netto JP, Petterson D, Rooney WD, Schwartz D, Szidonya L, Neuwelt EA (2017) Current and potential imaging applications of ferumoxytol for magnetic resonance imaging. Kidney Int 92(1):47–66. https://doi.org/10.1016/j.kint.2016.12.037
9. Feng Q, Liu Y, Huang J, Chen K, Huang J, Xiao K (2018) Uptake, distribution, clearance, and toxicity of iron oxide nanoparticles with different sizes and coatings. Sci Rep 8 (1):2082. https://doi.org/10.1038/s41598-018-19628-z
10. Longmire M, Choyke PL, Kobayashi H (2008) Clearance properties of nano-sized particles and molecules as imaging agents: considerations and caveats. Nanomedicine (Lond) 3(5):703–717. https://doi.org/10.2217/17435889.3.5.703
11. O'Connor PM (2006) Renal oxygen delivery: matching delivery to metabolic demand. Clin Exp Pharmacol Physiol 33(10):961–967. https://doi.org/10.1111/j.1440-1681.2006.04475.x
12. Hansell P, Welch WJ, Blantz RC, Palm F (2013) Determinants of kidney oxygen consumption and their relationship to tissue oxygen tension in diabetes and hypertension. Clin Exp Pharmacol Physiol 40(2):123–137. https://doi.org/10.1111/1440-1681.12034
13. Le Dorze M, Legrand M, Payen D, Ince C (2009) The role of the microcirculation in acute kidney injury. Curr Opin Crit Care 15 (6):503–508. https://doi.org/10.1097/MCC.0b013e328332f6cf
14. Ries M, Basseau F, Tyndal B, Jones R, Deminière C, Catargi B, Combe C, Moonen CWT, Grenier N (2003) Renal diffusion and BOLD MRI in experimental diabetic nephropathy. J Magn Reson Imaging 17 (1):104–113. https://doi.org/10.1002/jmri.10224
15. Prasad PV (2006) Evaluation of intra-renal oxygenation by BOLD MRI. Nephron Clin Pract 103(2):c58–c65. https://doi.org/10.1159/000090610
16. Niendorf T, Pohlmann A, Arakelyan K, Flemming B, Cantow K, Hentschel J, Grosenick D, Ladwig M, Reimann H, Klix S, Waiczies S, Seeliger E (2015) How bold is blood oxygenation level-dependent (BOLD) magnetic resonance imaging of the kidney? Opportunities, challenges and future directions. Acta Physiol 213(1):19–38. https://doi.org/10.1111/apha.12393
17. Dardzinski BJ, Sotak CH (1994) Rapid tissue oxygen tension mapping using 19F inversion-recovery echo-planar imaging of P erfluoro-15-crown-5-ether. Magn Reson Med 32 (1):88–97
18. Noth U, Morrissey SP, Deichmann R, Adolf H, Schwarzbauer C, Lutz J, Haase A (1995) In vivo measurement of partial oxygen pressure in large vessels and in the reticuloendothelial system using fast 19F-MRI. Magn Reson Med 34(5):738–745
19. Chen J, Vemuri C, Palekar RU, Gaut JP, Goette M, Hu L, Cui G, Zhang H, Wickline SA (2015) Antithrombin nanoparticles improve kidney reperfusion and protect kidney function after ischemia-reperfusion injury. Am J Physiol Renal Physiol 308(7):28
20. Hu L, Chen J, Yang X, Senpan A, Allen JS, Yanaba N, Caruthers SD, Lanza GM, Hammerman MR, Wickline SA (2013) Assessing intrarenal nonperfusion and vascular leakage in acute kidney injury with multinuclear 1H/19F MRI and perfluorocarbon nanoparticles. Magn Reson Med. https://doi.org/10.1002/mrm.24851
21. Riess JG (2005) Understanding the fundamentals of perfluorocarbons and perfluorocarbon emulsions relevant to in vivo oxygen

delivery. Artif Cell Blood Sub Biotechnol 33 (1):47–63

22. Schmieder AH, Caruthers SD, Keupp J, Wickline SA, Lanza GM (2015) Recent advances in (19)fluorine magnetic resonance imaging with perfluorocarbon emulsions. Engineering (Beijing, China) 1(4):475–489. https://doi.org/10.15302/j-eng-2015103
23. Mitsuno T, Ohyanagi H, Naito R (1982) Clinical studies of a perfluorochemical whole blood substitute (Fluosol-DA) summary of 186 cases. Ann Surg 195(1):60–69. https://doi.org/10.1097/00000658-198201001-00010
24. Gould SA, Rosen AL, Sehgal LR, Sehgal HL, Langdale LA, Krause LM, Rice CL, Chamberlin WH, Moss GS (1986) Fluosol-DA as a red-cell substitute in acute anemia. N Engl J Med 314(26):1653–1656. https://doi.org/10.1056/nejm198606263142601
25. McFarland E, Koutcher JA, Rosen BR, Teicher B, Brady TJ (1985) In vivo 19F NMR imaging. J Comput Assist Tomogr 9 (1):8–15
26. Jacoby C, Temme S, Mayenfels F, Benoit N, Krafft MP, Schubert R, Schrader J, Flögel U (2014) Probing different perfluorocarbons for in vivo inflammation imaging by 19F MRI: image reconstruction, biological half-lives and sensitivity. NMR Biomed 27 (3):261–271. https://doi.org/10.1002/nbm.3059
27. Parhami P, Fung B (1983) Fluorine-19 relaxation study of perfluoro chemicals as oxygen carriers. J Phys Chem 87(11):1928–1931
28. Mason RP, Nunnally RL, Antich PP (1991) Tissue oxygenation: a novel determination using 19F surface coil NMR spectroscopy of sequestered perfluorocarbon emulsion. Magn Reson Med 18(1):71–79. https://doi.org/10.1002/mrm.1910180109
29. Mason RP, Jeffrey FMH, Malloy CR, Babcock EE, Antich PP (1992) A noninvasive assessment of myocardial oxygen tension: 19f nmr spectroscopy of sequestered perfluorocarbon emulsion. Magn Reson Med 27(2):310–317. https://doi.org/10.1002/mrm.1910270210
30. Pereira PCB, Miranda DM, Oliveira EA, Silva ACSE (2009) Molecular pathophysiology of renal tubular acidosis. Curr Genomics 10 (1):51–59. https://doi.org/10.2174/138920209787581262
31. Zhang S, Wu K, Sherry AD (1999) A novel pH-sensitive MRI contrast agent. Angew Chem Int Ed 38(21):3192–3194. https://doi.org/10.1002/(sici)1521-3773(19991102)38:21<3192::aid-anie3192>3.0.co;2-#
32. Longo DL, Busato A, Lanzardo S, Antico F, Aime S (2013) Imaging the pH evolution of an acute kidney injury model by means of iopamidol, a MRI-CEST pH-responsive contrast agent. Magn Reson Med 70 (3):859–864. https://doi.org/10.1002/mrm.24513
33. Raghunand N, Gatenby RA, Gillies RJ (2003) Microenvironmental and cellular consequences of altered blood flow in tumours. Br J Radiol 76(Suppl_1):S11–S22. https://doi.org/10.1259/bjr/12913493
34. Gianolio E, Napolitano R, Fedeli F, Arena F, Aime S (2009) Poly-β-cyclodextrin based platform for pH mapping via a ratiometric 19F/1H MRI method. Chem Commun 40:6044–6046. https://doi.org/10.1039/B914540K
35. Chang YC, Graves DJ (1985) Use of 6-fluoroderivatives of pyridoxal and pyridoxal phosphate in the study of the coenzyme function in glycogen phosphorylase. J Biol Chem 260(5):2709–2714
36. Mehta VD, Kulkarni PV, Mason RP, Constantinescu A, Aravind S, Goomer N, Antich PP (1994) 6-Fluoropyridoxol: a novel probe of cellular pH using 19F NMR spectroscopy. FEBS Lett 349(2):234–238. https://doi.org/10.1016/0014-5793(94)00675-x
37. He S, Mason RP, Hunjan S, Mehta VD, Arora V, Katipally R, Kulkarni PV, Antich PP (1998) Development of novel 19F NMR pH indicators: synthesis and evaluation of a series of fluorinated vitamin B6 analogues. Bioorg Med Chem 6(9):1631–1639. https://doi.org/10.1016/S0968-0896(98)00104-7
38. Neubauer AM, Myerson J, Caruthers SD, Hockett FD, Winter PM, Chen J, Gaffney PJ, Robertson JD, Lanza GM, Wickline SA (2008) Gadolinium-modulated 19F signals from perfluorocarbon nanoparticles as a new strategy for molecular imaging. Magn Reson Med 60(5):1066–1072
39. Chalmers KH, De Luca E, Hogg NHM, Kenwright AM, Kuprov I, Parker D, Botta M, Wilson JI, Blamire AM (2010) Design principles and theory of paramagnetic fluorine-labelled lanthanide complexes as probes for 19F magnetic resonance: a proof-of-concept study. Chem Eur J 16(1):134–148. https://doi.org/10.1002/chem.200902300
40. Gaudette AI, Thorarinsdottir AE, Harris TD (2017) pH-dependent spin state population and 19F NMR chemical shift via remote ligand protonation in an iron(ii) complex.

Chem Commun 53(96):12962–12965. https://doi.org/10.1039/C7CC08158H

41. Xie D, Ohman LE, Que EL (2018) Towards Ni(II) complexes with spin switches for 19F MR-based pH sensing. MAGMA. https://doi.org/10.1007/s10334-018-0698-4
42. Preslar AT, Tantakitti F, Park K, Zhang S, Stupp SI, Meade TJ (2016) 19F magnetic resonance imaging signals from peptide amphiphile nanostructures are strongly affected by their shape. ACS Nano 10 (8):7376–7384. https://doi.org/10.1021/acsnano.6b00267
43. Liu KD, Glidden DV, Eisner MD, Parsons PE, Ware LB, Wheeler A, Korpak A, Thompson BT, Chertow GM, Matthay MA (2007) Predictive and pathogenetic value of plasma biomarkers for acute kidney injury in patients with acute lung injury. Crit Care Med 35 (12):2755–2761
44. Levy EM, Viscoli CM, Horwitz RI (1996) The effect of acute renal failure on mortality. A cohort analysis. JAMA 275 (19):1489–1494
45. Jorres A, Gahl GM, Dobis C, Polenakovic MH, Cakalaroski K, Rutkowski B, Kisielnicka E, Krieter DH, Rumpf KW, Guenther C, Gaus W, Hoegel J (1999) Haemodialysis-membrane biocompatibility and mortality of patients with dialysis-dependent acute renal failure: a prospective randomised multicentre trial. International Multicentre Study Group. Lancet 354 (9187):1337–1341
46. Brouns R, De Deyn PP (2004) Neurological complications in renal failure: a review. Clin Neurol Neurosurg 107(1):1–16. https://doi.org/10.1016/j.clineuro.2004.07.012
47. Flögel U, Ding Z, Hardung H, Jander S, Reichmann G, Jacoby C, Schubert R, Schrader J (2008) In vivo monitoring of inflammation after cardiac and cerebral ischemia by fluorine magnetic resonance imaging. Circulation 118(2):140–148
48. Hitchens TK, Ye Q, Eytan DF, Janjic JM, Ahrens ET, Ho C (2011) 19F MRI detection of acute allograft rejection with in vivo perfluorocarbon labeling of immune cells. Magn Reson Med 65(4):1144–1153. https://doi.org/10.1002/mrm.22702
49. Temme S, Bonner F, Schrader J, Flögel U (2012) 19F magnetic resonance imaging of endogenous macrophages in inflammation. Wiley Interdiscip Rev Nanomed Nanobiotechnol 4(3):329–343. https://doi.org/10.1002/wnan.1163
50. Waiczies H, Lepore S, Drechsler S, Qadri F, Purfurst B, Sydow K, Dathe M, Kuhne A, Lindel T, Hoffmann W, Pohlmann A, Niendorf T, Waiczies S (2013) Visualizing brain inflammation with a shingled-leg radiofrequency head probe for 19F/1H MRI. Sci Rep 3:1280. https://doi.org/10.1038/srep01280
51. Flögel U, Burghoff S, van Lent PL, Temme S, Galbarz L, Ding Z, El-Tayeb A, Huels S, Bonner F, Borg N, Jacoby C, Muller CE, van den Berg WB, Schrader J (2012) Selective activation of adenosine A2A receptors on immune cells by a CD73-dependent prodrug suppresses joint inflammation in experimental rheumatoid arthritis. Sci Transl Med 4 (146):146ra108. https://doi.org/10.1126/scitranslmed.3003717
52. Ahrens ET, Flores R, Xu H, Morel PA (2005) In vivo imaging platform for tracking immunotherapeutic cells. Nat Biotechnol 23 (8):983–987
53. Waiczies H, Lepore S, Janitzek N, Hagen U, Seifert F, Ittermann B, Purfurst B, Pezzutto A, Paul F, Niendorf T, Waiczies S (2011) Perfluorocarbon particle size influences magnetic resonance signal and immunological properties of dendritic cells. PLoS One 6(7):e21981
54. Waiczies H, Guenther M, Skodowski J, Lepore S, Pohlmann A, Niendorf T, Waiczies S (2013) Monitoring dendritic cell migration using 19F/1H magnetic resonance imaging. J Vis Exp 73:e50251. https://doi.org/10.3791/50251
55. Ahrens ET, Helfer BM, O'Hanlon CF, Schirda C (2014) Clinical cell therapy imaging using a perfluorocarbon tracer and fluorine-19 MRI. Magn Reson Med 72 (6):1696-1701. https://doi.org/10.1002/mrm.25454
56. Ten Brinke A, Hilkens CMU, Cools N, Geissler EK, Hutchinson JA, Lombardi G, Lord P, Sawitzki B, Trzonkowski P, Van Ham SM, Martinez-Caceres EM (2015) Clinical use of tolerogenic dendritic cells-harmonization approach in european collaborative effort. Mediat Inflamm 2015:8. https://doi.org/10.1155/2015/471719
57. Hutchinson JA, Riquelme P, Sawitzki B, Tomiuk S, Miqueu P, Zuhayra M, Oberg HH, Pascher A, Lützen U, Janßen U, Broichhausen C, Renders L, Thaiss F, Scheuermann E, Henze E, Volk H-D, Chatenoud L, Lechler RI, Wood KJ, Kabelitz D, Schlitt HJ, Geissler EK, Fändrich F (2011) Cutting edge: immunological consequences and trafficking of human regulatory

macrophages administered to renal transplant recipients. J Immunol 187(5):2072–2078. https://doi.org/10.4049/jimmunol.1100762

58. Ruiz-Cabello J, Barnett BP, Bottomley PA, Bulte JW (2011) Fluorine (19F) MRS and MRI in biomedicine. NMR Biomed 24 (2):114–129. https://doi.org/10.1002/nbm.1570
59. Jirak D, Galisova A, Kolouchova K, Babuka D, Hruby M (2018) Fluorine polymer probes for magnetic resonance imaging: quo vadis? MAGMA. https://doi.org/10.1007/s10334-018-0724-6
60. Helfer BM, Balducci A, Nelson AD, Janjic JM, Gil RR, Kalinski P, de Vries IJ, Ahrens ET, Mailliard RB (2010) Functional assessment of human dendritic cells labeled for in vivo (19)F magnetic resonance imaging cell tracking. Cytotherapy 12(2):238–250. https://doi.org/10.3109/14653240903446902
61. Bonetto F, Srinivas M, Heerschap A, Mailliard R, Ahrens ET, Figdor CG, de Vries IJ (2011) A novel (19)F agent for detection and quantification of human dendritic cells using magnetic resonance imaging. Int J Cancer 129(2):365–373. https://doi.org/10.1002/ijc.25672
62. Waiczies S, Lepore S, Sydow K, Drechsler S, Ku MC, Martin C, Lorenz D, Schutz I, Reimann HM, Purfurst B, Dieringer MA, Waiczies H, Dathe M, Pohlmann A, Niendorf T (2015) Anchoring dipalmitoyl phosphoethanolamine to nanoparticles boosts cellular uptake and fluorine-19 magnetic resonance signal. Sci Rep 5:8427. https://doi.org/10.1038/srep08427
63. Hutchinson JA, Ahrens N, Riquelme P, Walter L, Gruber M, Böger CA, Farkas S, Scherer MN, Broichhausen C, Bein T, Schlitt H-J, Fändrich F, Banas B, Geissler EK (2014) Clinical management of patients receiving cell-based immunoregulatory therapy. Transfusion 54(9):2336–2343. https://doi.org/10.1111/trf.12641
64. Bagalkot V, Deiuliis JA, Rajagopalan S, Maiseyeu A (2016) "Eat me" imaging and therapy. Adv Drug Deliv Rev 99(Pt A):2–11. https://doi.org/10.1016/j.addr.2016.01.009
65. Lindner JR, Song J, Xu F, Klibanov AL, Singbartl K, Ley K, Kaul S (2000) Noninvasive ultrasound imaging of inflammation using microbubbles targeted to activated leukocytes. Inflammation 102:2745–2750
66. Steinman RM, Mellman IS, Muller WA, Cohn ZA (1983) Endocytosis and the recycling of plasma membrane. J Cell Biol 96(1):1–27
67. Kaneda MM, Sasaki Y, Lanza GM, Milbrandt J, Wickline SA (2010) Mechanisms of nucleotide trafficking during siRNA delivery to endothelial cells using perfluorocarbon nanoemulsions. Biomaterials 31 (11):3079–3086
68. Partlow KC, Lanza GM, Wickline SA (2008) Exploiting lipid raft transport with membrane targeted nanoparticles: a strategy for cytosolic drug delivery. Biomaterials 29 (23):3367–3375
69. Chapelin F, Capitini CM, Ahrens ET (2018) Fluorine-19 MRI for detection and quantification of immune cell therapy for cancer. J Immunother Cancer 6(1):105. https://doi.org/10.1186/s40425-018-0416-9
70. Chapelin F, Gao S, Okada H, Weber TG, Messer K, Ahrens ET (2017) Fluorine-19 nuclear magnetic resonance of chimeric antigen receptor T cell biodistribution in murine cancer model. Sci Rep 7(1):17748. https://doi.org/10.1038/s41598-017-17669-4
71. Sanz-Ortega L, Rojas JM, Marcos A, Portilla Y, Stein JV, Barber DF (2019) T cells loaded with magnetic nanoparticles are retained in peripheral lymph nodes by the application of a magnetic field. J Nanobiotechnol 17(1):14. https://doi.org/10.1186/s12951-019-0440-z
72. Stephens DJ, Allan VJ (2003) Light microscopy techniques for live cell imaging. Science 300(5616):82–86. https://doi.org/10.1126/science.1082160
73. Bouvain P, Flocke V, Krämer W, Schubert R, Schrader J, Flögel U, Temme S (2018) Dissociation of 19F and fluorescence signal upon cellular uptake of dual-contrast perfluorocarbon nanoemulsions. MAGMA. https://doi.org/10.1007/s10334-018-0723-7
74. Gustafson HH, Holt-Casper D, Grainger DW, Ghandehari H (2015) Nanoparticle uptake: the phagocyte problem. Nano Today 10(4):487–510. https://doi.org/10.1016/j.nantod.2015.06.006
75. Waiczies S, Niendorf T, Lombardi G (2017) Labeling of cell therapies: how can we get it right? Oncoimmunology 2017:e1345403. https://doi.org/10.1080/2162402x.2017.1345403
76. Tirotta I, Dichiarante V, Pigliacelli C, Cavallo G, Terraneo G, Bombelli FB, Metrangolo P, Resnati G (2015) 19F magnetic resonance imaging (MRI): from design of materials to clinical applications. Chem Rev 115(2):1106–1129. https://doi.org/10.1021/cr500286d
77. Jiang ZX, Liu X, Jeong EK, Yu YB (2009) Symmetry-guided design and fluorous synthesis of a stable and rapidly excreted imaging

tracer for 19F MRI. Angew Chem Int Edn 48 (26):4755–4758. https://doi.org/10.1002/anie.200901005

78. Tirotta I, Mastropietro A, Cordiglieri C, Gazzera L, Baggi F, Baselli G, Bruzzone MG, Zucca I, Cavallo G, Terraneo G, Baldelli Bombelli F, Metrangolo P, Resnati G (2014) A superfluorinated molecular probe for highly sensitive in vivo(19)F-MRI. J Am Chem Soc 136(24):8524–8527. https://doi.org/10.1021/ja503270n
79. Peterson KL, Srivastava K, Pierre VC (2018) Fluorinated paramagnetic complexes: sensitive and responsive probes for magnetic resonance spectroscopy and imaging. Front Chem 6:160–160. https://doi.org/10.3389/fchem.2018.00160
80. Kislukhin AA, Xu H, Adams SR, Narsinh KH, Tsien RY, Ahrens ET (2016) Paramagnetic fluorinated nanoemulsions for sensitive cellular fluorine-19 magnetic resonance imaging. Nat Mater 15:662. https://doi.org/10.1038/nmat4585. https://www.nature.com/articles/nmat4585#supplementary-information
81. Harvey P, Kuprov I, Parker D (2012) Lanthanide complexes as paramagnetic probes for 19F magnetic resonance. Eur J Inorg Chem 2012(12):2015–2022
82. Jiang Z-X, Feng Y, Yu YB (2011) Fluorinated paramagnetic chelates as potential multichromic 19 F tracer agents. Chem Commun 47(25):7233–7235
83. Hu L, Zhang L, Chen J, Lanza GM, Wickline SA (2011) Diffusional mechanisms augment the fluorine MR relaxation in paramagnetic perfluorocarbon nanoparticles that provides a "relaxation switch" for detecting cellular endosomal activation. J Magn Reson Imaging 34(3):653–661
84. Srivastava K, Ferrauto G, Young VG, Aime S, Pierre VC (2017) Eight-coordinate, stable Fe (II) complex as a dual 19F and CEST contrast agent for ratiometric pH imaging. Inorg Chem 56(20):12206–12213. https://doi.org/10.1021/acs.inorgchem.7b01629
85. Yu M, Bouley BS, Xie D, Que EL (2019) Highly fluorinated metal complexes as dual 19F and PARACEST imaging agents. Dalton Trans. https://doi.org/10.1039/C9DT01852B
86. Faber C, Schmid F (2016) Pulse sequence considerations and schemes. Fluorine magnetic resonance imaging. Pan Stanford Publishing, Singapore, pp 1–28
87. Chalmers KH, Kenwright AM, Parker D, Blamire AM (2011) 19F-lanthanide complexes with increased sensitivity for 19F-MRI: optimization of the MR acquisition. Magn Reson Med 66(4):931–936. https://doi.org/10.1002/mrm.22881
88. Schmid F, Höltke C, Parker D, Faber C (2013) Boosting 19F MRI—SNR efficient detection of paramagnetic contrast agents using ultrafast sequences. Magn Reson Med 69(4):1056–1062. https://doi.org/10.1002/mrm.24341
89. Goette MJ, Keupp J, Rahmer J, Lanza GM, Wickline SA, Caruthers SD (2015) Balanced UTE-SSFP for 19F MR imaging of complex spectra. Magn Reson Med 74(2):537–543. https://doi.org/10.1002/mrm.25437
90. Mastropietro A, De Bernardi E, Breschi GL, Zucca I, Cametti M, Soffientini CD, de Curtis M, Terraneo G, Metrangolo P, Spreafico R, Resnati G, Baselli G (2014) Optimization of rapid acquisition with relaxation enhancement (RARE) pulse sequence parameters for (1)(9)F-MRI studies. J Magn Reson Imaging 40(1):162–170
91. Srinivas M, Morel PA, Ernst LA, Laidlaw DH, Ahrens ET (2007) Fluorine-19 MRI for visualization and quantification of cell migration in a diabetes model. Magn Reson Med 58 (4):725–734. https://doi.org/10.1002/mrm.21352
92. Hennig J, Nauerth A, Friedburg H (1986) RARE imaging: a fast imaging method for clinical MR. Magn Reson Med 3:823–833. https://doi.org/10.1002/mrm.1910030602
93. Rahmer J, Börnert P, Groen J, Bos C (2006) Three-dimensional radial ultrashort echo-time imaging with T2 adapted sampling. Magn Reson Med 55(5):1075–1082. https://doi.org/10.1002/mrm.20868
94. Hennig J (1999) K-space sampling strategies. Eur Radiol 9(6):1020–1031. https://doi.org/10.1007/s003300050788
95. Keupp J, Rahmer J, Grässlin I, Mazurkewitz PC, Schaeffter T, Lanza GM, Wickline SA, Caruthers SD (2011) Simultaneous dual-nuclei imaging for motion corrected detection and quantification of 19F imaging agents. Magn Reson Med 66(4):1116–1122. https://doi.org/10.1002/mrm.22877
96. Hu L, Hockett FD, Chen J, Zhang L, Caruthers SD, Lanza GM, Wickline SA (2011) A generalized strategy for designing (19)F/(1) H dual-frequency MRI coil for small animal imaging at 4.7 Tesla. J Magn Reson Imaging 34(1):245–252
97. Hoult DI, Richards RE (1976) The signal-to-noise ratio of the nuclear magnetic resonance experiment. J Magn Reson 24(1):71–85
98. Kovacs H, Moskau D, Spraul M (2005) Cryogenically cooled probes – a leap in NMR

technology. Prog Nucl Magn Reson Spectrosc 46(2–3):131–155

99. Baltes C, Radzwill N, Bosshard S, Marek D, Rudin M (2009) Micro MRI of the mouse brain using a novel 400 MHz cryogenic quadrature RF probe. NMR Biomed 22 (8):834–842
100. Waiczies S, Millward JM, Starke L, Delgado PR, Huelnhagen T, Prinz C, Marek D, Wecker D, Wissmann R, Koch SP, Boehm-Sturm P, Waiczies H, Niendorf T, Pohlmann A (2017) Enhanced fluorine-19 MRI sensitivity using a cryogenic radiofrequency probe: technical developments and ex vivo demonstration in a mouse model of neuroinflammation. Sci Rep 7(1):9808. https://doi.org/10.1038/s41598-017-09622-2
101. Sack M, Wetterling F, Sartorius A, Ende G, Weber-Fahr W (2014) Signal-to-noise ratio of a mouse brain 13C CryoProbe™ system in comparison with room temperature coils: spectroscopic phantom and in vivo results. NMR Biomed 27(6):709–715. https://doi.org/10.1002/nbm.3110
102. Axel L, Hayes C (1985) Surface coil magnetic resonance imaging. Arch Int Physiol Biochim 93(5):11–18. https://doi.org/10.3109/13813458509080620
103. Crowley MG, Evelhoch JL, JJH A (1985) The surface-coil NMR receiver in the presence of homogeneous B1 excitation. J Magn Reson 64(1):20–31. https://doi.org/10.1016/0022-2364(85)90026-5
104. Goette MJ, Lanza GM, Caruthers SD, Wickline SA (2015) Improved quantitative (19) F MR molecular imaging with flip angle calibration and B1 -mapping compensation. J Magn Reson Imaging 42(2):488–494. https://doi.org/10.1002/jmri.24812
105. Vernikouskaya I, Pochert A, Lindén M, Rasche V (2018) Quantitative 19F MRI of perfluoro-15-crown-5-ether using uniformity correction of the spin excitation and signal reception. MAGMA. https://doi.org/10.1007/s10334-018-0696-6
106. Ladd ME (2018) The quest for higher sensitivity in MRI through higher magnetic fields. Z Med Phys 28(1):1–3. https://doi.org/10.1016/j.zemedi.2017.12.001
107. Niendorf T, Barth M, Kober F, Trattnig S (2016) From ultrahigh to extreme field magnetic resonance: where physics, biology and medicine meet. Magma (New York, NY) 29 (3):309–311. https://doi.org/10.1007/s10334-016-0564-1
108. Hoult DI, Lauterbur PC (1979) Sensitivity of the zeugmatographic experiment involving human samples. J Magn Reson 34 (2):425–433
109. Pohmann R, Speck O, Scheffler K (2016) Signal-to-noise ratio and MR tissue parameters in human brain imaging at 3, 7, and 9.4 tesla using current receive coil arrays. Magn Reson Med 75(2):801–809. https://doi.org/10.1002/mrm.25677
110. Hoult DI (2000) The principle of reciprocity in signal strength calculations—a mathematical guide. Concept Magn Reson 12 (4):173–187. https://doi.org/10.1002/1099-0534(2000)12:4<173::AID-CMR1>3.0.CO;2-Q
111. Guérin B, Villena JF, Polimeridis AG, Adalsteinsson E, Daniel L, White JK, Wald LL (2017) The ultimate signal-to-noise ratio in realistic body models. Magn Reson Med 78 (5):1969–1980. https://doi.org/10.1002/mrm.26564
112. Schepkin VD, Brey WW, Gor'kov PL, Grant SC (2010) Initial in vivo rodent sodium and proton MR imaging at 21.1 T. Magn Reson Imaging 28(3):400–407. https://doi.org/10.1016/j.mri.2009.10.002
113. Waiczies S, Rosenberg JT, Prinz C, Starke L, Millward JM, Ramos Delgado P, Pohlmann A, Kühne A, Waiczies H, Niendorf T (2018) Fluorine-19 magnetic resonance at 21.1 Tesla to detect brain inflammation. Proc Intl Soc Mag Reson Med 26:3314

3

Essential Practical Steps for MRI of the Kidney in Experimental Research

Andreas Pohlmann, João S. Periquito, and Thoralf Niendorf

Abstract

Magnetic resonance imaging (MRI) is an emerging method to obtain valuable functional and structural information about the kidney noninvasively. Before performing specialized MR measurements for probing tissue structure and function, some essential practical steps are needed, which are common for most applications. Here we describe in a step-by-step manner how to (1) achieve the double-oblique slice orientation coronal-to-the-kidney, (2) adapt the scan protocol for avoiding aortic flow artifacts and covering both kidneys, (3) perform localized shimming on the kidney, and (4) check perfusion in the large renal blood vessels using time-of-flight (TOF) angiography. The procedures are tailored to preclinical MRI but conceptionally are also applicable to human MRI.

This chapter is based upon work from the COST Action PARENCHIMA, a community-driven network funded by the European Cooperation in Science and Technology (COST) program of the European Union, which aims to improve the reproducibility and standardization of renal MRI biomarkers. This experimental protocol chapter explains the initial and essential MRI steps that precede specific functional and structural MR imaging techniques (T_1- and T_2*-mapping, DWI, ASL, etc.), which are described in separate chapters.

Key words Magnetic resonance imaging (MRI), Kidney, Mice, Rats, Shimming, Time-of-flight (TOF) angiography

1 Introduction

Magnetic resonance imaging (MRI) is a state-of-the-art noninvasive method to obtain valuable functional and structural information about the kidney. The wide range of available contrast agent mechanisms and the corresponding MR techniques can enable a comprehensive characterization of the kidney. This includes morphology (e.g., kidney size), tissue microstructure (e.g., diffusion-weighted MRI, T1 mapping, elastography), and function (e.g., arterial spin labeling MRI for perfusion mapping or mapping of T_2* for probing blood oxygenation).

Before carrying out these specialized MR measurements, some essential practical steps are required, which are common for most

Andreas Pohlmann and Thoralf Niendorf (eds.), *Preclinical MRI of the Kidney: Methods and Protocols*, Methods in Molecular Biology, vol. 2216, https://doi.org/10.1007/978-1-0716-0978-1_20,

applications. Here we describe in a step-by-step manner how to (1) achieve the double oblique slice orientation coronal-to-the-kidney, (2) adapt the scan protocol for avoiding aortic flow artifacts and covering both kidneys, (3) perform localized shimming on the kidney, and (4) check perfusion in the large renal blood vessels using time-of-flight (TOF) angiography. The procedures are tailored to preclinical MRI but are also conceptually applicable to human MRI.

This experimental protocol chapter is complemented by separate chapters describing the basic concepts, experimental protocol and data analysis of numerous renal MR techniques, which are part of this book.

This chapter is part of the book Pohlmann A, Niendorf T (eds) (2020) Preclinical MRI of the Kidney—Methods and Protocols. Springer, New York.

2 Materials

2.1 Animals

These experimental protocols are tailored for rats (e.g., Wistar, Sprague-Dawley, or Lewis) with a body mass of 250–350 g. Advice for adaptation to mice is given where necessary.

2.2 Lab Equipment

Anesthesia: For nonrecovery experiments urethane solution (Sigma-Aldrich, Steinheim, Germany; 20% in distilled water) can provide anesthesia for several hours with comparatively little side effects on renal physiology, which is an important issue. For an in-depth description and discussion of the anesthesia please refer to the chapter by Kaucsar T et al. "Preparation and Monitoring of Small Animals in Renal MRI."

Monitoring several physiological parameters of the animal is essential to ensure the anesthesia works and while the animal is unconscious and does not feel pain, it is physiologically as close to the normal nonanesthetized state as possible. For an in-depth description of physiological monitoring please refer to the chapter by Kaucsar T et al. "Preparation and Monitoring of Small Animals in Renal MRI."

2.3 MRI Hardware

The general hardware requirements for renal ^{1}H MRI on mice and rats are described in the chapter by Ramos Delgado P et al. "Hardware Considerations for Preclinical Magnetic Resonance of the Kidney." The techniques described in this chapter are tailored for a 9.4 T MR system (Biospec 94/20, Bruker Biospin, Ettlingen, Germany), but advice for adaptation to other field strengths and systems is given where necessary. No special or additional hardware is required, except for the following:

A physiological monitoring system that can track the respiration, and which is connected to the MR system such that it can be used to trigger the image acquisition.

2.4 MRI Techniques

This protocol requires only standard MR techniques that should be available on any commercial system. The shimming capabilities and procedure are specific to the MR hardware and each vendors software platform; in this protocol we focus on describing the shimming on a Bruker BioSpec system running ParaVision 6.0.1.

1. 2D spoiled gradient-echo sequence ("FLASH" on Bruker systems).
2. 2D spoiled gradient-echo sequence with flow compensation and angio-mode (only one slice excitation per TR) ("FcFLASH" on Bruker systems).
3. 2D fast spin echo sequence ("RARE" on Bruker systems).

3 Methods

3.1 MR Protocol Setup

The basic protocols described here are based on default protocols available in Bruker ParaVision, which have been adapted to the geometry of the rat abdomen. Although it is one of the aims of this book to also describe the reasons for the choice of parameters, we have refrained from doing so here because the choice of parameters is not crucial for these protocols. Here we present working protocols for rats on a Bruker 9.4 T system. For MRI at lower field strengths the reduced signal-to-noise ratio (SNR) may be compensated by signal averaging and/or reducing the spatial resolution. For MRI of mice a good starting point is to reduce the FOV used in the rat protocols to the smaller body size of the mouse while keeping the matrix size the same. In this way the relative resolution (voxels per animal/organ dimensions) is similar. Despite the smaller voxel size the SNR is often not much worse than for the rat protocol, because the smaller size of the mouse RF coil improves the SNR (e.g., mouse heart four-element surface coil vs rat heart four-element surface coil).

3.1.1 Multislice Tripilot Scan (R01_TriPilotmulti)

1. Pulse sequence: 2D spoiled gradient-echo sequence (FLASH).
2. Contrast: TR = 126 ms, TE = 2 ms, flip angle = 90°, averages = 3.
3. Spatial resolution: in plane of (234 × 234) μm^2; three packages of seven slices with 1.0 mm thickness, slice distances of 5.0/4.5/4.0 mm and hence slice gaps of 4.0/3.5/3.0 mm (axial/coronal/sagittal); FOV = (60 × 60) mm^2; matrix size = 256 × 256 derived from a 85 × 128 acquisition matrix.

4. Acceleration: 2.0 in phase encoding and frequency encoding directions by zero-filling, 1.72 in frequency encoding direction by partial-Fourier.
5. Sequence: bandwidth = 89 kHz, trigger = off, fat suppression = off, flip-back = on, dummy scans = 10, motion suppression = on, duration: TA = 49 s.

3.1.2 Axial Multislice Pilot Scan

1. Pulse sequence: 2D fast spin echo sequence (RARE).
2. Contrast: TR = 540 ms, TE = 12 ms, effective TE = 24, flip angle = 90°, averages = 1.
3. Spatial resolution: in plane of (407 × 406) μm^2; eight slices of 1.0 mm thickness, a slice distance of 2.2 mm and hence a slice gap of 1.2 mm; FOV = (70 × 52) mm^2; matrix size = 172 × 128 identical to the 172 × 128 acquisition matrix.
4. Acceleration: RARE factor (echo train length or number of echoes per excitation) = 4.
5. Sequence: bandwidth = 63 kHz, trigger = on (per phase step), fat suppression = on, flip-back = on, dummy scans = 2, duration: TA = 17 s.

3.1.3 Coronal Pilot Scan

1. Pulse sequence: 2D fast spin echo sequence (RARE).
2. Contrast: TR = 540 ms, TE = 12 ms, effective TE = 24, flip angle = 90°, averages = 1.
3. Spatial resolution: in plane of (407 × 406) μm^2; one slice of 1.0 mm thickness; FOV = (70 × 52) mm^2; matrix size = 172 × 128 identical to the 172 × 128 acquisition matrix.
4. Acceleration: RARE factor = 4.
5. Sequence: bandwidth = 63 kHz, trigger = on (per phase step), fat suppression = on, flip-back = on, duration: TA = 17 s.

3.1.4 Abdominal Time-of-Flight (TOF) Angiography

1. Pulse sequence: Flow compensated 2D spoiled gradient-echo sequence (FcFLASH).
2. Contrast: TR = 13 ms, TE = 2.3 ms, flip angle = 80°, averages = 1.
3. Spatial resolution: in plane of (200 × 200) μm^2; nine slices of 1.4 mm thickness, a slice distance of 2.1 mm and hence a slice gap of 0.7 mm; FOV = (51.2 × 51.2) mm^2; matrix size = 256 × 256 derived from a 183 × 172 acquisition matrix.
4. Acceleration: 1.5 in phase encoding direction by zero-filling, 1.4 in frequency encoding direction by partial-Fourier.
5. Sequence: bandwidth = 75 kHz, angio mode = yes, trigger = off, fat suppression = off, duration: TA = 20 s.

3.1.5 Kidney TOF-Angiography

1. Pulse sequence: Flow compensated 2D spoiled gradient-echo sequence (FcFLASH).
2. Contrast: TR = 7 ms, TE = 3 ms, flip angle = 80°, averages = 1.
3. Spatial resolution: in plane of (200 × 208) μm^2; 15 slices of 1.0 mm thickness, a slice distance of 0.5 mm and hence a slice gap of −0.5 mm (overlapping); FOV = (60 × 40) mm^2; matrix size = 300 × 192 derived from a 214 × 128 acquisition matrix.
4. Acceleration: 1.5 in phase encoding direction by zero-filling, 1.4 in frequency encoding direction by partial-Fourier.
5. Sequence: bandwidth = 75 kHz, angio mode = yes, trigger = off, fat suppression = off, duration: TA = 14 s.

3.2 Animal Preparation

Anesthetize the animal and transfer it to scanner. For more information on the choice and use of anesthesia please refer to the chapter by Kaucsar T et al. "Preparation and Monitoring of Small Animals in Renal MRI".

Start the temperature monitoring system, apply some surgical lubricant to the temperature probe and place it in the rectum of the animal.

Attach the respiration sensor (e.g., balloon) to the abdomen of the animal using adhesive tape. Start and setup the respiratory monitoring system. If necessary, adjust the position of the respiration sensor until the amplitude of the respiration trace is sufficiently large for the system to reliably detect the trigger points at the beginning of expiration.

3.3 Pilot Scans and Slice Positioning Coronal to tthe Kidney

Here we describe how to acquire a single image slice in coronal-to-the-kidney orientation, which is the best approach if only one kidney is of interest. If both kidneys are of interest, each kidney may be imaged separately using the steps described below.

3.3.1 Slice Planning: From Pilot Scan to the Coronal-to-the-Kidney Image

However, if the experimental conditions do not allow for imaging each kidney separately, then a compromise must be made. This could be the case if, for instance, the available scan time is limited: slice planning, shimming, and acquiring images twice may take too long. Also, the experimental procedure might demand acquisition of the images for both kidneys simultaneously (multislice scan), for example when monitoring dynamic physiological processes. In these cases shimming should be performed on a voxel enclosing both kidneys and the image slice package orientation should be chosen such that it depicts both kidneys in a view that is as close as possible to coronal-to-the-kidney orientation.

1. Start with acquiring a fast pilot scan to obtain images in the three orthogonal planes x, y, and z: load the *multislice tripilot* protocol and run it with the default slice geometry and the usual automatic adjustments (shimming and adjustments of the

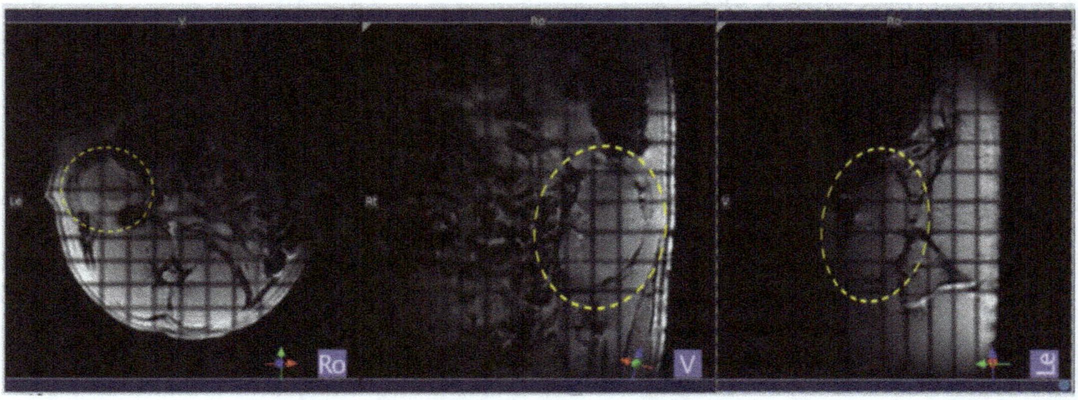

Fig. 1 Slice planning on a small animal MR system (here 9.4 T Bruker Biospec with ParaVision 6. Images obtained from the very first MR scan, a fast *multislice tripilot*. Shown are three selected image slices in strictly axial (left), coronal (center), and sagittal (right) orientation with respect to the scanner coordinates. The location of the left kidney is highlighted by the dashed yellow line. The dark stripes are saturation effects occurring at the intersection of the slices (*see* **Note 1**)

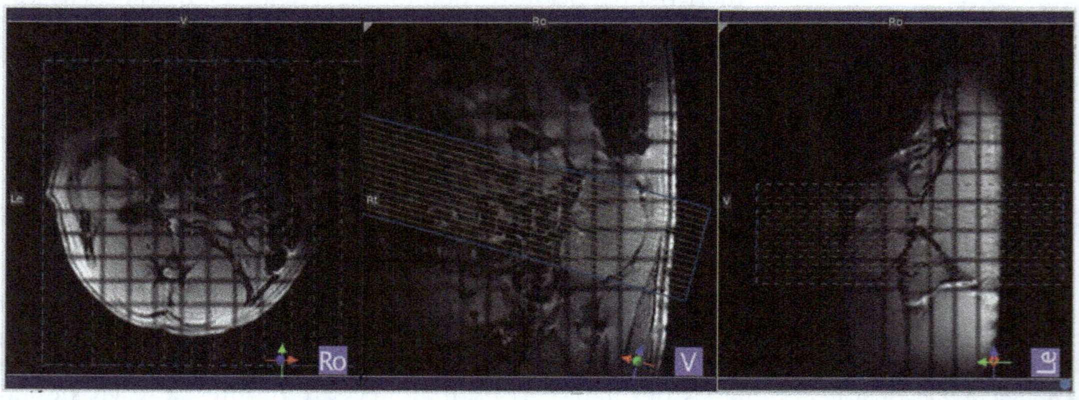

Fig. 2 Images obtained from the fast *multislice tripilot* showing the planning of the *axial multislice pilot scan*: The slice package should be rotated such that it is axial to the kidney in the coronal *multislice tripilot* images (center)

base frequency, the RF pulse reference power, and the receiver gain). Example images are shown in Fig. 1 (*see* **Note 1**).

2. Keep a record of the reference power in the lab notebook for later reference. Comparing the reference power to those used in previous studies with the same setup is very helpful for early identifying possible technical issues in an in-vivo study.
3. Load the *axial multislice pilot scan*, adapt the slice package position and orientation such that it is centered on the kidney and axial to the kidney (not to the animal's body) (Fig. 2).
4. In the monitoring unit set the trigger delay so that the trigger starts at the beginning of the expiratory plateau and the

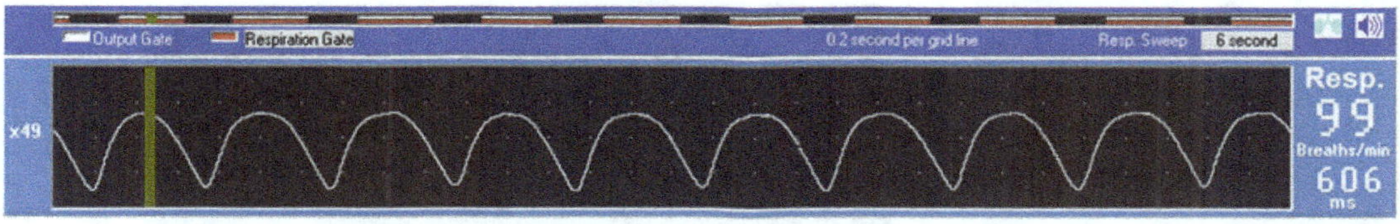

Fig. 3 Setup of the respiratory triggering in the physiological monitoring system. The respiratory gate is defined such that it spans across the expiratory phase and avoids the inspiratory motion. The above trace is for a urethane anesthetized rat. With isoflurane anesthesia the respiratory rate is lower and a long expiratory plateau is typical

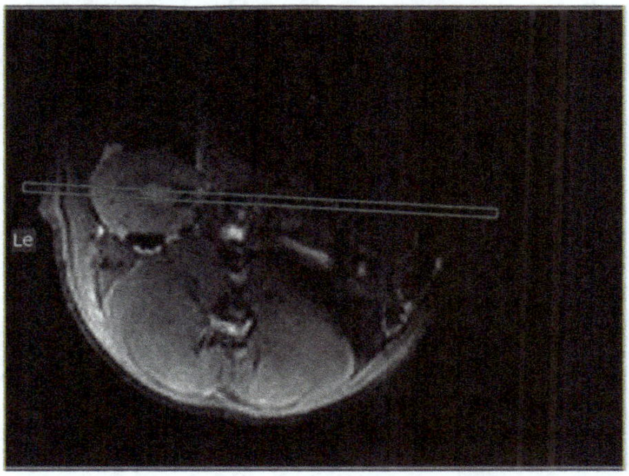

Fig. 4 Image obtained from the fast *axial multislice pilot scan* showing the planning of the *coronal pilot scan*: The slice should be perpendicular to the *axial multislice pilot scan* and rotated such that it runs through the center of the kidney

duration such that it covers the entire expiratory phase (Fig. 3, *see* **Note 2**).

5. If you use a RARE protocol like described here, adjust the TR so that it is longer that the respiratory trigger window but shorter than the current respiration period. For the example shown in Fig. 3, TR should be set to a value within the range 400–570 ms, in order to lie safely between 370 ms (respiratory trigger window) and 606 ms (respiration period). Run the scan. An example image slice is shown in Fig. 4.
6. Load the *coronal pilot scan* protocol and adjust the geometry: the slice should be perpendicular to the *axial multislice pilot scan* and rotated such that it runs through the center of the kidney (Fig. 4). The frequency encoding direction should be rostral–caudal in order to avoid aliasing. Run the scan. An example image is shown in Fig. 5.

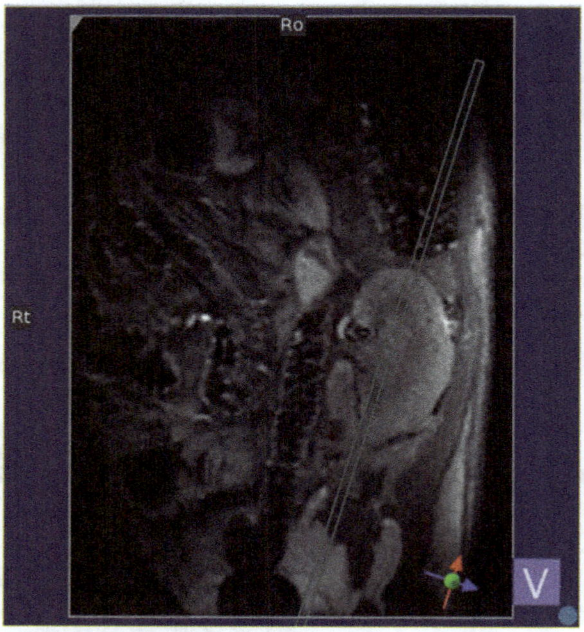

Fig. 5 Image obtained from the *coronal pilot scan* showing the planning of the *sagittal pilot scan*: The slice should be perpendicular to the *coronal pilot scan* and rotated such that it runs along the long axis of the kidney

7. To acquire a *sagittal pilot scan*, duplicate the previous scan protocol and adapt the slice orientation: The slice should be perpendicular to the *coronal pilot scan* and rotated such that it runs along the long axis of the kidney (Fig. 5). Run the scan. An example image is shown in Fig. 6.
8. For the *coronal-to-the-kidney scan*, duplicate the *coronal pilot scan* protocol and fine-adjust the slice orientation: The slice should be rotated such that it runs along the long axis of the kidney in the *sagittal pilot scan* (Fig. 6). Run the scan. An example of the final image acquired in double-oblique *coronal-to-the-kidney* orientation is shown in Fig. 7.

3.3.2 Transferring the Coronal-to-the-Kidney Geometry to Other Scans

1. Start from the pilot scan with coronal-to-the-kidney geometry (Fig. 7).
2. From this protocol copy the slice orientation (*see* **Note 3**) to the first of your special scans (e.g., DWI, T_2*-mapping). Pay attention not to copy the entire slice package geometry, because this typically would include the FOV, slice thickness, and number of slices, which are usually different between the pilot scans and functional scans.
3. To illustrate how a typical result should look like, Fig. 8 shows an example of a coronal-to-the-kidney T_2-weighted image from a multispin echo scan.

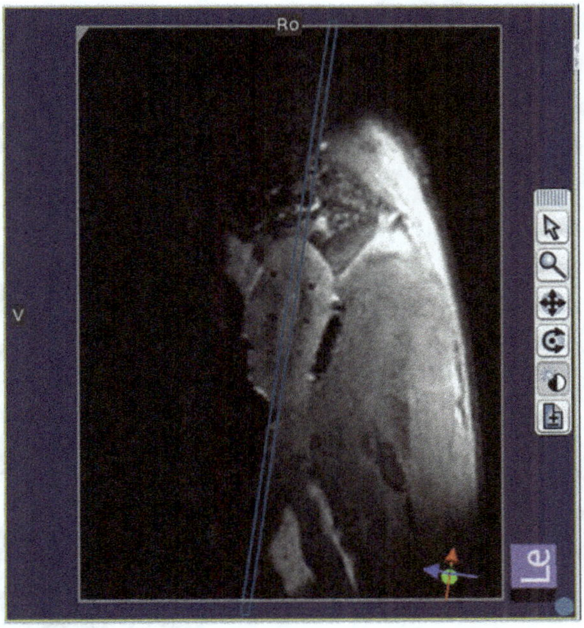

Fig. 6 Image obtained from the *sagittal pilot scan* showing the planning of the *coronal-to-the-kidney scan*: The slice should be rotated such that it runs along the long axis of the kidney

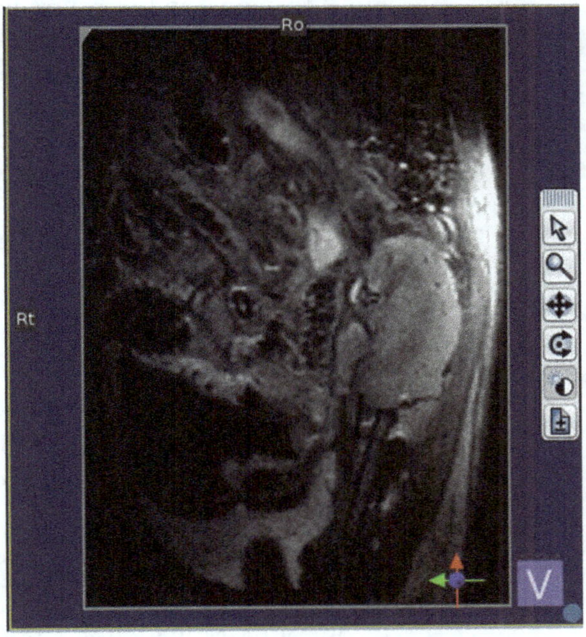

Fig. 7 Final image acquired in double-oblique *coronal-to-the-kidney* orientation (The black tubular structures caudal to the kidney are implanted probes that are not relevant in this context)

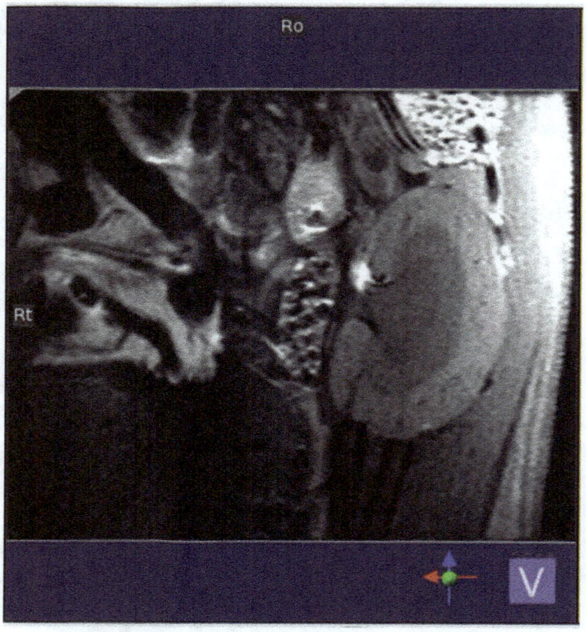

Fig. 8 T_2-weighted image acquired in double-oblique *coronal-to-the-kidney* orientation

3.3.3 Reducing Aortic Flow Artifacts (Optional)

The coronal-to-the-kidney slice orientation will naturally vary from animal to animal and of course between the right and left kidney. Sometimes the aorta lies within the image slice, which can result in unwanted flow artifacts. These artifacts can be reduced using a saturation slice, where a block of repeated excitation and spoiling is applied just before the imaging block in order to suppress the signal:

1. In the protocol setup look for the field-of-view saturation option (e.g., “FOV sat”) and enable it. This will add a saturation slice with default geometry.
2. Load the *abdominal TOF-angiography* scan. Copy the slice orientation (*see* **Note 3**) from the *axial multislice pilot* and run the scan. An example image is shown in Fig. 9.
3. Load the following images to the viewer: the *axial pilot* scan, *coronal-to-the-kidney* scan, and the *abdominal TOF-angiography* scan (Fig. 9).
4. In the image viewer enable the display of saturation slices (gray in Fig. 9).
5. Adjust the saturation slice thickness and orientation: place it in approximately sagittal orientation and rotate it such that it covers the aorta without intersecting the kidney(!).

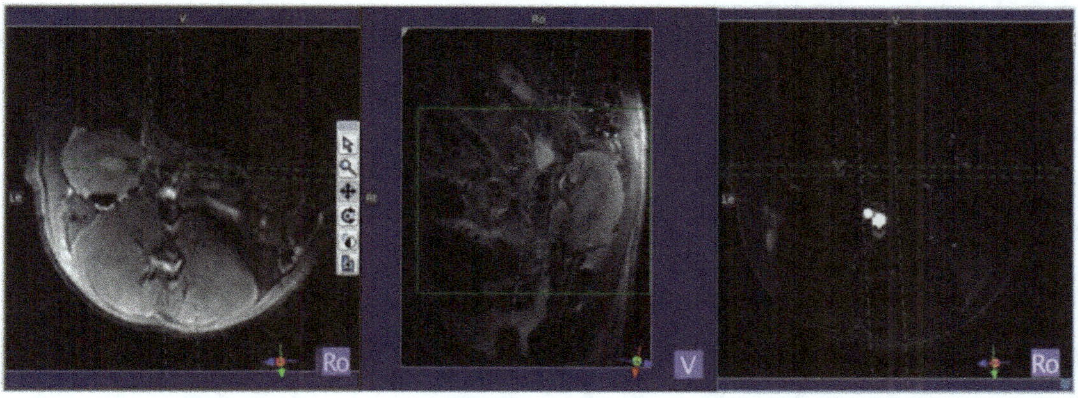

Fig. 9 Images obtained from the *axial pilot* scan (left), *coronal-to-the-kidney* scan (center), and an *abdominal TOF-angiography* scan (right) showing the planning of an optional *FOV saturation slice* (gray dashed lines). The saturation slice has the purpose of reducing possible flow artifacts from the aorta, and hence should be placed in approximately sagittal orientation and rotated such that it covers the aorta without intersecting the kidney. Please note that in this example the aorta was not within the kidney image slice, but, nevertheless, placing a saturation slice was performed as part of our standard operating procedure (SOP)

3.3.4 Multislice and Covering Both Kidneys (Optional)

1. To set up a multislice protocol, simply follow the steps for a single slice and subsequently change the number of slices to the desired number. This should be an odd number (3,5,7, . . .), so that the original single slice remains in the center.
2. For acquiring coronal-to-the-kidney images from both kidneys with the same scan protocol add a second slice package. This allows you to acquire two slice packages with arbitrary orientation, one coronal to the left kidney and one coronal to the right kidney.
3. First plan the geometry of the slice package for one kidney and afterward repeat the same steps for the other kidney.
4. Pay attention to where the two slice packages intersect. In the rare case when the slices of the right and left kidney cross within the kidney, adjust the slice orientation slightly to move the intersection to outside of the kidney. This is important, because otherwise the saturation effect would lead to a dark stripe artifact in the kidney. Alternatively, split the protocol into two, one for each kidney. This will permit acquiring images in the desired orientations without artifacts; however, it also doubles the scan time.

3.4 Localized Shimming

Shimming is particularly important for T_2*-mapping, since macroscopic magnetic field inhomogeneities shorten T_2*, but provide no tissue specific information—rather they overshadow the microscopic T_2* effects of interest and hinder quantitative intra- and intersubject comparisons. But a good shim is also relevant for other imaging techniques, such diffusion weighted imaging

(DWI) or perfusion measurements with arterial-spin-labeling (ASL), because they are commonly based on an echo-planar-imaging (EPI) sequence due to its fast imaging speed. EPI is prone to magnetic susceptibility artifacts, which increase with the number of echoes acquired after each excitation. Hence, this can particularly become a problem when the number of segments is small or one in the case of single-shot acquisition. These artifacts appear as T_2* induced signal loss (or even signal voids) in areas with very high B_0 gradients, image distortion due to the inherently low phase encoding bandwidth, and off-resonance effects caused by frequency dispersions. Therefore, EPI is in kidney regions adjacent to bowels or in close proximity to skin/fat/muscle boundaries is particularly challenging. To this end, it is often beneficial not to use the default standard shim (usually on the entire field-of-view), but to perform additional shimming tailored to the kidney.

Ideally, shimming is performed on a voxel enclosing only the kidney of interest. When a good shim is crucial, the shim volume may be reduced even further to a volume that is smaller than the kidney and just a little thicker than the slice package (*see* **Note 4**). This is the procedure we describe in the following.

However, if both kidneys are of interest and the available scan time or experimental procedure does not allow for imaging each kidney separately, then shimming should be performed instead on a voxel enclosing both kidneys.

Field map-based shimming has become the standard shimming method on preclinical and clinical MR systems. It consists of (1) the manual definition of a shim volume, (2) the acquisition of a 3D B_0 field map (usually with a dual-echo gradient-echo method), and (3) the calculation of the shim currents needed to make the B_0 field within the shim volume as homogeneous as possible. This is the approach we recommend and describe in the following step-by-step instructions. Yet, in our experience, simple iterative linear (first-order) shimming on the selected volume is usually sufficient.

The main limiting factor for achieving a good shim is the capability of the shim coil set. For first-order (linear) shimming no additional shim coils are needed, since the standard *x*/*y*/*z* gradient coils used for imaging can double as shim coils. Higher-order shimming (nonlinear spatial harmonics) requires additional coils, typically one for each spatial harmonic (newer designs are more efficient), that is, a minimum of five separate coils are employed for second-order field correction. Therefore, it is usually impossible to correct complex and small B_0 inhomogeneities caused by for example by bowel gas, invasive measurement probes, or trapped air bubbles (from surgery). Considering the very small size of a rat and mouse kidney, in practice the shimming cannot compensate much more than a linear B_0 gradient within the rodent kidney.

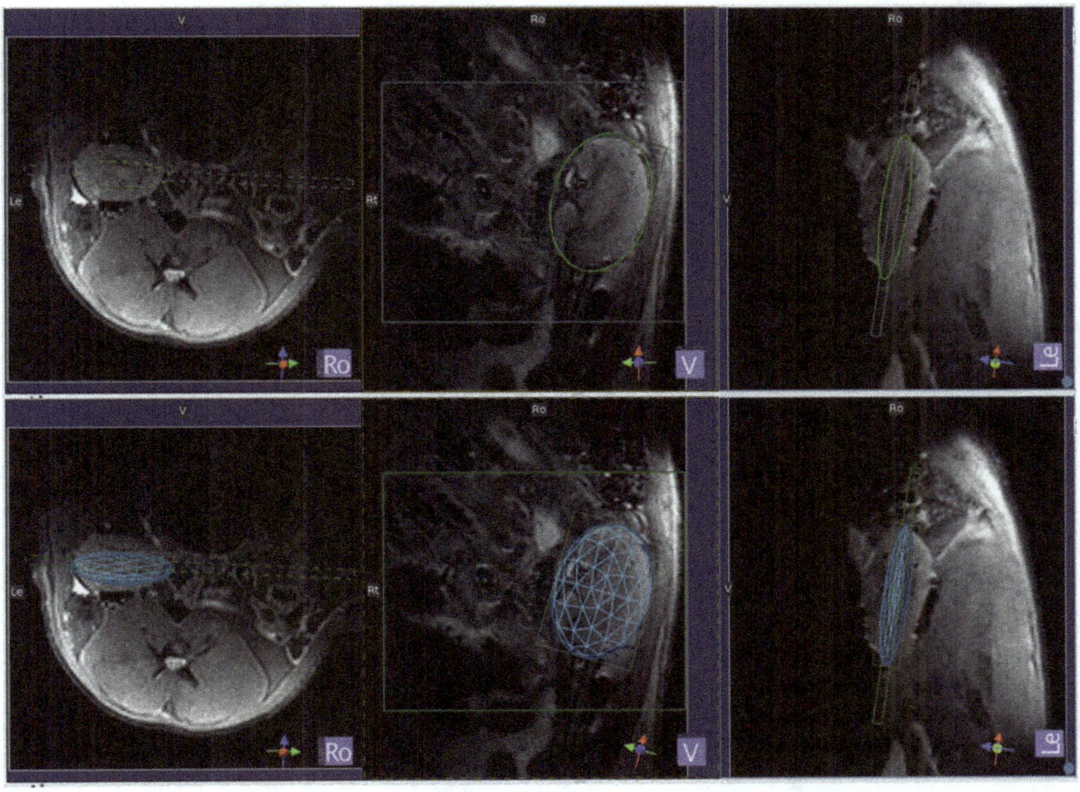

Fig. 10 Shimming on a rat kidney on a small animal MR system (here 9.4 T Bruker Biospec with ParaVision 6). Images obtained from the *axial pilot* scan (left), *coronal-to-the-kidney* scan (center), and an *sagittal pilot* scan (right) showing the planning of the double-oblique *shim volume*. The shim volume tightly encloses the kidney in "coronal" view and is about twice as thick as the imaging slice. Top panel: green outline of the ellipsoid shim volume. Bottom panel: ellipsoid shim volume shown as blue 2D grid

3.4.1 Planning the Shim Volume (Bruker ParaVision)

1. Load into the viewer the images obtained from the *axial pilot* scan, *coronal-to-the-kidney* scan, and *sagittal pilot* scan, as shown in Fig. 10.
2. Open the scan protocol for which the shimming should be performed and go to the *Adjustment* section of the protocol.
3. In the *Adjustment* > *Automatic Shim* tab select *Mapshim*.
4. In the *Adjustment* > *Automatic Shim* tab select *Default Shim Volume*, then deselect it again. You now have a shim volume geometry that is identical to the slice geometry.
5. In the *Adjustment* > *Automatic Shim* tab select a cuboid or better the *ellipsoid* volume, which fits very well to the shape of the kidney.
6. Adjust the geometry of the double-oblique shim volume, such that the volume tightly encloses the kidney in the "coronal" view and that it is about twice as thick as the image slice

package. Figure 10 shows the ellipsoid shim volume with a thickness of 4 mm for one image slice of 1.5 mm).

3.4.2 Shimming (Bruker ParaVision)

1. Finish all other changes you may want to make to the scan protocol.
2. In the *Adjustment Platform* select the *B0 map* and in the protocol parameters enable the respiratory triggering. It is usually OK to use the default FOV, but check that all the visible part of the animal lies within in (*see* **Note 5**).
3. Start the acquisition of the B_0 map, this usually takes a couple of minutes. When the acquisition has finished, exit the *Adjustment Platform* and return to the scan protocol.
4. In the *Adjustment* > *Automatic Shim* tab select *Mapshim* (you probably did that already during the shim volume planning).
5. In the *Adjustment* > *Automatic Shim* tab enable *Iterative Correction* of the first order shims.
6. It should be displayed that a B_0 map is available (if it does not, go back to acquiring the B_0 map).
7. *Apply* the changes to the protocol and run the scan—shimming will be performed as the first step of the data acquisition, followed by a frequency adjustment (necessary after shimming).
8. For repeating the same scan later in the experiment, copy this protocol and make sure to change the selection of *Mapshim* to *Current Shim* in the *Adjustment* > *Automatic Shim* tab.
9. To use the new shim for subsequent measurements, select *Current Shim* in the *Adjustment* > *Automatic Shim* tab of each of these protocols.

3.4.3 Shimming on a Clinical MR System (Siemens Syngo)

1. Load into the viewer localizer images acquired in the *coronal-to-the-kidney* orientation, and the *sagittal-to-the-kidney* orientation.
2. Open the scan protocol for which the shimming should be performed.
3. Click on the icon for the *Position Toolbar* to open it.
4. In the *Position Toolbar* click on the *Adjust Volume on/off* button. The default shim volume geometry that is identical to the slice geometry is now displayed as a green frame (Fig. 11).
5. Adjust the geometry of the shim volume, such that the volume encloses the kidney in the "coronal" view and that it is about twice as thick as the image slice package. Figure 11 shows the cuboid shim volume with a thickness of 4 mm.

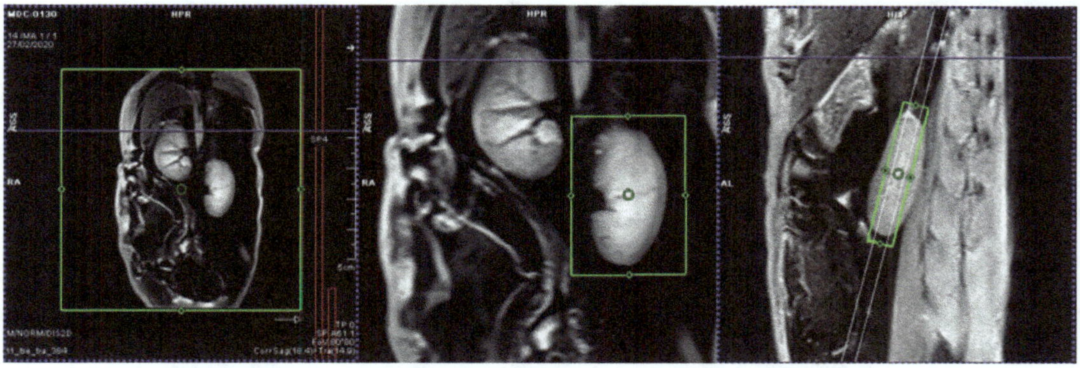

Fig. 11 Shimming on a rat kidney on a clinical MR system (here 3 T Siemens Skyra with Syngo). After clicking on the *Adjust Volume on/off* button in the *Position Toolbar* the default shim volume geometry is displayed as a green frame (left). Then the geometry of the shim volume was adjusted, such that it encloses the kidney in the coronal-to-the-kidney view (center) and that it is about twice as thick as the image slice, as can be seen in the *sagittal-to-the-kidney* scan (right). Here the size of the shim volume was (20 × 16 × 4) mm^3

6. In the scan protocol parameter setup click on the *System* tab and then the *Adjustments* tab. Select as the *B0 Shim Mode* = *Standard* or *Abdominal.*
7. *Apply* the changes to the protocol and start the scan—B_0 mapping (if not already done) and shimming will be performed as the first step of the data acquisition, followed by a frequency adjustment (necessary after shimming).

3.5 Fast and Simple Test of Renal Blood Flow (Optional)

Time-of-flight (TOF) angiography is a simple technique to check the perfusion in the large renal blood vessels. Acquiring a TOF angiogram only requires a few seconds and it can provide very valuable information in experiments that involve major changes in renal blood flow, such as short-time reversible occlusions of the renal artery, renal vein, or aorta as well as ischemia–reperfusion. One can confirm that the vessel occlusion and reperfusion are successful, or otherwise repeat the procedure. TOF angiography is also essential in MRI experiments that include implanted invasive probes (e.g., fiber-optical pO_2 probes, ultrasound flow probes, near-infrared probes) or devices for physiological interventions, such as inflatable balloons that serve as remotely controllable blood-vessel occluders. The reason is that these devices are relatively large and if they are placed in proximity to a blood vessel they may apply too much pressure on it, hindering or even stopping the blood flow within it. TOF angiography can help to detect such hypoperfusion early in the experiment, when a surgical correction may still be possible.

3.5.1 Measurement Concept

For correct interpretation of the TOF angiogram it is important to understand the measurement concept. The measurement uses a conventional gradient echo (GRE) pulse sequence with a high flip angle (FA) and very short repetition time (TR). After a few excitations this results in saturation, that is, a suppression of the signal (from stationary protons), because there is too little time for T_1 recovery from the previous excitation leading to almost no signal being available for the next excitation. However, the fast-moving spins of blood flowing in large vessels that cross the image slice are not stationary—under normal blood flow conditions the blood present in the image slice during one excitation has been entirely replaced with new blood (from outside of the slice) before the next excitation. That means that the water protons of the blood are still fully "relaxed" when the excitation RF pulse is applied—these spins have never seen an RF pulse before and hence give maximum signal. The signal of the blood is not suppressed, because the effective TR is infinitely long—unlike for stationary protons in tissue to which the very short nominal TR applies.

The TOF contrast is not a quantitative measure. While in theory there is a window of flow velocities that will create intermediate blood signal intensities (between maximum signal from fresh blood to almost no signal from stationary blood), in practice the TOF contrast has an approximately binary character: you see signal or you do not. What flow velocity is needed to see the maximum blood signal can be roughly estimated from the distance that blood needs to flow (i.e., the image slice/slab thickness) and the available time (i.e., TR). However, the vessel orientation and flow profile in the vessel also play a role, so one cannot draw conclusions about the actual blood flow velocity; it rather serves as a simple tool for qualitative comparison of blood flow between (patho)physiological states.

3.5.2 Protocol

Here we describe how to perform a TOF angiography to check for (ab)normal perfusion in the large renal blood vessels.

Please note that this protocol is not designed for creating a 3D depiction of the renal vascular architecture via maximum-intensity projections (MPIs)—this would require whole kidney coverage, a higher spatial resolution, and hence a longer acquisition time.

1. In the viewer open the images obtained from the *axial pilot* scan, *coronal-to-the-kidney* scan, and the *sagittal pilot* scan (Fig. 12).
2. Load the *kidney TOF-angiography* protocol.
3. If you have acquired a *sagittal pilot scan* at the beginning of the experiment, then copy the slice orientation from that scan (*see* **Note 3**). Otherwise start with a default sagittal slice orientation.
4. Plan the slice geometry sagittal with regard to the kidney, as shown in Fig. 12.
5. Start the scan. Figure 13 shows an example image in which six major vessels are clearly visible (in Wistar rat kidneys typically 6 or 8 vessels are seen). During temporary occlusions of the

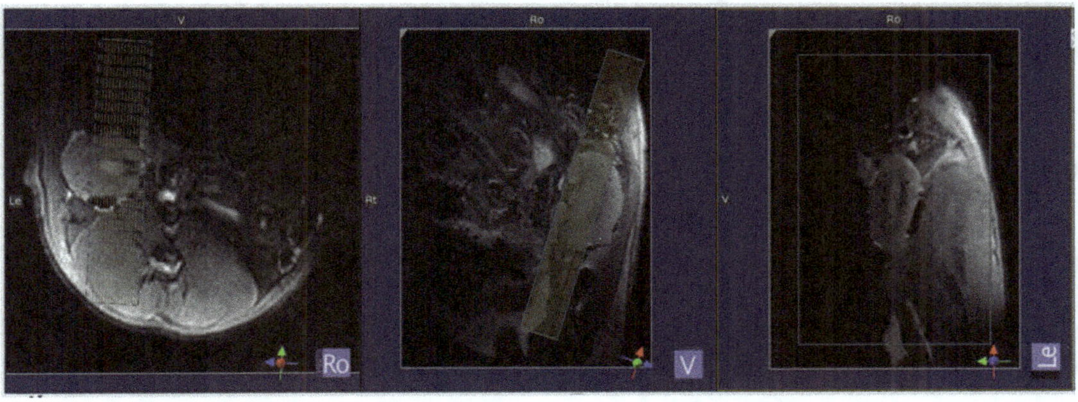

Fig. 12 Basic TOF angiography of a rat kidney on a small animal MR system (here 9.4 T Bruker Biospec with ParaVision 6). Images obtained from the *axial pilot* scan (left), *coronal-to-the-kidney* scan (center), and an *sagittal pilot* scan (right) showing the planning of the *kidney TOF-angiography*. The slice package is positioned sagittal with regard to the kidney

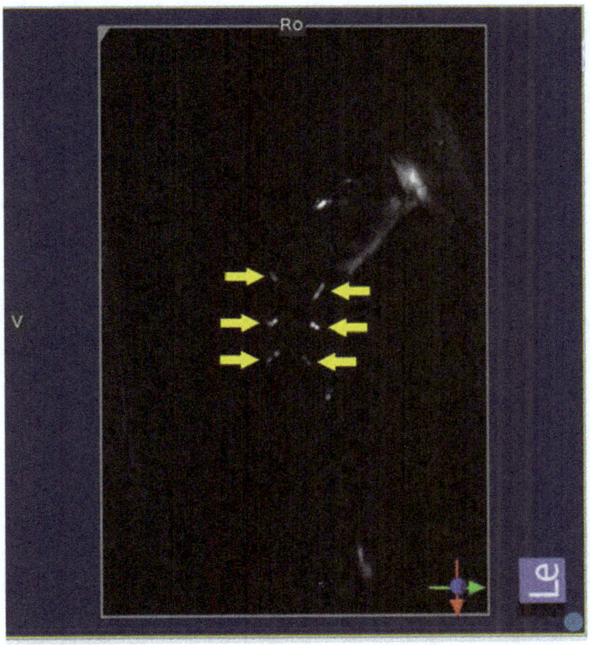

Fig. 13 Selected images slice obtained from the *kidney TOF-angiography*. Six major vessels can be clearly seen. In experiments where a temporary occlusion of the renal artery, vein, or aorta via a remote controlled hydraulic occluder is performed, this scan is very useful to confirm vessel occlusion was successful (vessels are not visible anymore) and reperfusion was successful (vessels are visible again like above)

renal artery, vein, or aorta (via a remote controlled hydraulic occluder) the vessels will disappear and reappear after successful reperfusion.

4 Notes

1. The saturation effect is an inevitable artifact that occurs when several crossing slices are acquired in an interleaved manner, that is, excitation of all slices during one TR. This effect can be avoided be acquiring all slices consecutively, however, that significantly increases the scan time. For the initial scan this artifact is acceptable because it only serves to localize the kidney, so speed is given preference.
2. If you use a RARE protocol like described here, the TR needs to be relatively long to allow for sufficient T_1-recovery and hence acceptable signal-to-noise ratio (SNR). Due to the long TR it is advisable to have only one excitation per breath. To ensure that there will be only one triggered acquisition per breath, adjust the TR so that it is longer than the respiratory trigger window but shorter than the current respiration period. Alternatively, you could adjust the trigger window in the monitoring software to be very short (e.g., 10 ms), but then you will have to reverse this change for every gradient echo scan. You must monitor the respiration continuously throughout the entire experiment and, if necessary, adapt the TR accordingly.
3. With "copying the slice orientation" we mean copying the spatial location of the center of the slice package as well as copying its spatial orientation, that is, the angulation in all three directions x, y, and z (or left–right, anterior–posterior, rostral–caudal). On a system running Bruker ParaVision this is achieved by copying the slice orientation; in contrast, copying the slice geometry includes the FOV, slice thickness, and number of slices.
4. Considering the small size of a rat and mouse kidney and the limited capabilities of shim coils, it is unrealistic to expect that a "perfect" shim on the kidney can be achieved. In practice, one aims to remove a linear B_0 gradient in the kidney. Nonlinear B_0 gradients within the kidney are very challenging to compensate for, because they are only a few millimeters in size. This would require a high-end gradient set with very high-order shims.
5. For rats the default shim volume has a reasonable size, but you must check for your particular setup (RF coil, rat size) that it is large enough so that there will be no aliasing artifacts in the two phase encoding directions. If the default shim volume is much larger than the object (possible for small mice) one can reduce the size of the shim volume. As this will reduce the signal-to-

noise ratio of the B_0 map and hence it may be useful to increase the number of averages. When you modify the shim volume FOV try to maintain the *isotropic* voxel size, as this permits capturing the B_0 inhomogeneities in all spatial directions with equal accuracy.

Acknowledgments

This work was funded in part (Thoralf Niendorf, Andreas Pohlmann, Joao Periquito) by the German Research Foundation (Gefoerdert durch die Deutsche Forschungsgemeinschaft (DFG), Projektnummer 394046635, SFB 1365, RENOPROTECTION. Funded by the Deutsche Forschungsgemeinschaft (DFG, German Research Foundation), Project number 394046635, SFB 1365, RENOPROTECTION).

This chapter is based upon work from COST Action PARENCHIMA, supported by European Cooperation in Science and Technology (COST). COST (www.cost.eu) is a funding agency for research and innovation networks. COST Actions help connect research initiatives across Europe and enable scientists to grow their ideas by sharing them with their peers. This boosts their research, career and innovation.

PARENCHIMA (renalmri.org) is a community-driven Action in the COST program of the European Union, which unites more than 200 experts in renal MRI from 30 countries with the aim to improve the reproducibility and standardization of renal MRI biomarkers.

4

Hyperpolarized Carbon (^{13}C) MRI of the Kidney: Experimental Protocol

Christoffer Laustsen, Cornelius von Morze, and Galen D. Reed

Abstract

Alterations in renal metabolism are associated with both physiological and pathophysiologic events. The existing noninvasive analytic tools including medical imaging have limited capability for investigating these processes, which potentially limits current understanding of kidney disease and the precision of its clinical diagnosis. Hyperpolarized ^{13}C MRI is a new medical imaging modality that can capture changes in the metabolic processing of certain rapidly metabolized substrates, as well as changes in kidney function. Here we describe experimental protocols for renal metabolic [1-^{13}C]pyruvate and functional ^{13}C-urea imaging step-by-step. These methods and protocols are useful for investigating renal blood flow and function as well as the renal metabolic status of rodents in vivo under various experimental (patho)physiological conditions.

This chapter is based upon work from the COST Action PARENCHIMA, a community-driven network funded by the European Cooperation in Science and Technology (COST) program of the European Union, which aims to improve the reproducibility and standardization of renal MRI biomarkers. This experimental protocol is complemented by two separate chapters describing the basic concept and data analysis.

Key words Magnetic resonance imaging (MRI), Kidney, Mice, Rats, Hyperpolarization, 13C, DNP

1 Introduction

The causal link between renal blood flow (RBF) and glomerular filtration rate (GFR), tubular reabsorption and thus oxygen/metabolic demand and the development of renal dysfunction is well-known [1]. Therefore, diagnostic modalities able to image RBF, GFR, and the metabolic effects have long been sought for.

One such method is hyperpolarized ^{13}C MR, described in the chapter by von Morze C et al. “Hyperpolarized Carbon (^{13}C) MRI of the Kidneys: Basic Concept.” In short, a transient enhancement of more than 10.000 times in spin polarization of a substrate molecule, such as [1-^{13}C]pyruvate, is achieved by irradiating a supercooled mixture of ^{13}C spins and electron spins with a microwave frequency obeying the nuclear Overhauser condition—and subsequently rapidly dissolved by superheated water [2]. The

Andreas Pohlmann and Thoralf Niendorf (eds.), *Preclinical MRI of the Kidney: Methods and Protocols*, Methods in Molecular Biology, vol. 2216, https://doi.org/10.1007/978-1-0716-0978-1_29,

resulting mixture retains the high polarization and allows injection of metabolic and functional active molecules and subsequent imaging of the substrate and potential metabolic derivatives following cellular uptake and enzymatic conversion [3, 4]. We will describe basic experiments using hyperpolarized ^{13}C MRS and MRI for monitoring of the metabolic conversion of [1-^{13}C]pyruvate and the intra-renal distribution of ^{13}C-urea in the kidney of rodents in a step-by-step experimental protocol. The rationale for choosing acquisition parameters is given in generic terms, together with specific parameter examples for 3 T, 4.7 T and 9.4 T MRI. Several imaging sequences to map renal metabolism and function are described as optional components of the experiment.

This experimental protocol chapter is complemented by two separate chapters describing the basic concept and data analysis, which are part of this book.

This chapter is part of the book Pohlmann A, Niendorf T (eds) (2020) Preclinical MRI of the Kidney—Methods and Protocols. Springer, New York.

2 Materials

2.1 Animals

This experimental protocol is tailored for rats (Wistar, Sprague-Dawley, or Lewis) with a body mass of 200–350 g. Advice for adaptation to mice is given as *Notes* where necessary.

2.2 Lab Equipment

1. Anesthesia has been shown to impact renal metabolism using hyperpolarized MRI [5]; An appropriate and convenient choice is the use of gas anesthesia. For in-depth description, *see* the chapter by Kaucsar T et al. “Preparation and Monitoring of Small Animals in Renal MRI.”
2. Gases: O_2 with or without additional N_2, as well as a gas-mixing system to achieve required blood oxygen saturation level.
3. Hyperpolarizer equipment, typically the commercial preclinical polarizer HyperSense (Oxford Instruments Molecular Biotools, Oxford, United Kingdom) or newer variants of this design [6, 7] as well as the clinical intent polarizer, the so-called SPINLAB (GE Healthcare, Milwaukee, WI, USA).
4. Vein or artery access, typically tail vein access for fast bolus infusion of the hyperpolarized substrate either by manual injection or by infusion pumps [7] (*see* **Note 1**).
5. Phantom: A ^{13}C containing phantom is needed to confirm center frequency and power calibration. A typical phantom used: 8 M ^{13}C-urea (Sigma, St. Louis, MO, USA) in 90% H_2O and 10% Glycerol with 3 μl/ml Gd contrast agent (Dotarem; Guerbet, Roissy, France) (*see* **Note 2**).

2.3 MRI Hardware

The general hardware requirements for renal ^{1}H MRI on mice and rats are described in the chapter by Ramos Delgado P et al. "Hardware Considerations for Preclinical Magnetic Resonance of the Kidney." The technique described in this chapter was tailored for a 3 T clinical system (GE Healthcare, Milwaukee, WI, USA) and a 9.4 Tesla MR system (Agilent, Yarnton, UK) but advice for adaptation to other field strengths is given where necessary. Additional hardware is required, for excitation and reception of ^{13}C: X-band RF amplifiers and signal preamplifiers supporting the resonance frequency of ^{13}C, ^{13}C transmit and receive RF coils, such as $^{1}H/^{13}C$ volume RF coils [8–10] as well as transmit/receive switches adjusted to the resonance frequency of ^{13}C.

1. A physiological monitoring system that can track the respiration, and which is connected to the MR system such that it can be used to trigger the image acquisition.

3 Methods

3.1 MRI Protocol Setup

3.1.1 Prescan

1. Single pulse and acquire sequence to identify ^{13}C phantom frequency and calibration of the ^{13}C transmitter power for a given pulse shape, width, and amplitude (*see* **Note 3**).

3.1.2 2D/3D Slice Selective Chemical Shift Imaging (CSI)

1. Sequence type: 2D or 3D chemical shift imaging sequence. This is a standard sequence on preclinical MRI and clinical MRI systems [9, 11, 12].
2. Repetition time (TR): choose the shortest possible with sufficient spectral resolution (which is inversely related to the duration of the data sampling window), for efficient temporal resolution.
3. Echo time (TE): choose the shortest possible for good signal-to-noise and reduction of first order phase effects (*see* **Note 4**).
4. Flip angle (FA): adapt to ensure a good compromise between SNR, T_1 relaxation and sufficient signal following repeated excitations. FA is often a low flip angle of $\Theta = 5–10°$ leaving a factor of $\cos(\theta)^n$ longitudinal magnetization remaining, with n being the number of excitations (*see* **Note 5**).
5. Acquisition bandwidth (BW): set to a value in the typically range of 4000–20,000 Hz, Number of acquisition points (NP): 256–2048 [9, 11, 12]. Choose BW and NP to ensure sufficient resolution and acquisition time of approximately $2.5 \times T_2^*$.

6. K-space ordering: use conventional view ordering, which will result in the center of k-space being sampled late in the acquisition (*see* **Note 6**).
7. For an example of a specific parameter set, please *see* **Note 7**.

3.1.3 2D/3D Echo-Planar Spectroscopic Imaging (EPSI)

1. Sequence type: 2D or 3D echo-planar spectroscopic imaging (EPSI) with or without double spin echo refocusing. This approach superimposes an oscillating readout gradient onto CSI acquisition, replacing one of the phase encoding dimensions needed for CSI. This is not a standard sequence on most preclinical or clinical MRI systems [9, 13, 14].
2. Spectral bandwidth (BW): set spectral BW in the order of 500–600 Hz. The EPSI readout is limited by gradient switching and thus only much lower spectral acquisition bandwidths than CSI are achievable, with outside resonances potentially aliasing into the spectral window. Spectral bandwidth can be traded for spatial resolution but is typically in the order of 500–600 Hz (*see* **Note 8**) for a spatial resolution of ~5 mm.
3. Flip angle (FA): adapt to ensure a good compromise between SNR, T_1 relaxation, and sufficient signal following repeated excitations. FA is often a low flip of $\Theta = 5–10°$ leaving a factor of $\cos(\theta)^n$ longitudinal magnetization remaining, with n being the number of excitations (*see* **Note 5**).
4. Respiration trigger: can be added to improve the spatial localization.
5. Geometry: adapt so that animal fits into FOV and both kidneys are covered. Axial or coronal directions are most often used.
6. For an example of a specific parameter set, please *see* **Note 9**.

3.1.4 Multi-echo Gradient-Echo Sequence for IDEAL Mapping

1. Sequence type: 2D multi-gradient echo sequence. This is a standard sequence on preclinical MRI systems; alternatively, single timepoint acquisitions such as EPI or spiral readout can be used [15–18] (*see* **Note 10**).
2. Repetition time (TR): choose the shortest possible with sufficient distinct echo times, for highest temporal resolution.
3. Flip angle (FA): adapt to ensure a good compromise between SNR, T_1 relaxation and sufficient signal following repeated excitations. FA is often a low flip of $\Theta = 5–10°$ utilizing cos $(\theta)^n$ of excitations of the nonrecoverable magnetization. n being the number of excitations.
4. Echo time (TE): set the number of echoes to $N + 1$ echoes with N being the number of peaks to be resolved. TE is determined by the ability to separate the a priori known peaks to resolve. This can be calculated using the number of signal averages

(NSA) [17]. A rule of thumb is that minimally $N + 1$ echoes are needed to accurately resolve N peaks.

5. Acquisition bandwidth (BW): use a high BW to shorten ΔTE, to ensure good separation of the peaks according to NSA.
6. Respiration trigger: on (per slice), can be added to improve the spatial localization.
7. Geometry: adapt so that animal fits into FOV and both kidneys are covered. Axial or coronal directions are most often used.
8. For an example of a specific parameter set, please *see* **Note 11**.
9. Use double spin echo (DSE) or flow gradients to suppress flowing spins [19, 20] (optional).

3.1.5 Spectral-Spatial Imaging

1. Sequence type: 2D spectral-spatial excitation with Cartesian, EPI or spiral trajectory readout [8, 21–23] or 3D sequences with or without slice selection and thus spectrally selective narrow band pulses [24] (*see* **Note 12**).
2. Repetition time (TR): adapt to the respiration. If respiration is triggered, the effective TR will be given by the respiration trigger and will be the respiration interval, that is, one excitation per breath. Choose TR to be a little shorter (about 100 ms) than the average respiration interval that is displayed on the physiological monitoring unit (*see* **Note 13**).
3. Flip angle (FA): use a low FA (in the range of 3–8°) on the substrate peak ([1-^{13}C]pyruvate) and high FA (in the range of 30–90°) on the metabolic derivatives, to preserve magnetization for metabolic conversions allowing a longer temporal window in dynamic studies, and allowing saturation recovery kinetics to be fitted.
4. For an example of a specific parameter set, please *see* **Note 14**.

3.1.6 Perfusion Imaging

1. Sequence type: 2D/3D balanced steady state free precession (bSSFP) sequence [25–27].
2. Repetition time (TR): use shortest possible TR for high temporal resolution. If triggering respiration, adapt to the respiration. The effective TR will be given by the respiration trigger and will be the respiration interval, that is, one frame per breath. Ideally choose NP × TR to be shorter (about 100 ms) than the average respiration interval that is displayed on the physiological monitoring unit.
3. For perfusion assessment use full saturation of the inflowing spins or (optional) a lower flip angle (in the range of 10–30°) [28, 29].

Table 1
bSSFP sequence parameters [23–25]

Sequence	TR/TE, ms	Matrix size	FOV, mm	Acquisition bandwidth, kHz	Flip angle (°)	Preparation	References
2D at 3 T	11.5/5.7	32 × 32	80	20	15	$\alpha/2$	[23]
2D at 9.4 T	4.8/2.4	32 × 32	60		15	–	[24]
3D at 9.4 T	5.4/2.7	48 × 48 × 48	60	20	15	–	[25]

4. Use preparation pulses (optional) to improve magnetization utilization; typically, $\alpha/2$ pulses before and after the bSSFP train to achieve faster pseudo-steady state and to retain the magnetization for subsequent scans [30].
5. For an example of a specific parameter set, please *see* Table 1.

3.2 In Vivo ^{13}C MR

3.2.1 Preparations

1. Anesthetize the animal and transfer it to the scanner.
2. Place ^{13}C enriched phantom in the FOV (*see* **Note 15**).
3. Set up the temperature monitoring (rectal probe) and respiratory monitoring (balloon on chest) unit.
4. Perform anatomical imaging as described in the chapter by Pohlmann A et al. "Essential Practical Steps for MRI of the Kidney in Experimental Research."
5. Perform localized shimming on the kidney imaging as described in the chapter by Pohlmann A et al. "Essential Practical Steps for MRI of the Kidney in Experimental Research" (*see* **Note 16**).
6. Perform ^{13}C frequency calibration and ^{13}C power calibration (*see* **Note 17**).

3.2.2 Hyperpolarized ^{13}C Metabolic and Functional Imaging

1. Load the ^{13}C sequence of choice, adapt the slice orientation to provide a coronal or axial view with respect to the kidney (in scanner coordinates this is double-oblique).
2. Triggering (^{13}C): in the monitoring unit set the trigger delay so that the trigger starts at the beginning of the expiratory plateau (no chest motion) and the duration such that it covers the entire expiratory phase, that is, until just before inhalation starts.
3. Run the ^{13}C imaging scan (*see* **Note 18**). Examples of images are shown in Figs. 1, 2, 3, and 4.

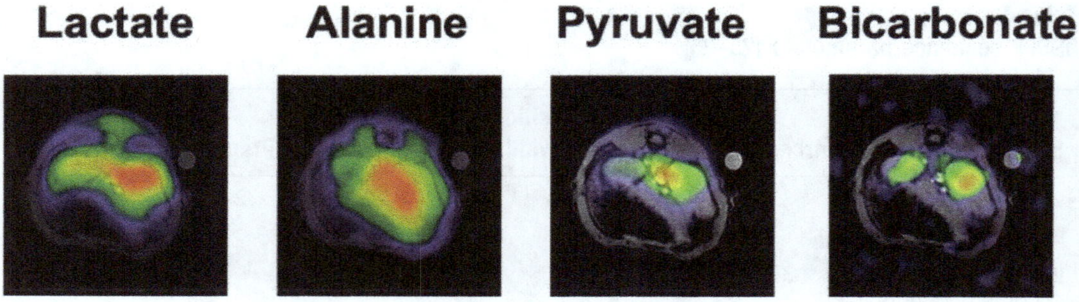

Fig. 1 Series of axial metabolic maps (color) from a 2D CSI overlaid on ^{1}H anatomical scans (grayscale), showing the individual metabolites after integration of the individual peaks

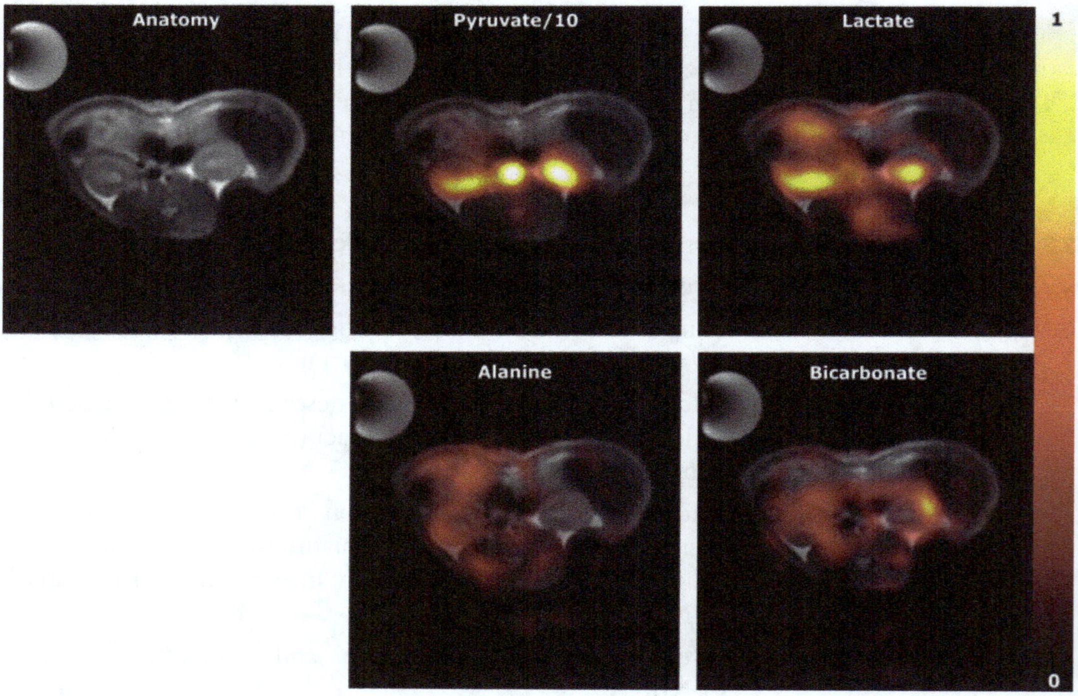

Fig. 2 Examples of axial IDEAL spiral sequence in the kidney at 3 T

3.3 Emerging Sequences

Several novel alternative strategies have been proposed for various imaging applications and just to mention a few there are control of the inflowing spins with bolus tracking [31, 32], spatiotemporal encoding [33], improved resolution by spatially shaped excitations [32, 34]. Variations of the balanced steady state sequences [35, 36] hold potential for further improvement by optimally designing the imaging strategy toward the long T_2's seen in most ^{13}C molecules. Relaxation contrast is another potential renal contrast mechanism, showing substantial promise to improve the diagnostic potential of hyperpolarized MR [37–40].

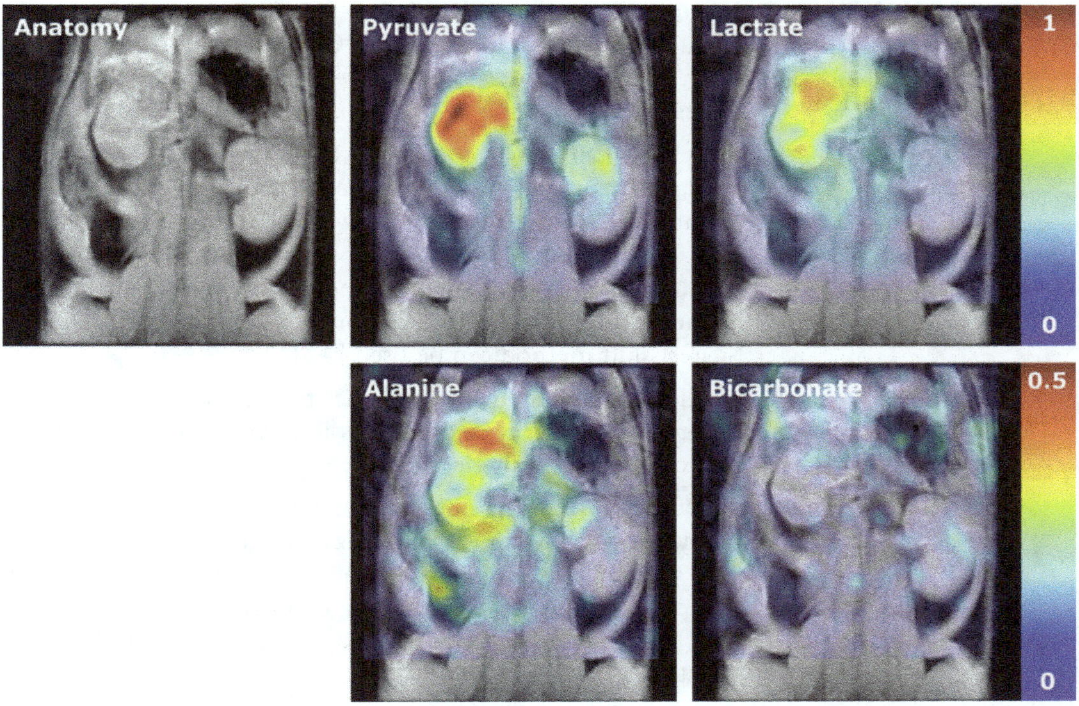

Fig. 3 Examples of coronal spectral spatial (spsp) excitation sequence in the kidney at 3 T

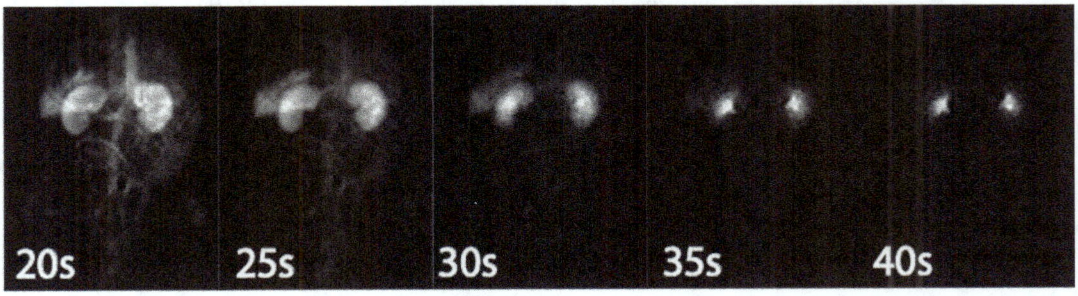

Fig. 4 2D BSSFP dynamic coronal imaging of hyperpolarized [$^{13}C,^{15}N_2$]urea at 3 T. Using a 180 flip angle, 0.92 mm in plane resolution, no slice select. The imaging durations were 1 s separated by 4 s delays, with catalyzation/decatalyzation pulses before and after each image

4 Notes

1. In order to allow optimal usage of the substrate, keep dead-volume as small as possible for injection line; injection speed is typically 0.1 ml/s and up to 2 ml for a rat. If the sequence is single timepoint imaging method or flow artifacts are corrupting the images with a minimum of 20 s time delay from start of injection it is an appropriate choice for intrarenal metabolism and function of the rodent kidneys.

2. Ensure short enough T_1 of the ^{13}C phantom to allow rapid frequency and power calibration. Caution, due to B_0 variation the reference ^{13}C peak is not always representative of the in vivo position.
3. Frequency calibration and power calibration can be done in a similar manner as any ^1H experiment with a centering on the phantom peak and running a power calibration using a standard nutation experiment. Calibrating with a 180 pulse is desirable as the signal changes more rapidly as a function of applied power than with a 90 pulse. Alternatively, a Bloch–Siegert shift method can be used [41].
4. As the RF pulse length contributes to the TE and the RF flip often is very low, it is often possible to shorten the TE by reducing the RF pulse length.
5. Signal decay over the phase encoding steps, either due to T_1 decay or consumption of magnetization due to RF pulses (i.e., T_2). Constant flip angle excitation constitutes a k-space filter that can introduce significant image blurring. Alternatively, an increasing flip angle can be employed to compensate for such effects [42].
6. A variety of CSI sampling patterns can be adopted to optimize temporal constraints, SNR, and partial volume effects [9].
7. Example *for a 300 g rat at 9.4 T*: TR = 70 ms; TE = 0.68 ms, flip angle = 10°; pulse length 500 us; receiver bandwidth = 8 kHz; number of points = 512 complex points (i.e., 1024), averages = 1; slice orientation = axial oblique; FOV = (60 × 60) mm; matrix size = 16 × 16 zero-filled to 32 × 32; 1 slice with 1–2 cm thickness; TA = 17 s (without triggering).
8. The low bandwidth will typically require prior knowledge of the peaks of interest and their folding patterns to fully recover the spectral information [9].
9. Example 3D EPSI for a 300 g rat at 3 T: An EPSI sequence with double spin echo refocusing (13). Images are acquired with (8 × 8 × 8) mm^3 voxel size and a matrix size of 18 × 10 × 8, coronal view, with a TR of 215 ms, TE of 140 ms, and a spectral width 543 Hz.
10. The multispectral signals are resolved by fitting to a signal model with unknown components at known frequency offsets. B_0 offset is typically an important component of the model and is fitted along with the spectral components or estimated separately (see https://github.com/LarsonLab/hyperpolarized-mri-toolbox).
11. Example: *2D IDEAL-spiral for a 300 g rat at 3 T (18)*: TR = 100 ms; TE = 0.9 ms; flip angle = 10°; 11 IDEAL

echoes with ΔTE values 0.9 ms, determined by the NSA formalism to resolve [1-^{13}C]pyruvate, [1-^{13}C]lactate, [1-^{13}C]alanine, [1-^{13}C]pyruvate hydrate, [^{13}C]bicarbonate. Slice orientation = axial oblique; FOV = (80 × 80) mm^2; matrix size = 32 × 32; 5 mm × 5 mm real spatial resolution; 1 slice with 1–2 cm thickness covering both kidneys. Dynamic acquisition over 60–80 s.

12. Offset frequencies for individual metabolites must be specified a priori. It is important to note that the frequency might be different than the in vivo version of a given phantom metabolite and thus it is important to verify the correct frequency.
13. Monitor the respiration continuously throughout the entire experiment and if necessary adapt the TR accordingly for the ^{13}C examination.
14. Example: *2D spectral-spatial for a 300 g rat at 3 T (20)*: TR = 1 s; TE = 10 ms; flip angle = 90° on [1-^{13}C]lactate, flip angle = 15° on [1-^{13}C]pyruvate;, flip angle = 90° on [^{13}C] bicarbonate and flip angle = 90° on [1-^{13}C]alanine; slice orientation = axial oblique; FOV = (80 × 80) mm; matrix size = 32 × 32; 5 mm × 5 mm real spatial resolution; 1 slice with 1–2 cm thickness covering both kidneys. Dynamic acquisition over 60–80 s.
15. Be careful with the frequency shift between in vivo and ex vivo phantom conditions.
16. B_0 shimming is particularly important, since macroscopic magnetic field inhomogeneities shorten T_2*, and potentially shift the peak positions relative to the main magnetic field. Shimming should be performed on a voxel enclosing only the kidney using either the default iterative shimming method or manual shimming.
17. It is often possible to retain a similar B_1 amplitude for similar sized animals. ^{13}C Tx gain and Tx/Rx frequency is largely similar in rats and mice and thus the differences should be small between experiments (typically below 1 dB and 50 Hz).
18. A good starting point is to use the same relative resolution as for rats. For this, reduce the FOV to the mouse body width and keep the matrix size the same.

Acknowledgments

This chapter is based upon work from COST Action PARENCH IMA, supported by European Cooperation in Science and Technology (COST). COST (www.cost.eu) is a funding agency for research and innovation networks. COST Actions help connect research initiatives across Europe and enable scientists to enrich their ideas by sharing them with their peers. This boosts their research, career, and innovation.

PARENCHIMA (renalmri.org) is a community-driven Action in the COST program of the European Union, which unites more than 200 experts in renal MRI from 30 countries with the aim to improve the reproducibility and standardization of renal MRI biomarkers.

References

1. Blantz RC, Deng A, Miracle CM, Thomson SC (2007) Regulation of kidney function and metabolism: a question of supply and demand. Trans Am Clin Climatol Assoc 118:23–43
2. Ardenkjaer-Larsen JH, Fridlund B, Gram A, Hansson G, Hansson L, Lerche MH, Servin R, Thaning M, Golman K (2003) Increase in signal-to-noise ratio of > 10,000 times in liquid-state NMR. Proc Natl Acad Sci U S A 100(18):10158–10163. https://doi.org/10.1073/pnas.1733835100
3. Kurhanewicz J, Vigneron DB, Ardenkjaer-Larsen JH, Bankson JA, Brindle K, Cunningham CH, Gallagher FA, Keshari KR, Kjaer A, Laustsen C, Mankoff DA, Merritt ME, Nelson SJ, Pauly JM, Lee P, Ronen S, Tyler DJ, Rajan SS, Spielman DM, Wald L, Zhang X, Malloy CR, Rizi R (2018) Hyperpolarized (13)C MRI: path to clinical translation in oncology. Neoplasia 21(1):1–16. https://doi.org/10.1016/j.neo.2018.09.006
4. Laustsen C (2016) Hyperpolarized renal magnetic resonance imaging: potential and pitfalls. Front Physiol 7:72. https://doi.org/10.3389/fphys.2016.00072
5. Qi H, Mariager CO, Lindhardt J, Nielsen PM, Stodkilde-Jorgensen H, Laustsen C (2018) Effects of anesthesia on renal function and metabolism in rats assessed by hyperpolarized MRI. Magn Reson Med 80(5):2073–2080. https://doi.org/10.1002/mrm.27165
6. Ardenkjaer-Larsen JH, Bowen S, Petersen JR, Rybalko O, Vinding MS, Ullisch M, Nielsen NC (2018) Cryogen-free dissolution dynamic nuclear polarization polarizer operating at 3.35 T, 6.70 T, and 10.1 T. Magn Reson Med. https://doi.org/10.1002/mrm.27537
7. Comment A, van den Brandt B, Uffmann K, Kurdzesau F, Jannin S, Konter JA, Hautle P, Wenckebach WT, Gruetter R, van der Klink JJ (2007) Design and performance of a DNP prepolarizer coupled to a rodent MRI scanner. Concepts Magn Reson B Magn Reson Eng 31B(4):255–269. https://doi.org/10.1002/cmr.b.20099
8. Xu T, Mayer D, Gu M, Yen YF, Josan S, Tropp J, Pfefferbaum A, Hurd R, Spielman D (2011) Quantification of in vivo metabolic kinetics of hyperpolarized pyruvate in rat kidneys using dynamic 13C MRSI. NMR Biomed 24(8):997–1005. https://doi.org/10.1002/nbm.1719
9. Yen YF, Kohler SJ, Chen AP, Tropp J, Bok R, Wolber J, Albers MJ, Gram KA, Zierhut ML, Park I, Zhang V, Hu S, Nelson SJ, Vigneron DB, Kurhanewicz J, Dirven HA, Hurd RE (2009) Imaging considerations for in vivo 13C metabolic mapping using hyperpolarized 13C-pyruvate. Magn Reson Med 62(1):1–10. https://doi.org/10.1002/mrm.21987
10. Bertelsen LB, Nielsen PM, Qi H, Norlinger TS, Zhang X, Stodkilde-Jorgensen H, Laustsen C (2016) Diabetes induced renal urea transport alterations assessed with 3D hyperpolarized 13 C,15 N-Urea. Magn Reson Med. https://doi.org/10.1002/mrm.26256
11. Laustsen C, Østergaard JA, Lauritzen MH, Nørregaard R, Bowen S, Søgaard LV, Flyvbjerg A, Pedersen M, Ardenkjær-Larsen JH (2013) Assessment of early diabetic renal changes with hyperpolarized [1-13C]pyruvate. Diabetes Metab Res Rev 29(2):125–129. https://doi.org/10.1002/dmrr.2370
12. Laustsen C, Hansen ES, Kjaergaard U, Bertelsen LB, Ringgaard S, Stodkilde-Jorgensen H (2015) Acute porcine renal metabolic effect of endogastric soft drink administration assessed with hyperpolarized [1-13c]pyruvate. Magn Reson Med. https://doi.org/10.1002/mrm.25692
13. Ohliger MA, von Morze C, Marco-Rius I, Gordon J, Larson PEZ, Bok R, Chen HY, Kurhanewicz J, Vigneron D (2017) Combining hyperpolarized (13) C MRI with a liver-specific gadolinium contrast agent for selective assessment of hepatocyte metabolism. Magn Reson Med 77(6):2356–2363. https://doi.org/10.1002/mrm.26296
14. Cunningham CH, Chen AP, Albers MJ, Kurhanewicz J, Hurd RE, Yen YF, Pauly JM, Nelson SJ, Vigneron DB (2007) Double spin-echo sequence for rapid spectroscopic imaging of hyperpolarized 13C. J Magn Reson 187

(2):357–362. https://doi.org/10.1016/j.jmr.2007.05.014

15. Leupold J, Månsson S, Stefan Petersson J, Hennig J, Wieben O (2009) Fast multiecho balanced SSFP metabolite mapping of 1H and hyperpolarized 13C compounds. Magn Reson Mater Phys 22(4):251–256
16. Niles DJ, Gordon JW, Huang G, Reese S, Adamson EB, Djamali A, Fain SB (2018) Evaluation of renal metabolic response to partial ureteral obstruction with hyperpolarized (13) C MRI. NMR Biomed 31(1). https://doi.org/10.1002/nbm.3846
17. Wiesinger F, Weidl E, Menzel MI, Janich MA, Khegai O, Glaser SJ, Haase A, Schwaiger M, Schulte RF (2012) IDEAL spiral CSI for dynamic metabolic MR imaging of hyperpolarized [1-13C]pyruvate. Magn Reson Med 68 (1):8–16. https://doi.org/10.1002/mrm.23212
18. Qi H, Nielsen PM, Schroeder M, Bertelsen LB, Palm F, Laustsen C (2018) Acute renal metabolic effect of metformin assessed with hyperpolarised MRI in rats. Diabetologia 61 (2):445–454. https://doi.org/10.1007/s00125-017-4445-6
19. Josan S, Yen Y-F, Hurd R, Pfefferbaum A, Spielman D, Mayer D (2011) Application of double spin echo spiral chemical shift imaging to rapid metabolic mapping of hyperpolarized [1-^{13}C]-pyruvate. J Magn Reson 209 (2):332–336. https://doi.org/10.1016/j.jmr.2011.01.010
20. Gordon JW, Niles DJ, Adamson EB, Johnson KM, Fain SB (2016) Application of flow sensitive gradients for improved measures of metabolism using hyperpolarized (13) c MRI. Magn Reson Med 75(3):1242–1248. https://doi.org/10.1002/mrm.25584
21. Shang H, Sukumar S, von Morze C, Bok RA, Marco-Rius I, Kerr A, Reed GD, Milshteyn E, Ohliger MA, Kurhanewicz J, Larson PEZ, Pauly JM, Vigneron DB (2017) Spectrally selective three-dimensional dynamic balanced steady-state free precession for hyperpolarized C-13 metabolic imaging with spectrally selective radiofrequency pulses. Magn Reson Med 78(3):963–975. https://doi.org/10.1002/mrm.26480
22. Schulte RF, Sperl JI, Weidl E, Menzel MI, Janich MA, Khegai O, Durst M, Ardenkjaer-Larsen JH, Glaser SJ, Haase A, Schwaiger M, Wiesinger F (2013) Saturation-recovery metabolic-exchange rate imaging with hyperpolarized [1-13C] pyruvate using spectral-spatial excitation. Magn Reson Med 69 (5):1209–1216. https://doi.org/10.1002/mrm.24353
23. Lau AZ, Chen AP, Hurd RE, Cunningham CH (2011) Spectral-spatial excitation for rapid imaging of DNP compounds. NMR Biomed 24(8):988–996. https://doi.org/10.1002/nbm.1743
24. Eichhorn TR, Takado Y, Salameh N, Capozzi A, Cheng T, Hyacinthe JN, Mishkovsky M, Roussel C, Comment A (2013) Hyperpolarization without persistent radicals for in vivo real-time metabolic imaging. Proc Natl Acad Sci U S A 110 (45):18064–18069. https://doi.org/10.1073/pnas.1314928110
25. von Morze C, Bok RA, Sands JM, Kurhanewicz J, Vigneron DB (2012) Monitoring urea transport in rat kidney in vivo using hyperpolarized 13C magnetic resonance imaging. Am J Physiol Ren Physiol. https://doi.org/10.1152/ajprenal.00640.2011
26. Qi H, Norlinger TS, Nielsen PM, Bertelsen LB, Mikkelsen E, Xu Y, Stodkilde Jorgensen H, Laustsen C (2016) Early diabetic kidney maintains the corticomedullary urea and sodium gradient. Physiol Rep 4(5). https://doi.org/10.14814/phy2.12714
27. Nielsen PM, Szocska Hansen ES, Norlinger TS, Norregaard R, Bonde Bertelsen L, Stodkilde Jorgensen H, Laustsen C (2016) Renal ischemia and reperfusion assessment with three-dimensional hyperpolarized (13) C, (15) N2-urea. Magn Reson Med 76 (5):1524–1530. https://doi.org/10.1002/mrm.26377
28. Johansson E, Olsson LE, Månsson S, Petersson JS, Golman K, Ståhlberg F, Wirestam R (2004) Perfusion assessment with bolus differentiation: a technique applicable to hyperpolarized tracers. Magn Reson Med 52(5):1043–1051. https://doi.org/10.1002/mrm.20247
29. von Morze C, Larson PE, Hu S, Keshari K, Wilson DM, Ardenkjaer-Larsen JH, Goga A, Bok R, Kurhanewicz J, Vigneron DB (2011) Imaging of blood flow using hyperpolarized [(13)C]urea in preclinical cancer models. J Magn Reson Imaging 33(3):692–697. https://doi.org/10.1002/jmri.22484
30. Svensson J, Mansson S, Johansson E, Petersson JS, Olsson LE (2003) Hyperpolarized 13C MR angiography using trueFISP. Magn Reson Med 50(2):256–262. https://doi.org/10.1002/mrm.10530
31. Durst M, Koellisch U, Gringeri C, Janich MA, Rancan G, Frank A, Wiesinger F, Menzel MI, Haase A, Schulte RF (2014) Bolus tracking for improved metabolic imaging of hyperpolarised compounds. J Magn Reson (San Diego, CA: 1997) 243:40–46. https://doi.org/10.1016/j.jmr.2014.02.011

32. Tang S, Jiang W, Chen HY, Bok R, Vigneron DB, Larson PE (2015) A 2DRF pulse sequence for bolus tracking in hyperpolarized 13C imaging. Magn Reson Med 74(2):506–512. https://doi.org/10.1002/mrm.25427
33. Schmidt R, Laustsen C, Dumez J-N, Kettunen MI, Serrao EM, Marco-Rius I, Brindle KM, Ardenkjaer-Larsen JH, Frydman L (2014) In vivo single-shot 13C spectroscopic imaging of hyperpolarized metabolites by spatiotemporal encoding. J Magn Reson 240:8–15. https://doi.org/10.1016/j.jmr.2013.12.013
34. Vinding MS, Laustsen C, Maximov II, Sogaard LV, Ardenkjaer-Larsen JH, Nielsen NC (2013) Dynamic nuclear polarization and optimal control spatial-selective 13C MRI and MRS. J Magn Reson (San Diego, CA: 1997) 227:57–61. https://doi.org/10.1016/j.jmr.2012.12.002
35. Varma G, Wang X, Vinogradov E, Bhatt RS, Sukhatme VP, Seth P, Lenkinski RE, Alsop DC, Grant AK (2016) Selective spectroscopic imaging of hyperpolarized pyruvate and its metabolites using a single-echo variable phase advance method in balanced SSFP. Magn Reson Med 76(4):1102–1115. https://doi.org/10.1002/mrm.26004
36. Mansson S, Petersson JS, Scheffler K (2012) Fast metabolite mapping in the pig heart after injection of hyperpolarized 13C-pyruvate with low-flip angle balanced steady-state free precession imaging. Magn Reson Med 68 (6):1894–1899. https://doi.org/10.1002/mrm.24183
37. Reed GD, von Morze C, Bok R, Koelsch BL, Van Criekinge M, Smith KJ, Hong S, PEZ L, Kurhanewicz J, Vigneron DB (2014) High resolution ^{13}C MRI with hyperpolarized urea: in vivo T_2 mapping and ^{15}N labeling effects. IEEE Trans Med Imaging 33(2):362–371. https://doi.org/10.1109/TMI.2013.2285120
38. Reed GD, von Morze C, Verkman AS, Koelsch BL, Chaumeil MM, Lustig M, Ronen SM, Sands JM, Larson PEZ, Wang ZJ, Ardenkjær Larsen JH, Kurhanewicz J, Vigneron DB (2015) Imaging renal urea handling in rats at millimeter resolution using hyperpolarized magnetic resonance relaxometry. ArXiv 1511:200
39. Laustsen C, Stokholm Norlinger T, Christoffer Hansen D, Qi H, Mose Nielsen P, Bonde Bertelsen L, Henrik Ardenkjaer-Larsen J, Stodkilde Jorgensen H (2015) Hyperpolarized C urea relaxation mechanism reveals renal changes in diabetic nephropathy. Magn Reson Med. https://doi.org/10.1002/mrm.26036
40. Qi H, Mariager CO, Nielsen PM, Schroeder M, Lindhardt J, Norregaard R, Klein JD, Sands JM, Laustsen C (2019) Glucagon infusion alters the hyperpolarized (13) C-urea renal hemodynamic signature. NMR Biomed 32(1):e4028. https://doi.org/10.1002/nbm.4028
41. Schulte RF, Sacolick L, Deppe MH, Janich MA, Schwaiger M, Wild JM, Wiesinger F (2011) Transmit gain calibration for nonproton MR using the Bloch-Siegert shift. NMR Biomed 24(9):1068–1072. https://doi.org/10.1002/nbm.1657
42. Zhao L, Mulkern R, Tseng CH, Williamson D, Patz S, Kraft R, Walsworth RL, Jolesz FA, Albert MS (1996) Gradient-echo imaging considerations for hyperpolarized 129Xe MR. J Magn Reson B 113:179–183

5

Dynamic Contrast Enhanced (DCE) MRI-Derived Renal Perfusion and Filtration: Experimental Protocol

Pietro Irrera, Lorena Consolino, Walter Dastrù, Michael Pedersen, Frank G. Zöllner, and Dario Livio Longo

Abstract

Dynamic contrast-enhanced magnetic resonance imaging (DCE-MRI) can provide a noninvasive way for assessing renal functional information following the administration of a small molecular weight gadolinium-based contrast agent. This method may be useful for investigating renal perfusion and glomerular filtration rates of rodents in vivo under various experimental (patho)physiological conditions. Here we describe a step-by-step protocol for DCE-MRI studies in small animals providing practical notes on acquisition parameters, sequences, T_1 mapping approaches and procedures.

This chapters is based upon work from the COST Action PARENCHIMA, a community-driven network funded by the European Cooperation in Science and Technology (COST) program of the European Union, which aims to improve the reproducibility and standardization of renal MRI biomarkers. This experimental protocol chapter is complemented by two separate chapters describing the basic concept and data analysis.

Key words Magnetic resonance imaging (MRI), Kidney, Mice, Rats, Dynamic contrast-enhanced (DCE), Contrast agent, T_1 map

1 Introduction

Kidneys play an important role in fluid regulation, waste products elimination, and homeostasis of salts and pH. Therefore, accurate measurement of kidney function is essential for monitoring early renal injuries, disease progression, renal transplantation and in assessing therapeutic efficacy after renal failure [1, 2]. Magnetic resonance imaging (MRI) has emerged as a powerful technique that combines anatomical details with functional information. In recent years, various MRI techniques have been investigated for assessing renal function, including dynamic contrast-enhanced (DCE) MRI, arterial spin labelling (ASL), blood oxygenation level dependent (BOLD), diffusion weighted imaging (DWI), sodium imaging, chemical exchange saturation

Andreas Pohlmann and Thoralf Niendorf (eds.), *Preclinical MRI of the Kidney: Methods and Protocols*, Methods in Molecular Biology, vol. 2216, https://doi.org/10.1007/978-1-0716-0978-1_25,

transfer (CEST), and hyperpolarized MRI [3–9]. These techniques have shown promising results for the noninvasive evaluation of several renal function, including filtration, perfusion, oxygenation, pH, homeostasis, and others [10–27]. Among them, DCE-MRI or MR renography has emerged as a reliable method to reveal renal pathophysiology, functional and hemodynamic parameters. DCE-MRI relies on bolus administration of a gadolinium-based contrast agent (CA) [16], which changes the intrinsic longitudinal (T_1) and transversal (T_2) relaxation rates of protons in tissue. This means that administration of CA leads to an increased signal intensity on T_1-weighted images or decreased signal intensity on T_2-weighted images. DCE-MRI usually refers to T_1-weighted MR imaging techniques combined with a gadolinium-based CA using an acquisition scheme with a high temporal resolution. In the kidney the acquired signal over time leads to an MRI renogram, where the absolute signal intensity, in complex manner, depends on the native T_1 value, MRI sequence parameters, the specific magnetic relaxivity constant of the CA (the contrast agent efficiency, dependent also on its chemical structure [28–34]) and the concentration of the CA residing in the tissue [35, 36].

The main purpose of DCE-MRI is to reveal information about extravascular permeability, blood perfusion and compartmental kinetics. In practice, this method provides images prior and following the administration of the CA using a continuous image acquisition protocol. In kidneys, DCE-MRI is suitable for assessing kidney function in terms of filtration and perfusion [17]. Different post-processing methods allow estimations of kidney function and perfusion, either from simple semiquantitative approaches to more elaborated model-based analyses [37–42].

Here we describe step-by-step an experimental dynamic contrast enhanced (DCE) MRI protocol for monitoring the passage of a Gd-based tracer in the kidneys of rodents. The rationale for the choosing acquisition parameters is given in generic terms, together with specific parameter examples.

This experimental protocol chapter is complemented by two separate chapters describing the basic concepts and data analysis, which are part of this book.

This chapter is part of the book Pohlmann A, Niendorf T (eds) (2020) Preclinical MRI of the Kidney—Methods and Protocols. Springer, New York.

2 Materials

2.1 Animals

This experimental protocol was tailored for immune-competent (typically C57BL/6 and Balb/C) or immune-compromised (nude, NOD-SCID) mice with a body mass of 15–35 g. Advice for adaptation to rats is given as *Notes* where necessary. All animal studies have to be carried out in compliance with specific legislation covering the use of animals for scientific purposes. Therefore, all experiments must be authorized under national regulations.

2.2 Lab Equipment and Chemicals

1. Mouse tail illuminator/restrainer for catheterizing the tail vein.
2. Saline solution or heparin solution, 1-ml syringe, catheter (e.g., PE 20 polyethylene tubing) of known inner diameter to hold the saline flush and for contrast agent bolus is required.
3. Anesthesia: please refer to the chapter by Kaucsar T et al. "Preparation and Monitoring of Small Animals in Renal MRI" for an in-depth description and discussion of the anesthesia. Typically, 0.5–1.5% isoflurane is used for anesthesia administered to the mice using an anesthetic gas vaporizer (Leica Biosystems, Maryland, USA). For nonrecovery experiments, urethane solution (Sigma–Aldrich, Steinheim, Germany; 20% in distilled water) can provide anesthesia for several hours with comparatively fewer side effects on renal physiology, which is an important issue. For intramuscular anesthesia, please refer to **Note 1**.
4. Gases: O_2, N_2, and compressed air, as well as a gas-mixing system or general inhalation anesthesia equipment, including an anesthetic vaporizer, a flow meter, and an induction chamber.
5. Mouse cradle.
6. Gd-based contrast agents: typically, small molecular weight FDA-approved gadolinium-based contrast agents are employed, such as gadoteridol (Prohance®, Bracco Imaging SpA, Milano, Italy), gadobutrol (Gadovist®, Bayer Healthcare Pharmaceuticals, Germany), or gadoteric acid (Dotarem®, Guerbert, France). Such clinically available contrast agents have stock concentrations of 0.5–1.0 mol/l that need to be diluted for handling volumes with less error (*see* **Note 2**).
7. Small animal ventilator: animals (rats) needs to be ventilated so the DCE-MRI acquisition can be gated to minimize the respiratory motion artifacts.
8. Syringe infusion pump: an MRI-compatible single syringe pump (Harvard Bioscience, Holliston, USA) for contrast agent administration for allowing precise timing infusion.

2.3 MRI Hardware

The general hardware requirements for renal 1H MRI on mice and rats are described in the chapter by Ramos Delgado P et al. "Hardware Considerations for Preclinical Magnetic Resonance of the Kidney." The technique described in this chapter was tailored for MRI preclinical systems at a magnetic field strength of 7 T but advice for adaptation to other magnetic field strengths is given where necessary (*see* **Note 3**). No special or additional hardware is required, except for the following:

1. A physiological monitoring system that can track the respiration and which is connected to the MRI system such that it can be used to synchronize DCE-MRI with respiration. Typically, we use an MRI-compatible rodent monitoring and gating system equipped with an air-pillow to monitor breath rate (Small Animal Instruments, New York, USA).

2.4 MRI Techniques

DCE-MRI experiments are performed by dynamic acquisitions of a strongly T_1-weighted imaging technique. The acquired signal following the CA administration is converted to relative concentrations of the gadolinium agent using either phantom calibration scales or by mathematical calculation of the sequence equation that describes the relationship between signal and MRI sequence parameters. The MRI sequence parameters, required volume coverage, spatial resolution, and SNR will determine the final temporal resolution. Several T_1 mapping approaches can be exploited for measuring the longitudinal relation times, a detailed description of different methods is provided in the chapter by Garteiser P et al. "Experimental Protocols for MRI Mapping of Renal T_1."

3 Methods

3.1 MR Protocol Setup

3.1.1 Variable Repetition Time (VTR) Acquisition for T_1 Mapping

1. Use a 2D RARE (rapid acquisition with refocused echoes) sequence with variable repetition times (RAREVTR on a Bruker MR system).
2. Set the acceleration factor (RARE-factor or echo train length, ETL) to at least 4 in order to shorten the acquisition time; an acceleration factor of 8–16 can be used to further shorten the acquisition time by sampling more k-space lines within a single repetition period (TR). Centric encoding can be exploited to minimize T_2 effects with increasing doses, but at the expenses or "blurred" images.
3. Set the echo time (TE) as short as possible for pure T_1-weight; in our setup an effective TE of 25 ms (defined by the acquisition of the central k-space line) was used.
4. Choose enough averages in order to have a sufficient signal to noise ratio (SNR) of above 30.
5. Repeat the RARE acquisition a number of times by changing the value of the repetition time (TR) to sample changes in signal intensities according to the expected T_1 values of the kidneys.
6. Because of the variability of the T_1 values inside the kidney regions, choose the TRs values to span a range large enough to permit an accurate calculation of T_1 by selecting 3–7 TR values in the range 100–10,000 ms (*see* **Note 4**).

7. For in vivo experiments, keep the overall acquisition time as short as possible by considering a trade-off between number of TRs, averages and matrix size (or spatial resolution).
8. For an example of a specific parameter set please *see* **Note 5**.

3.1.2 Variable Flip Angle (VFA) Acquisition for T_1 Mapping

1. Use a 2D gradient-echo sequence (FLASH on a Bruker system).
2. Set the echo time (TE) as short as possible for heavily T_1 weighting; in our setup a TE of 1.5 ms was used.
3. In order to have a sufficient signal to noise ratio, at least two averages have been acquired or enough averages for SNR > 30.
4. Repeat the FLASH acquisition a number of times by changing the value of the flip angle (FA). The changes in signal intensities will follow a parabolic curve, thus low flip angles and higher flip angles are needed to sample both side of this curve. Acquire a minimum of 2–3 flip angles, considering that experiments with more flip angles will improve the goodness of the T_1 estimate.
5. Set the TR in the range 10–100 ms for providing good T_1 weighting. Shorter TR increases T_1 weighting, but with detrimental SNR values; thus, a trade-off must be chosen, even considering number of averages and overall acquisition time.
6. For an example of a specific parameter set please *see* **Note 6**.

3.1.3 Fast Low Angle Shot (FLASH) T1-Weighted Sequence for DCE-MRI Experiments

1. Use a T_1-weighted sequence as a fast low angle shot (FLASH) sequence (in Bruker systems, this sequence refers to a dubbed FLASH sequence).
2. Use short TR to increase T_1-weighting, but this will decrease SNR. Therefore, a good balance should be found between strongly T_1-weighted images and image quality with sufficient SNR. Besides, TE and FA affect T_1-weighting and SNR. A good TR range could be between 5 and 100 ms (usually shorter values for 3D imaging and longer for 2D multislice acquisition).
3. Use the shortest echo time (TE) possible for pure T_1 weight.
4. Flip Angle (FA): high FA corresponds to a strong T_1 weighting, but at expenses of reduced SNR, therefore a good balance may result in FAs in the range 10–60°.
5. Use Partial Fourier acceleration to reduce the size of the acquired matrix and improve the time efficiency of data acquisition.
6. Use a high acquisition bandwidth (BW) to shorten TE, while keeping an eye on the SNR, which decreases with the square root of the increasing BW. For the image with the shortest TE an SNR of at least 30 is recommended.

7. Employ Fat Saturation modules. It is important to avoid fat signal overlaying with the kidney due to chemical shift.
8. Respiration trigger: there is no need to use respiratory triggering (per slice).
9. Adapt the geometry (or slice position) so that animal fits into FOV in Left-Right direction (approximately 30–40 mm according to the inner coil diameter) and use frequency encoding in Head-Feet direction. Use a slice with the lowest thickness the SNR allows, typically around 1–2 mm. The thinner the slices the better, as this improves the resolution which can be readily found on the raw images.
10. Use the highest in-plane resolution that the SNR allows, typically around 96 × 96 to 128 × 128 for FOV of 30 × 30 mm^2 or 40 × 40 mm^2. This resolution should be balanced by the need for sufficient SNR in the images. Zero-filling or use of partial Fourier techniques in the phase encoding direction can be helpful to speed up acquisition to minimize motion artifacts and contrast agent concentration changes during the acquisition. One may use half-Fourier acquisition schemes in read direction (asymmetric echo) to further shorten the TE. Reducing the excitation and refocusing pulse lengths to below 1.5 ms can then also help to shorten TE.
11. For an example of specific parameter sets for a 7 T MRI system, please *see* **Notes 7** and **8**, whereas for a scanner operating at 3 T please *see* **Note 9.**

3.2 Preparations of the Contrast Agent Injection and of the Catheter

1. Fill the 1-ml syringe with the contrast agent solution (*see* **Note 2**).
2. Prepare the catheter by filling the PE20 tubing with the contrast agent solution, and with 20–40 μl of a heparin solution (or a saline solution), between the needle (the animal) and the contrast agent solution to prevent clotting before the contrast agent will be injected.
3. According to the length of the catheter (usually 60–100 cm to exit from the magnet bore) the contrast agent solution can be injected directly from the syringe containing the contrast agent or by changing the syringe with one filled with a (heparin-free) saline solution for the postinjection flush.

3.3 Preparations of the Mouse

1. Place the mouse on a mouse tail illuminator restrainer for catheterizing the tail vein. The tail vein can be catheterized by placing a 27/29-G needle in the animal.
2. Induce anesthesia in animals via isoflurane in an induction box. Then transfer the animal to the MRI system (*see* **Note 10**).
3. Set up the temperature monitoring (rectal probe) and respiratory monitoring (balloon on chest) unit. During imaging, keep

the animal's respiration rate at 35–80 breaths per min by adjusting the dose of anesthesia (approximately 1–1.5% isoflurane with air and oxygen mixed at a 3:1 ratio administered through a nose cone attached to the animal bed and ophthalmic ointment will be applied to the eyes) (*see* **Note 11**).

4. Perform anatomical imaging as described in the chapter by Pohlmann A et al. "Essential Practical Steps for MRI of the Kidney in Experimental Research."
5. Since the AIF should be sampled with the same temporal resolution of the DCE-MRI experiment, selection of anatomical slices including large vessels near the kidneys should be considered.
6. Perform localized shimming on the kidney imaging as described in the chapter by Pohlmann A et al. "Essential Practical Steps for MRI of the Kidney in Experimental Research."

3.4 In Vivo T_1 Mapping

Typically, a T_1 map is acquired before the injection of Gd-based agent.

1. Select the same geometry of the anatomical images, with the same number of slices and position.
2. Load or select one of the several T_1 mapping sequences previously described (3.1). Adapt the same slice orientation as for the anatomical image with coronal or axial view with respect to the kidneys.
3. Run the T_1-mapping scan. Examples images are shown in Fig. 1 and Fig. 2.

3.4.1 DCE-MRI Experiment

1. Load the T_1-weighted sequence, adapt the slice orientation to provide a coronal or axial view with respect to the kidney (in scanner coordinates this is double-oblique) by importing the same geometry as for the anatomical (and T_1 mapping sequence).
2. Set the required number of repetitions accordingly to the sampling time and to the duration of the dynamic acquisition. Typically, 50–100 repetitions provide enough points to be exploited by any of the analysis procedures.
3. Initiate the DCE-MRI scan.
4. After some baseline image acquisition (5–10 images before the injection are enough to derive average baseline values and signal oscillations) perform an intravenous bolus injection of the Gd-based CA through the tail vein at a dose of 0.02–0.1 mmol Gd /kg b.w. by using a power injector to maintain the exact administration rate for each imaged mouse.
5. A demonstration of the signal intensity changes that can be expected for the DCE-MRI experiment across the kidneys is

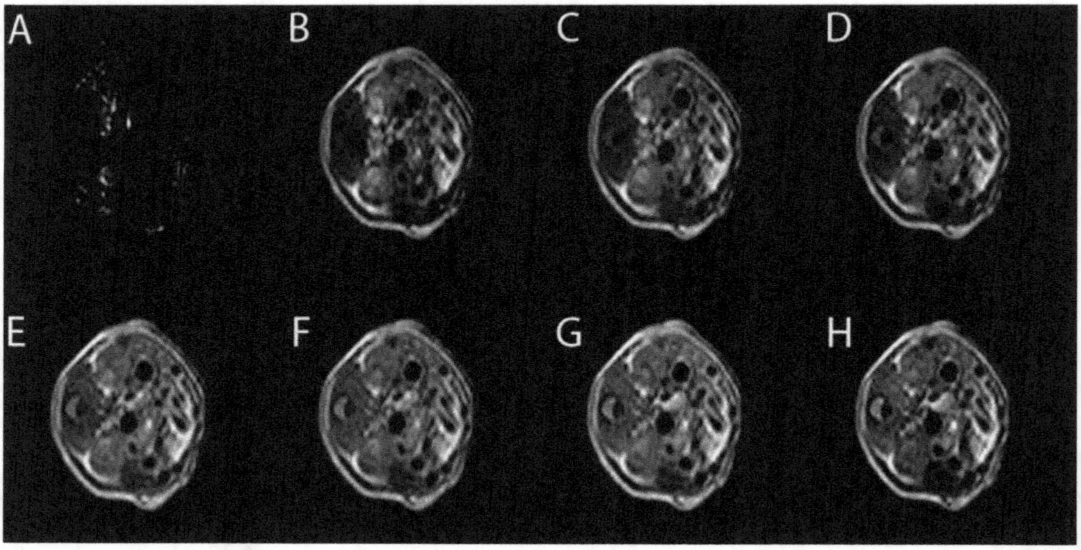

Fig. 1 Representative T_1-weighted images in kidneys obtained with the VTR scheme at different repetition times (TR) values: 75 ms (**a**), 534 ms (**b**), 1076 ms (**c**), 1738 ms (**d**), 2589 ms (**e**), 3782 ms (**f**), 5791 ms (**g**), and 15000 ms (**h**). Acquisition details are provided in **Note 5**

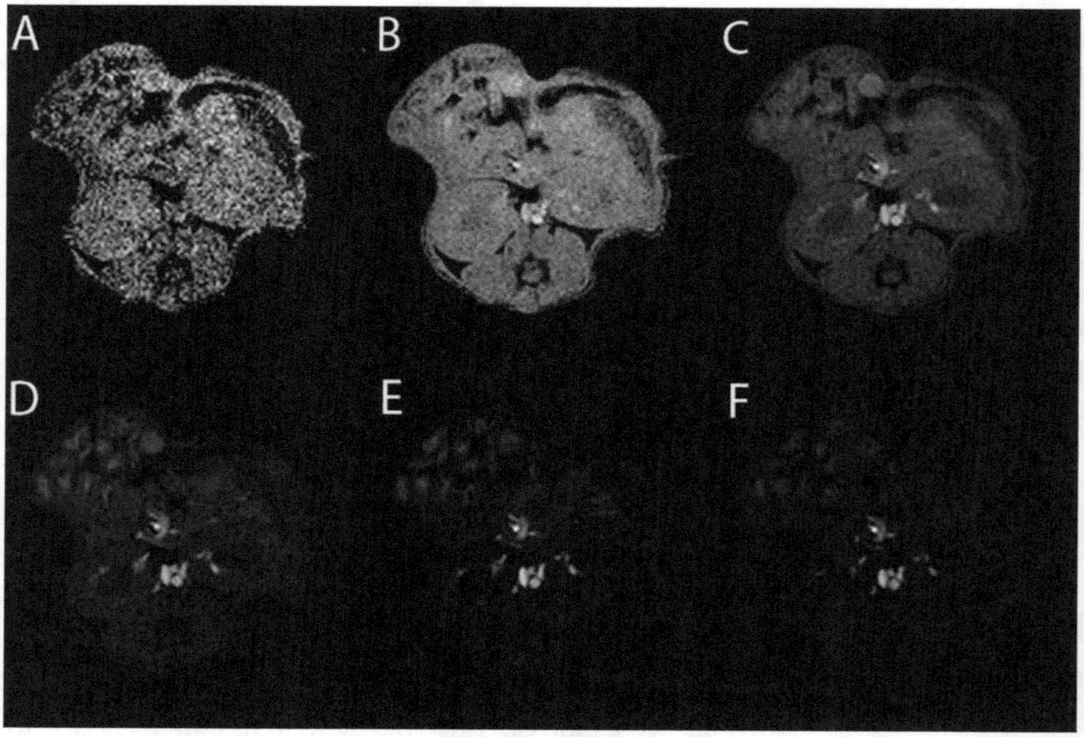

Fig. 2 Representative T_1-weighted images in kidneys obtained with VFA T_1 mapping approach by varying the excitation pulse flip angle values: 5° (**a**), 15° (**b**), 30° (**c**), 45° (**d**), 60° (**e**), and 75° (**f**) with a 7 T MRI system. Acquisition details are provided in **Note 6**

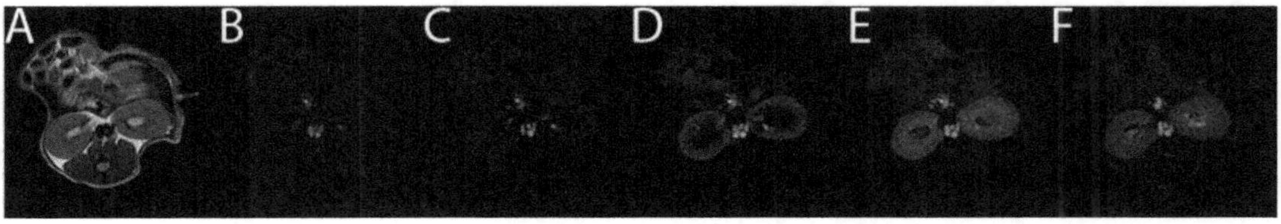

Fig. 3 Representative DCE-MRI images in kidneys (transversal orientation) at different time points following Gd-based contrast agent injection with a 7 T MRI scanner. Anatomical T_2-weighted (**a**) and GRE-FLASH T_1-weighted images before (**b**) and 4 s (**c**), 30 s (**d**), 5 min (**e**), and 10 min (**f**) after gadoteridol injection (dose 0.1 mmol Gd/kg b.w.). Acquisition details are provided in **Note 7**

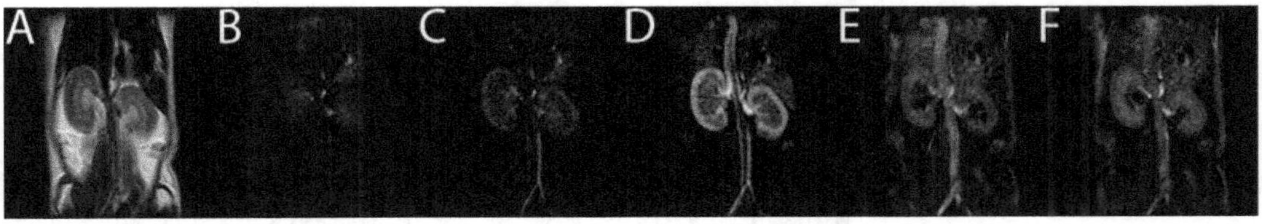

Fig. 4 Representative DCE-MRI images in kidneys (coronal orientation) at different time points following Gd-based contrast agent injection with a 7 T MRI scanner. Anatomical T_2-weighted (**a**) and GRE-FLASH T_1-weighted images before (**b**) and 4 s (bc), 30 s (**d**), 5 min (**e**), and 10 min (**f**) after gadoteridol injection (dose 0.1 mmol Gd/kg b.w.). Acquisition details are provided in **Note 8**

given in Fig. 3 (axial orientation) and Fig. 4 (coronal orientation).

4 Notes

1. Intramuscular anesthesia can be administered as a mixture of xylazine 5 mg/kg (Rompun, Bayer, Italy) and tiletamine/zolepan 20 mg/kg (Zoletil 100, Virbac, Italy) with a dose dependent on the length of the MRI session. Usually, a 40–80 μl volume allows for a sleeping time of 30–60 min for a 25 g mouse.
2. A required dose for DCE-MRI in the kidneys is in the range 0.01–0.1 mmol Gd/kg b.w. that would require too small volumes of the stock solution. Therefore, it is advisable to dilute stock solutions to ca. 50 mmol/l. For instance, a 25 g mouse would receive 50 μl of 50 mmol/l Gd-complex to achieve a dose of 0.1 mmol Gd/kg. Please avoid the inclusion of air bubbles in the catheter filled with the saline solution or with the contrast agent solution that will be injected into the animals.
3. DCE-MRI experiments are described for Bruker MRI systems, such as Avance 300 (7 T) and Biospec (3 T), (Bruker, Ettlingen, Germany) or for a Magnetom Skyra 3 T (Siemens Healthcare, Erlangen, Germany). Standard ^{1}H radiofrequency-coils

(birdcage, quadrature) or phased-array ^1H coils can be used for data reception.

4. Within the Bruker method, specific TR values can be suggested according to the estimated T_1 values of the tissue.
5. For estimated T_1 of 1–3 s, 10 TR values can be used (580, 810, 1075, 1380, 1740, 2180, 2740, 3525, 4830, and 10,000 ms) to correctly follow signal intensities recovery until plateau. With 10 TR values complete acquisition lasted 8:40 min (for 96 × 96 matrix and 8 slices).
6. For estimated T_1 values of 1–3 s, we used six different FA values (5°, 15°, 30°, 45°, 60°, and 75°). With a TR of 80 ms and matrix size of 96 × 96, the single image acquisition lasted more than 15 s (8 slices). The complete acquisition time of the VFA T_1 map with six FA values is approximately 2 min.
7. Example for DCE-MRI using a FLASH readout at 7 T: TR: 16 ms; TE: 1.6 ms; FA: 30°; scan averages: 2; slice thickness: 1.5 mm; slice number: 1; slice orientation: axial; frequency encoding: head-feet; FOV = 30 × 30 mm^2; matrix size = 128 × 128; fat suppression = on; acquisition time per image: 4 s; number of repetitions: 150.
8. Example for DCE-MRI using a FLASH readout at 7 T: TR: 15 ms; TE: 1.7 ms; FA: 30°; scan averages: 2; slice thickness: 1.5 mm; slice number: 1; slice orientation: coronal; frequency encoding: head-feet; FOV = 30 × 30 mm^2; matrix size = 128 × 128; fat suppression = on; acquisition time per image: 4 s; number of repetitions: 150.
9. Example for DCE-MRI using a 3D time-resolved angiography with stochastic trajectories (TWIST) sequence at 3 T: TR = 3.4 ms, TE = 1.4 ms, FA: 20°, FOV = 114 × 50 mm^2, generalized autocalibrating partially parallel acquisition (GRAPPA) of factor 2, matrix = 192 × 84; slice number: 2, voxel resolution = 0.6 × 0.6 × 1.2 mm^3. TWIST view sharing: 15% central region, 20% sampling density in the outer region, nominal temporal resolution 0.9 s per volume. Images were continuously acquired for 6 min.
10. Mice can be alternatively anesthetized with intramuscular anesthesia, tail veins heated with hot water/heater equipment at 37 °C and catheter placed in the animal.
11. It is important to monitor the respiration continuously throughout the entire experiment.

Acknowledgments

The Italian Ministry for Education and Research (MIUR) is gratefully acknowledged for yearly FOE funding to the Euro-BioImaging Multi-Modal Molecular Imaging Italian Node (MMMI).

This chapter is based upon work from COST Action PARENCHIMA, supported by European Cooperation in Science and Technology (COST). COST (www.cost.eu) is a funding agency for research and innovation networks. COST Actions help connect research initiatives across Europe and enable scientists to enrich their ideas by sharing them with their peers. This boosts their research, career, and innovation.

PARENCHIMA (renalmri.org) is a community-driven Action in the COST program of the European Union, which unites more than 200 experts in renal MRI from 30 countries with the aim to improve the reproducibility and standardization of renal MRI biomarkers.

References

1. Sawhney S, Mitchell M, Marks A, Fluck N, Black C (2015) Long-term prognosis after acute kidney injury (AKI): what is the role of baseline kidney function and recovery? A systematic review. BMJ Open 5(1):e006497. https://doi.org/10.1136/bmjopen-2014-006497
2. Joannidis M, Druml W, Forni LG, Groeneveld ABJ, Honore PM, Hoste E, Ostermann M, Oudemans-van Straaten HM, Schetz M (2017) Prevention of acute kidney injury and protection of renal function in the intensive care unit: update 2017: expert opinion of the Working Group on Prevention, AKI section, European Society of Intensive Care Medicine. Intensive Care Med 43(6):730–749. https://doi.org/10.1007/s00134-017-4832-y
3. Kline TL, Edwards ME, Garg I, Irazabal MV, Korfiatis P, Harris PC, King BF, Torres VE, Venkatesh SK, Erickson BJ (2018) Quantitative MRI of kidneys in renal disease. Abdom Radiol (NY) 43(3):629–638. https://doi.org/10.1007/s00261-017-1236-y
4. Zhang JL, Morrell G, Rusinek H, Sigmund EE, Chandarana H, Lerman LO, Prasad PV, Niles D, Artz N, Fain S, Vivier PH, Cheung AK, Lee VS (2014) New magnetic resonance imaging methods in nephrology. Kidney Int 85 (4):768–778. https://doi.org/10.1038/ki.2013.361
5. Zhang JL, Rusinek H, Chandarana H, Lee VS (2013) Functional MRI of the kidneys. J Magn Reson Imaging 37(2):282–293. https://doi.org/10.1002/jmri.23717
6. Mannelli L, Maki JH, Osman SF, Chandarana H, Lomas DJ, Shuman WP, Linnau KF, Green DE, Laffi G, Moshiri M (2012) Noncontrast functional MRI of the kidneys. Curr Urol Rep 13(1):99–107. https://doi.org/10.1007/s11934-011-0229-6
7. Attenberger UI, Morelli JN, Schoenberg SO, Michaely HJ (2011) Assessment of the kidneys: magnetic resonance angiography, perfusion and diffusion. J Cardiovasc Magn Reson 13:70. https://doi.org/10.1186/1532-429X-13-70
8. Grenier N, Pedersen M, Hauger O (2006) Contrast agents for functional and cellular MRI of the kidney. Eur J Radiol 60 (3):341–352. https://doi.org/10.1016/j.ejrad.2006.06.024
9. Ebrahimi B, Textor SC, Lerman LO (2014) Renal relevant radiology: renal functional magnetic resonance imaging. Clin J Am Soc Nephrol. https://doi.org/10.2215/CJN.02900313
10. Zollner FG, Konstandin S, Lommen J, Budjan J, Schoenberg SO, Schad LR, Haneder S (2016) Quantitative sodium MRI of kidney. NMR Biomed 29(2):197–205. https://doi.org/10.1002/nbm.3274
11. Zimmer F, Klotz S, Hoeger S, Yard BA, Kramer BK, Schad LR, Zollner FG (2017) Quantitative arterial spin labelling perfusion

measurements in rat models of renal transplantation and acute kidney injury at 3T. Z Med Phys 27(1):39–48. https://doi.org/10.1016/j.zemedi.2016.02.004

12. Hueper K, Peperhove M, Rong S, Gerstenberg J, Mengel M, Meier M, Gutberlet M, Tewes S, Barrmeyer A, Chen R, Haller H, Wacker F, Hartung D, Gueler F (2014) T1-mapping for assessment of ischemia-induced acute kidney injury and prediction of chronic kidney disease in mice. Eur Radiol 24(9):2252–2260. https://doi.org/10.1007/s00330-014-3250-6
13. Zollner FG, Schock-Kusch D, Backer S, Neudecker S, Gretz N, Schad LR (2013) Simultaneous measurement of kidney function by dynamic contrast enhanced MRI and FITC-sinistrin clearance in rats at 3 tesla: initial results. PLoS One 8(11):e79992. https://doi.org/10.1371/journal.pone.0079992
14. Hueper K, Rong S, Gutberlet M, Hartung D, Mengel M, Lu X, Haller H, Wacker F, Meier M, Gueler F (2013) T2 relaxation time and apparent diffusion coefficient for noninvasive assessment of renal pathology after acute kidney injury in mice: comparison with histopathology. Investig Radiol 48(12):834–842. https://doi.org/10.1097/RLI.0b013e31829d0414
15. Inoue T, Kozawa E, Okada H, Inukai K, Watanabe S, Kikuta T, Watanabe Y, Takenaka T, Katayama S, Tanaka J, Suzuki H (2011) Noninvasive evaluation of kidney hypoxia and fibrosis using magnetic resonance imaging. J Am Soc Nephrol 22(8):1429–1434. https://doi.org/10.1681/ASN.2010111143
16. Notohamiprodjo M, Reiser MF, Sourbron SP (2010) Diffusion and perfusion of the kidney. Eur J Radiol 76(3):337–347. https://doi.org/10.1016/j.ejrad.2010.05.033
17. Sourbron SP, Michaely HJ, Reiser MF, Schoenberg SO (2008) MRI-measurement of perfusion and glomerular filtration in the human kidney with a separable compartment model. Investig Radiol 43(1):40–48. https://doi.org/10.1097/RLI.0b013e31815597c5
18. Prasad PV (2006) Evaluation of intra-renal oxygenation by BOLD MRI. Nephron Clin Pract 103(2):c58–c65. https://doi.org/10.1159/000090610
19. Dujardin M, Sourbron S, Luypaert R, Verbeelen D, Stadnik T (2005) Quantification of renal perfusion and function on a voxel-by-voxel basis: a feasibility study. Magn Reson Med 54(4):841–849. https://doi.org/10.1002/mrm.20608
20. Longo DL, Dastru W, Digilio G, Keupp J, Langereis S, Lanzardo S, Prestigio S, Steinbach O, Terreno E, Uggeri F, Aime S (2011) Iopamidol as a responsive MRI-chemical exchange saturation transfer contrast agent for pH mapping of kidneys: in vivo studies in mice at 7 T. Magn Reson Med 65(1):202–211. https://doi.org/10.1002/mrm.22608
21. Longo DL, Busato A, Lanzardo S, Antico F, Aime S (2013) Imaging the pH evolution of an acute kidney injury model by means of iopamidol, a MRI-CEST pH-responsive contrast agent. Magn Reson Med 70(3):859–864. https://doi.org/10.1002/mrm.24513
22. Longo DL, Sun PZ, Consolino L, Michelotti FC, Uggeri F, Aime S (2014) A general MRI-CEST ratiometric approach for pH imaging: demonstration of in vivo pH mapping with iobitridol. J Am Chem Soc 136(41):14333–14336. https://doi.org/10.1021/ja5059313
23. Longo DL, Cutrin JC, Michelotti F, Irrera P, Aime S (2017) Noninvasive evaluation of renal pH homeostasis after ischemia reperfusion injury by CEST-MRI. NMR Biomed 30(7). https://doi.org/10.1002/nbm.3720
24. Longo D, Aime S (2017) Iodinated contrast media as pH-responsive CEST agents. In: Mcmahon MT, Gilad AA, JBM B, PCM VZ (eds) Chemical exchange saturation transfer imaging. Vol. Advances and applications. Pan Stanford Publishing, Singapore, pp 447–466. https://doi.org/10.1201/9781315364421-20
25. Wu Y, Zhou IY, Igarashi T, Longo DL, Aime S, Sun PZ (2018) A generalized ratiometric chemical exchange saturation transfer (CEST) MRI approach for mapping renal pH using iopamidol. Magn Reson Med 79(3):1553–1558. https://doi.org/10.1002/mrm.26817
26. Mariager CO, Nielsen PM, Qi HY, Schroeder M, Bertelsen LB, Laustsen C (2017) Can hyperpolarized C-13-urea be used to assess glomerular filtration rate? A retrospective study. Tomography 3(3):146–152. https://doi.org/10.18383/j.tom.2017.00010
27. Duwel S, Hundshammer C, Gersch M, Feuerecker B, Steiger K, Buck A, Walch A, Haase A, Glaser SJ, Schwaiger M, Schilling F (2017) Imaging of pH in vivo using hyperpolarized (13)C-labelled zymonic acid. Nat Commun 8:15126. https://doi.org/10.1038/ncomms15126
28. Aime S, Botta M, Terreno E (2005) Gd(III)-based contrast agents for MRI. Adv Inorgan

Chem 57(57):173–237. https://doi.org/10.1016/S0898-8838(05)57004-1

29. Sherry AD, Caravan P, Lenkinski RE (2009) Primer on gadolinium chemistry. J Magn Reson Imaging 30(6):1240–1248. https://doi.org/10.1002/jmri.21966
30. Longo DL, Arena F, Consolino L, Minazzi P, Geninatti-Crich S, Giovenzana GB, Aime S (2016) Gd-AAZTA-MADEC, an improved blood pool agent for DCE-MRI studies on mice on 1 T scanners. Biomaterials 75:47–57. https://doi.org/10.1016/j.biomaterials.2015.10.012
31. Geninatti-Crich S, Szabo I, Alberti D, Longo D, Aime S (2011) MRI of cells and mice at 1 and 7 Tesla with Gd-targeting agents: when the low field is better! Contrast Media Mol Imaging 6(6):421–425. https://doi.org/10.1002/cmmi.436
32. Avedano S, Botta M, Haigh JS, Longo DL, Woods M (2013) Coupling fast water exchange to slow molecular tumbling in Gd3+ chelates: why faster is not always better. Inorg Chem 52(15):8436–8450. https://doi.org/10.1021/ic400308a
33. Botta M, Avedano S, Giovenzana GB, Lombardi A, Longo D, Cassino C, Tei L, Aime S (2011) Relaxometric study of a series of monoaqua Gd-III complexes of rigidified EGTA-like chelators and their noncovalent interaction with human serum albumin. Eur J Inorg Chem 6:802–810. https://doi.org/10.1002/ejic.201001103
34. Botta M, Tei L (2012) Relaxivity enhancement in macromolecular and nanosized GdIII-based MRI contrast agents. Eur J Inorg Chem 12:1945–1960. https://doi.org/10.1002/ejic.201101305
35. Grenier N, Merville P, Combe C (2016) Radiologic imaging of the renal parenchyma structure and function. Nat Rev Nephrol 12(6):348–359. https://doi.org/10.1038/nrneph.2016.44
36. Winter KS, Helck AD, Ingrisch M, Staehler M, Stief C, Sommer WH, Braunagel M, Kazmierczak PM, Reiser MF, Nikolaou K, Notohamiprodjo M (2014) Dynamic contrast-enhanced magnetic resonance imaging assessment of kidney function and renal masses: single slice versus whole organ/tumor. Investig Radiol 49(11):720–727. https://doi.org/10.1097/RLI.0000000000000075
37. Sourbron SP, Buckley DL (2013) Classic models for dynamic contrast-enhanced MRI. NMR Biomed 26(8):1004–1027. https://doi.org/10.1002/nbm.2940
38. Zollner FG, Daab M, Sourbron SP, Schad LR, Schoenberg SO, Weisser G (2016) An open source software for analysis of dynamic contrast enhanced magnetic resonance images: UMM-Perfusion revisited. BMC Med Imaging 16:7. https://doi.org/10.1186/s12880-016-0109-0
39. Beeman SC, Osei-Owusu P, Duan C, Engelbach J, Bretthorst GL, JJH A, Blumer KJ, Garbow JR (2015) Renal DCE-MRI model selection using Bayesian Probability Theory. Tomography 1(1):61–68. https://doi.org/10.18383/j.tom.2015.00133
40. Zollner FG, Zimmer F, Klotz S, Hoeger S, Schad LR (2014) Renal perfusion in acute kidney injury with DCE-MRI: deconvolution analysis versus two-compartment filtration model. Magn Reson Imaging 32(6):781–785. https://doi.org/10.1016/j.mri.2014.02.014
41. Zöllner FG, Zimmer F, Klotz S, Hoeger S, Schad LR (2015) Functional imaging of acute kidney injury at 3 Tesla: investigating multiple parameters using DCE-MRI and a two-compartment filtration model. Z Med Phys 25(1):58–65. https://doi.org/10.1016/j.zemedi.2014.01.002
42. Zollner FG, Weisser G, Reich M, Kaiser S, Schoenberg SO, Sourbron SP, Schad LR (2013) UMMPerfusion: an open source software tool towards quantitative MRI perfusion analysis in clinical routine. J Digit Imaging 26(2):344–352. https://doi.org/10.1007/s10278-012-9510-6

6

MR Elastography of the Abdomen: Basic Concepts

Suraj D. Serai and Meng Yin

Abstract

Magnetic resonance elastography (MRE) is an emerging imaging modality that maps the elastic properties of tissue such as the shear modulus. It allows for noninvasive assessment of stiffness, which is a surrogate for fibrosis. MRE has been shown to accurately distinguish absent or low stage fibrosis from high stage fibrosis, primarily in the liver. Like other elasticity imaging modalities, it follows the general steps of elastography: (1) apply a known cyclic mechanical vibration to the tissue; (2) measure the internal tissue displacements caused by the mechanical wave using magnetic resonance phase encoding method; and (3) infer the mechanical properties from the measured mechanical response (displacement), by generating a simplified displacement map. The generated map is called an elastogram.

While the key interest of MRE has traditionally been in its application to liver, where in humans it is FDA approved and commercially available for clinical use to noninvasively assess degree of fibrosis, this is an area of active research and there are novel upcoming applications in brain, kidney, pancreas, spleen, heart, lungs, and so on. A detailed review of all the efforts is beyond the scope of this chapter, but a few specific examples are provided. Recent application of MRE for noninvasive evaluation of renal fibrosis has great potential for noninvasive assessment in patients with chronic kidney diseases. Development and applications of MRE in preclinical models is necessary primarily to validate the measurement against "gold-standard" invasive methods, to better understand physiology and pathophysiology, and to evaluate novel interventions. Application of MRE acquisitions in preclinical settings involves challenges in terms of available hardware, logistics, and data acquisition. This chapter will introduce the concepts of MRE and provide some illustrative applications.

This publication is based upon work from the COST Action PARENCHIMA, a community-driven network funded by the European Cooperation in Science and Technology (COST) program of the European Union, which aims to improve the reproducibility and standardization of renal MRI biomarkers. This introduction chapter is complemented by another separate chapter describing the experimental protocol and data analysis.

Key words Magnetic resonance elastography (MRE), Stiffness, Kidney, Preclinical imaging, MRI, Fibrosis

1 Introduction

Elastography based imaging techniques have received substantial attention in recent years for noninvasive assessment of tissue mechanical properties. These techniques take advantage of changed

Andreas Pohlmann and Thoralf Niendorf (eds.), *Preclinical MRI of the Kidney: Methods and Protocols*,
Methods in Molecular Biology, vol. 2216, https://doi.org/10.1007/978-1-0716-0978-1_18,

soft tissue elasticity in various pathologies to yield qualitative and quantitative information that can be used for diagnostic purposes. Measurements are acquired in specialized imaging modes that can detect tissue stiffness in response to an applied mechanical force (compression or shear wave). Elasticity reflects the ability of tissue to deform and resume its normal shape under an applied stress and relates to tissue stiffness. Tissue stiffness in turn reflects tissue composition and structure. The primary desired output is to measure the level of stiffness. The measurement that helps differentiate if the tissue is hard or soft can give diagnostic information about the presence of the disease.

In the liver, tissue stiffness has been shown to be elevated with advanced fibrosis and to correlate with various stage of fibrosis [1–3]. Tissue stiffness can be estimated by imaging with either ultrasound (US) or magnetic resonance imaging (MRI). US-based elastography techniques include strain-based imaging, transient elastography (TE), and shear wave elastography (SWE). MRI measures tissue stiffness with magnetic resonance elastography (MRE). Other than strain-based imaging, which has largely been abandoned in the liver, all of these techniques (TE, SWE, and MRE) estimate tissue stiffness by measuring the speed of a shear wave traversing the tissue. In MRI, elastography encompasses imaging techniques that noninvasively estimate tissue elasticity and related mechanical properties through the application of external forces [4]. MRE is a phase contrast-based MRI technique for observing strain waves propagating in soft tissues (e.g., brain, heart, liver, spleen, breast, kidney, and muscle). Mechanical shear waves with frequencies of 40 to 200 Hz are induced using either a piezoelectric transducer or speaker coil oscillator directly coupled to the region of interest. By using multiple phase offsets and motion encoding gradients, MRE acquires data that allows the generation of images that depict shear wave motion and the calculation of local values of the tissue viscoelastic properties. In this chapter, we will provide an overview of MRE including the basic concepts involved, and a few illustrative applications of MRE in preclinical imaging.

This introduction chapter is complemented by a separate publication describing the experimental procedure and data analysis, which is part of this book.

This chapter is part of the book Pohlmann A, Niendorf T (eds) (2020) Preclinical MRI of the Kidney—Methods and Protocols. Springer, New York.

2 Measurement Concept

2.1 Basic Concept of Stiffness Measured Using MRE

MRE uses mechanical shear waves to evaluate the viscoelastic properties of tissues. In the abdomen, mechanical shear waves produced by an external driver are propagated into the tissue using an abdominal driver placed over the region of interest and in contact with the

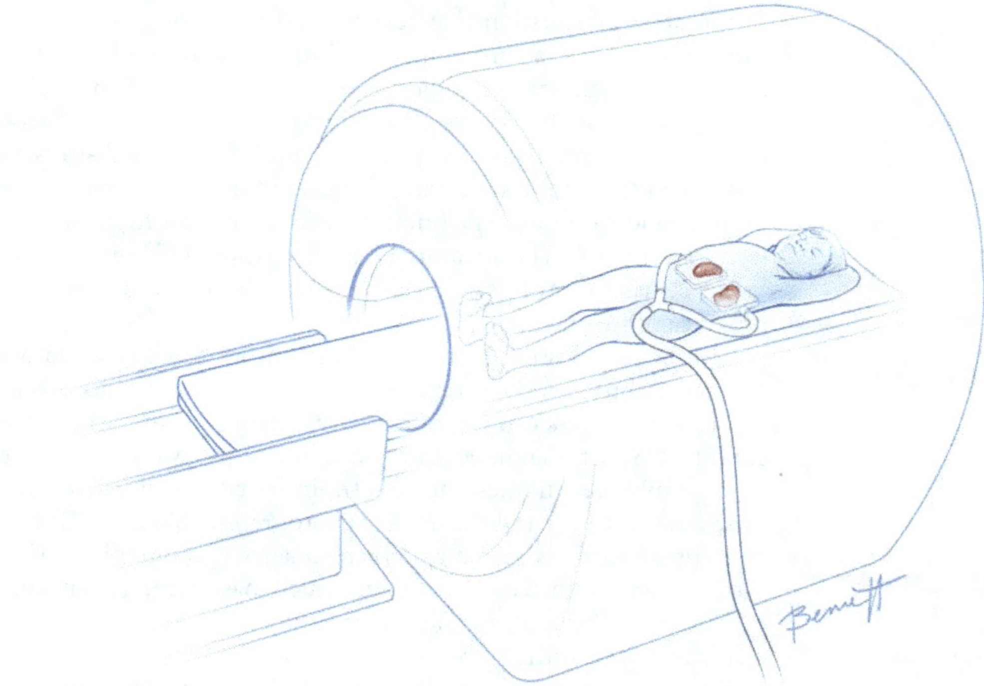

Fig. 1 Clinical MRE set up for the kidney

specific abdominal organ. Tissue displacements in the range of microns produced by propagating shear waves can be detected because phase shifts are encoded with motion encoding gradients in the MRE sequence. In liver, the typical frequency of shear waves used for clinical liver MRE is 60 Hz [5]. An accurate and reproducible stiffness measurement of organs such as pancreas and kidney, given their small size, complex geometry and boundary conditions, heterogeneous nature of the organ, and deeply seated location, requires 3D analysis of wave field data. For this reason, 3D MRE is recommended for such imaging. In 3D MRE, the propagating shear waves are imaged with a 2D multislice spin-echo echo-planar imaging (SE-EPI) pulse sequence modified to include the motion encoding gradients (MEG) in the X, Y, and Z directions. This is different from the 2D MRE typically utilized for liver imaging in which motion is encoded only in a single direction. An inversion algorithm automatically produces stiffness maps using the phase shift information. Shear stiffness values in kilopascals (kPa) are displayed for selected regions of interest in the target tissue. In renal MRE, the wave transmitting paddle is placed close to the kidney, preferably on the dorsal side (Fig. 1).

2.2 Generating Propagating Shear Waves

It is now well known that the MRE-measured shear modulus of soft tissue is dependent on the frequency of applied mechanical waves [6, 7]. That is why the term "shear stiffness" is often used to describe the shear modulus at a specific frequency. However, it should be fully understood that the formula that calculates the shear modulus from the measured velocity of the waves ($\mu = \rho c^2$, where μ = shear modulus, ρ = density of tissue, and c = wave speed) is valid only in purely elastic tissues.

In a typical MR elastography configuration, an active pneumatic mechanical wave driver is located outside the MR elastography room and is connected, by way of a flexible plastic (polyvinyl chloride) tube, to a passive driver that is fastened onto the abdominal wall or the abdominal organ or interest. The passive driver generates a continuous acoustic vibration that is transmitted through the abdomen, with a focus on the region of interest, at a fixed frequency, which typically lies in the range 40–400 Hz. A phase-contrast MRI pulse sequence with motion encoding gradients is synchronized to the frequency of mechanical waves created by the passive driver. This sequence is then used to image the micron-level cyclic displacements caused by the propagating shear waves to create a magnitude image, which provides anatomic information, and a phase difference image, which provides wave motion information. After the magnitude and phase images are created, an inversion algorithm can be used to processes these raw data images to create several additional images and maps. The gray-scale elastogram is commonly used to provide quantitative stiffness measurement, in kiloPascals. The color elastogram is generally used for qualitative tissue stiffness evaluation. The color elastogram used clinically has a stiffness range of 0–8 kPa. A 0–20 kPa color elastogram is also created and is useful for appreciating tissue stiffness heterogeneity. For research purposes, the range can also be adjusted as desired. More details on image acquisition, postprocessing, and analysis are included in the chapter by Serai SD et al. "MR Elastography of the Abdomen: Experimental Protocols."

2.3 Pulse Sequence for MRE Motion Encoding

The two types of acquisition sequences currently in use to obtain liver stiffness values are the gradient-recalled-echo (GRE) based (Fig. 2a) and the spin echo (SE) based with echo-planar readout (Fig. 2b); both of which have been shown to have excellent performance on both 1.5 and 3 T MRI scanners [8, 9]. The use of GRE-based sequence has been demonstrated to correlate with histological grading of liver fibrosis in previous studies and in a recent meta-analysis [8, 10]. The traditional GRE-based MRE acquisition works well on a 1.5 T scanner. However, the inherent limitations of GRE-based acquisition on field strengths at 3 T or higher are (1) enhanced sensitivity to susceptibility; T1 is longer at the higher field strength and hence signal drops off due to a longer echo time (TE); and (2) T2 and T2* are shorter at field strengths of 3 T and higher; hence, the relatively shorter T_2 and T_2* relaxation

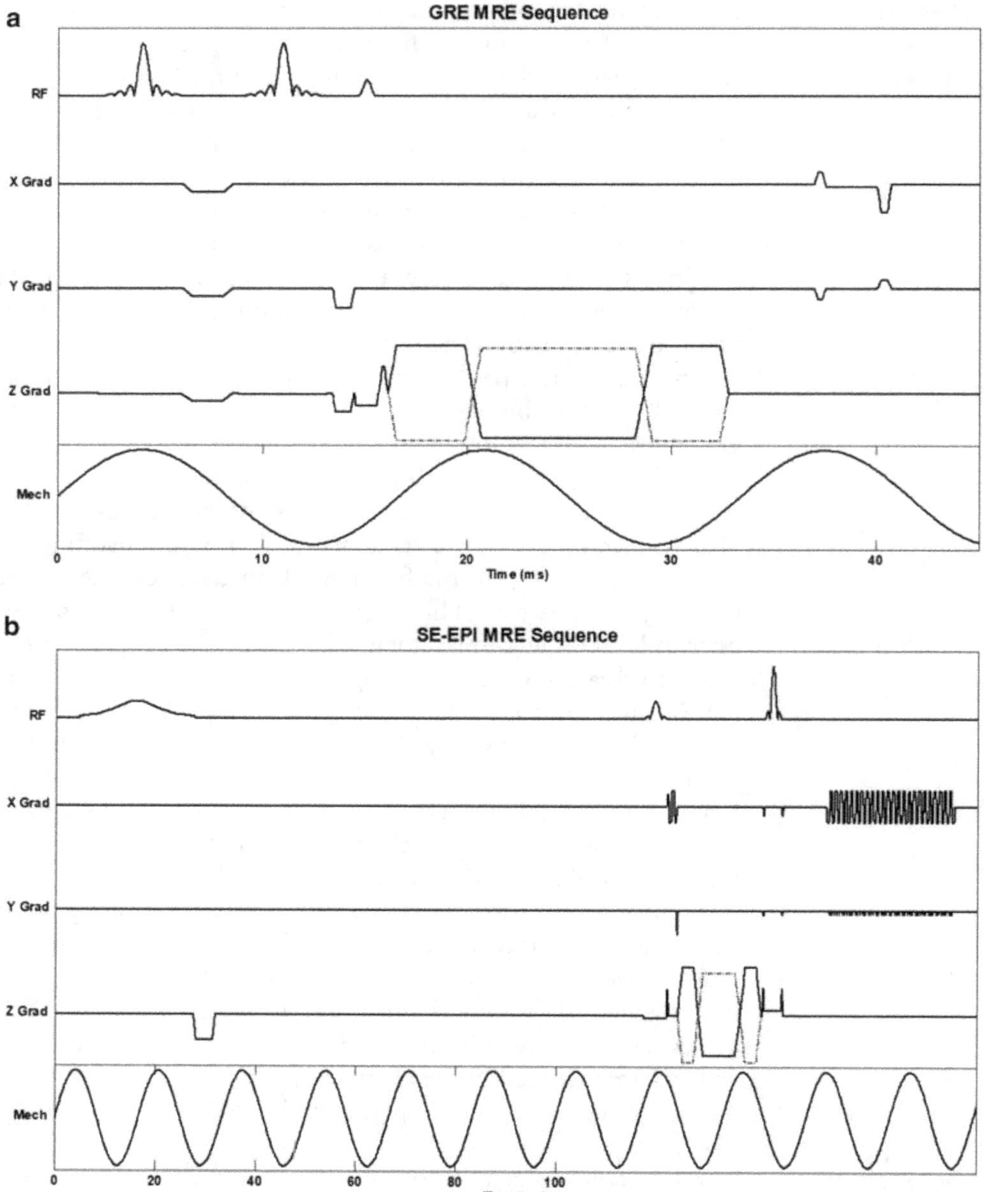

Fig. 2 (**a**) Pulse sequence diagram of a typical GRE-based MRE acquisition sequence and (**b**) SE-EPI-based MRE

time of the liver requires an even shorter TE. GRE-based MRE also has relatively lower accuracy in obese patients due to the increased distance from the driver to the liver. Thicker layers of fat can limit the acoustic penetration depth in the liver and produce limitations for encoding shear waves in the deeper areas of the liver, hence reducing the measurable area [9]. SE-EP–based acquisition overcomes this limitation by encoding more wavelengths per TR and hence can show more acoustic penetration. Since chronic liver disease is quite frequently associated with obesity, radiologists should be aware of the limitations of GRE-based acquisitions in such cases. GRE-based MRE acquisition also requires relatively longer periods of acquisition and have a higher susceptibility to breathing motion artifacts. The current GRE-based protocol for MRE image acquisition requires a breath hold of approximately 20 s for a single slice. Echo-planar imaging (EPI), on the other hand, is a faster magnetic resonance imaging technique that obtains all spatial-encoding information in a single radiofrequency (RF) pulse, allowing shorter acquisition times with reduced motion artifacts. SE-EPI-based images are advantageous in patients with limited breath-holding capacity because they allow image acquisition of multiple slices within only one breath hold, and also enable measuring larger areas of the liver due to the greater number of waves encoded per relaxation time (TR). The drawback of SE-EPI–based acquisition is the potential increase in susceptibility artifacts due to an EPI-based readout. While technically more demanding, 3D-MRE offers advantages that might provide even higher diagnostic performance [11, 12].

3 Applications of MRE to the Abdomen

3.1 MRE for Evaluation of Liver Fibrosis

Liver fibrosis is an important pathological and pathogenic feature, and the assessment of fibrosis is often necessary for prognosis, risk stratification, clinical decision-making, and disease severity monitoring. Hepatic fibrosis eventually leads to cirrhosis, which is associated with a 50% 5-year mortality due to severe complications including variceal bleeding, hepatic failure, and development of hepatocarcinoma. Approximately 170 million people world-wide (3% of the global population) are infected with chronic hepatitis C (HCV), and 10–15% will develop cirrhosis within 20 years of infection [13]. Needle liver biopsy analyzed with connective tissue stains has long been considered the "gold standard" to detect and quantify hepatic fibrosis. Because of the cost, sampling variability, need for sedation, and risk associated with biopsy, noninvasive methods to assess liver fibrosis such as elastography are needed [14, 15]. MRE uses low-frequency (40–80 Hz) sound waves to induce shear waves in the liver, visualizes the shear waves by tracking tissue displacement using a modified phase-contrast sequence, and measures the speed of the propagating wave with specialized software called an inversion algorithm (Fig. 3) [16]. In Fig. 3, it can be seen that the red to blue region is a wavelength and this wavelength becomes longer in the presence of a stiff region for a given excitation frequency (Fig. 4). Then these wave images are converted into spatial stiffness maps (elastograms) using an inversion algorithm. Clinically MRE of the liver is FDA approved for human use and available on major MRI scanners. In the commercial version, the sound waves are generated by an acoustic subwoofer

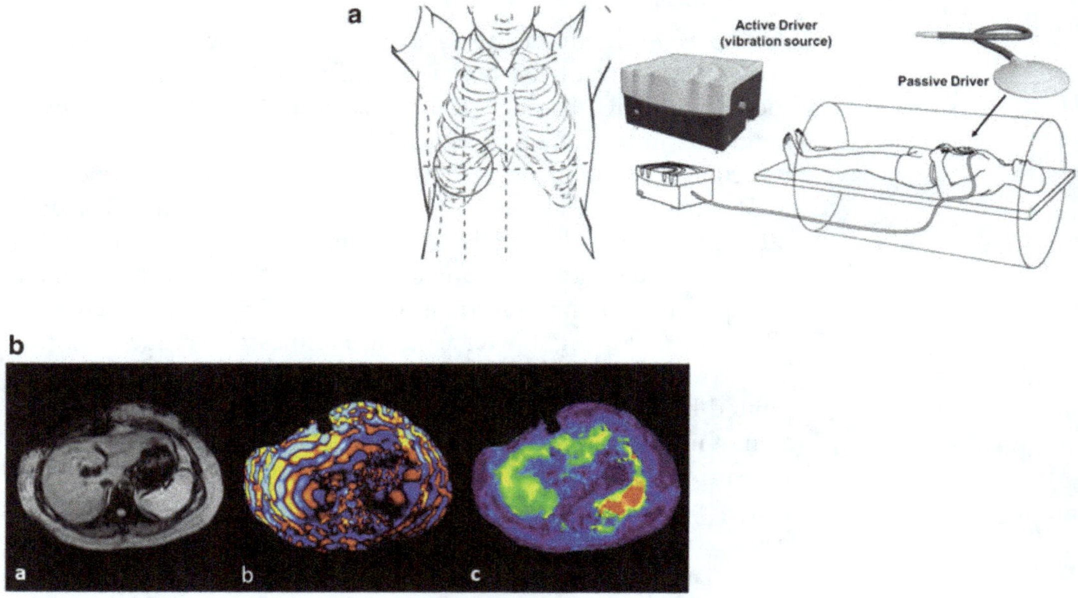

Fig. 3 Clinical MRE of the liver: (**A**) The passive driver should be placed over the right lower anterior chest wall at the level of the xiphisternum, centered on the mid-clavicular line. Once positioned, the passive driver should be held firmly against the chest wall by a wide elastic band, placed around the torso. Check to ensure that the band is stretched sufficiently so that the driver is not loose during full expiration. Note that the passive driver is connected via a plastic tube to the active driver (vibration source), which is located outside the scan room. (**B**) Magnitude and color-coded wave images of a successful MRE showing excellent illumination of waves through the liver. Stiffness map shows elevated liver stiffness consistent with significant fibrosis

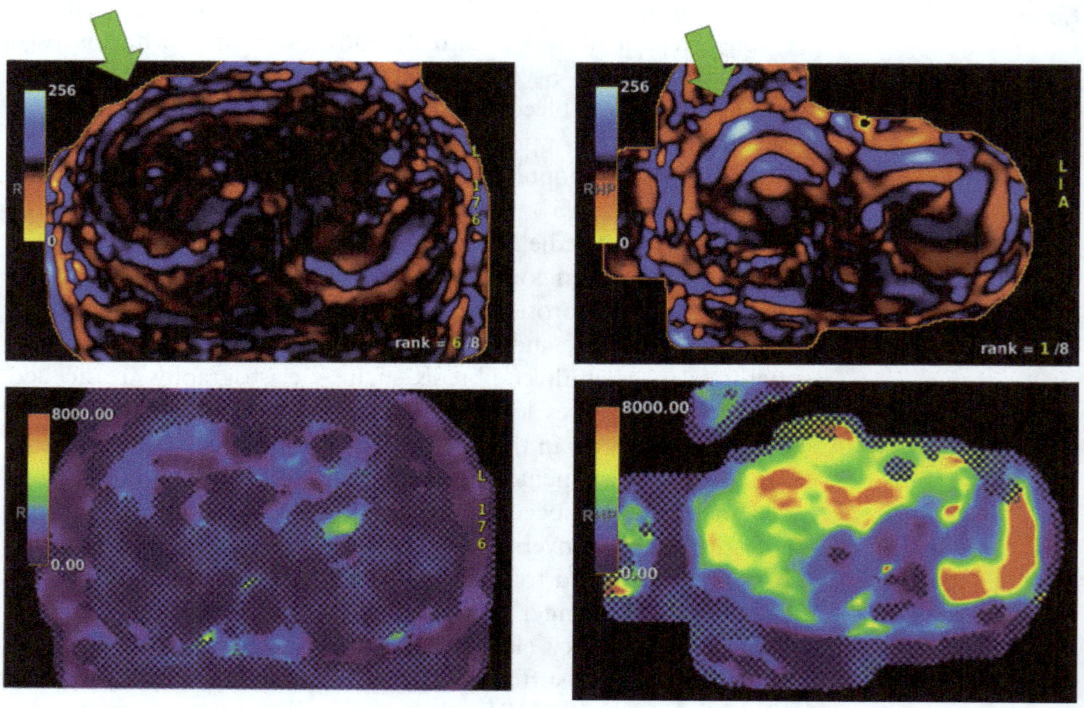

Fig. 4 Color (red and blue) wave images and its corresponding elastogram showing the difference in wavelength (green arrow) of a relatively "normal" subject vs. a patient with fibrosis

(called as "active driver") outside the scan room and are transmitted to a plastic disk (called as "passive driver") via a plastic tube passing through a wave guide [5]. During liver MRE image acquisition, the passive driver is secured by an elastic band over the right lower anterior chest wall. Most patients can feel the vibrations generated by the disk but do not find them uncomfortable. Identical MRE hardware and inversion algorithms are available on scanners manufactured by the three major MR vendors (GE, Philips, and Siemens) [10, 17]. MRE, as used clinically, currently has advantages over other tissue elastographic techniques. These advantages include the ability to further characterize tissue in terms of fat and iron content as well as standardization across manufacturer platforms, since the vast majority elastography hardware and software currently comes from a single manufacturer (Resoundant Inc.; Rochester, MN). Peer reviewed studies have shown that MRE is a robust, reliable, repeatable, and reproducible technique for detection and staging of liver fibrosis [10]. The accuracy of MRE has been reported to range from 0.85 to 0.99 for differentiating different stages of liver fibrosis [18]. The performance of MRE for differentiating mild fibrosis (stage 1) from normal liver or inflammation is lower and the performance is highest for diagnosis of cirrhosis (stage 4) [3, 10].

3.2 MRE for Evaluation of Liver Tumors

Motivated by the successful implementation of MRE for the study of diffuse changes in hepatic stiffness due to fibrosis, studies have been conducted to evaluate the potential role of MRE in characterizing hepatic tumors as malignant tumors appear to be stiffer than benign tumors [19–21]. In a preliminary work by Venkatesh et al., patients with 44 hepatic masses were evaluated with MRE and the results were correlated with pathological diagnosis or other accepted diagnostic criteria [20]. The stiffness of benign masses (nine hemangiomas, three focal nodular hyperplasia, and one hepatic adenoma) averaged 2.7 kPa, slightly higher than the mean stiffness of normal liver parenchyma (2.3 kPa). The mean stiffness of the malignant tumors was reported to be 10.1 kPa. The authors reported that a cutoff value of 5 kPa completely separated all benign liver masses from malignant lesions. Their results indicate that MRE shows substantial promise for aiding the characterization of liver tumors, which provides motivation for exploring the potential for evaluating other mass lesions in the abdomen as well.

3.3 MRE of the Spleen for Evaluation of Portal Hypertension

A study of 12 normal volunteers and 38 liver patients with biopsy-proven chronic liver diseases performed by Talwalkar et al., demonstrated higher spleen stiffness in patients with chronic liver disease and a very strong correlation between hepatic and splenic stiffness in these patients [22]. This may suggest that the bulk stiffness of the spleen is strongly affected by the portal venous pressure through a poroelasticity effect. A preclinical MRE study was performed on two adult mongrel dogs immediately after and 4 weeks after initiating cholestatic liver disease by common bile duct ligation [23]. This preclinical model is known to have portal hypertension within 4 weeks. In this study subcutaneous vascular access ports were placed with catheter tips in the portal vein and the right hepatic vein allowing measurement of hepatic venous pressure gradient [23]. The MRE-assessed splenic stiffness in these dogs rose from a mean value of 1.8 kPa to an average of 3.4 kPa. The MRE study from the authors provide evidence to support the hypothesis that in the absence of confounding effects, the MRE-assessed stiffness of the spleen reflects the magnitude of the hepatic venous pressure gradient. This also provides motivation for the development of improved MRE techniques for the assessment of the spleen as well as the development and validation of poroelastic models that may allow the hepatic venous pressure gradient to be estimated noninvasively from MRE-based measurements of splenic stiffness. This would be a very significant development because knowledge of the hepatic venous pressure gradient is considered to be very important in the management of chronic liver disease and is very difficult to determine noninvasively. In a cross-sectional study of 25 patients with autosomal recessive polycystic kidney disease (ARPKD) and 25 healthy controls, ARFI based elastography was able to distinguish between participants without and with clinical signs of portal hypertension, namely splenomegaly or low platelets [24].

3.4 MRE of the Kidney

Many different disease mechanisms induce glomerular injury, including glomerulonephritis, hypertensive nephrosclerosis and diabetic nephropathy [25]. However, once renal damage reaches a certain threshold, progression of renal disease is consistent, and largely independent of the initial insult. This common pathway to end-stage renal failure is mainly due to tubulointerstitial damage characterized by tubular atrophy, loss of peritubular capillaries, and interstitial fibrosis. Mechanisms leading to kidney failure via tubulointerstitial damage and development of fibrosis are mostly massive proteinuria and chronic hypoxia [26]. Fibrosis further impairs oxygen diffusion and supply to tubular cells. This in turn exacerbates fibrosis of the kidney, rendering it into a vicious cycle.

Renal fibrosis is the excessive accumulation and deposition of extracellular matrix in the interstitial space of the kidneys. The process of fibrogenesis in kidneys is very complicated and cannot be attributed to any single type of cellular activity. However, it can be described as an overall result of the kidney's incapability to properly regenerate the damaged tissues after renal injury. When kidneys suffer injury, extracellular matrix deposition is an integral part of the damage repair process. However, certain processes can lead to excessive matrix to be deposited in the interstitial space, which leads to scarring of the kidneys. This interferes with the normal functioning of the kidneys and causes progressive loss of renal function over time due to the reduction in the number of renal tubules. Renal fibrosis is a significant hallmark in the progression of CKD and can lead to end stage renal disease (ESRD), which necessitates dialysis or kidney transplant Thus, in the assessment of chronic renal failure, fibrosis is a major histological feature and may be an important surrogate endpoint for prognosis and monitoring of treatment response. Besides, some investigations suggest that fibrosis might be reversible, when the cause is treated, emphasizing the need for early detection and quantification of this fibrosis [27–33]. Currently, renal biopsy is the gold standard for diagnosing kidney fibrosis. In this procedure, the kidneys of the patient are located with help of ultrasonography or X-rays. After determining the location, a needle is inserted in the kidney either percutaneously (called percutaneous biopsy) or after performing a cut near the region of kidney being observed under local anesthesia (called open biopsy) to obtain tissue samples [32, 33]. These samples are used for histological analysis to determine the presence of renal fibrosis.

Kidney biopsy has several limitations. It is invasive and causes pain to the patients after the procedure is performed. It is also associated with a prolonged hospital stay and higher costs and the procedure suffers from intra- and inter- observer variability. Since, only a small region from the entire kidney is used to obtain samples leading to potential sampling error [34]. Thus a noninvasive, truly quantitative method of interstitial renal fibrosis monitoring would be desirable. Diffusion-weighted and Blood Oxygenation Level Dependent (BOLD) MRI findings have been shown to be correlated to renal function [35–39], but no data has been published as to their correlation with the degree of fibrosis. Blood or urinary markers of fibrosis are also currently evaluated but neither is used in clinical practice yet [40].

MRI and ultrasound (US)-based methods can estimate tissue stiffness (and thus the degree of fibrosis) by measuring the velocity of shear waves traveling through the organ of interest [41, 42]. US-based elastography techniques are mainly classified under strain imaging (SI) or shear wave imaging (SWI). The basic principle of SI is application of stress to the tissue and measuring the resulting normal strain which is reported as Young's modulus. SWI-based techniques use either a dynamic vibrating device or acoustic radiation force to generate shear waves in the tissues, which are reported either as shear wave speed or Young's modulus. Techniques based on SI include strain elastography (SE) and acoustic radiation force impulse strain imaging (ARFI), whereas SWI-based techniques include point shear wave elastography (pSWE), 2D shear wave elastography (SWE), and 1D transient elastography (TE).

Studies have used both SI and SWI to investigate renal fibrosis. SI-based techniques are found to be beneficial for diagnosing renal fibrosis in allografts than native kidneys [43]. This is because external compression can be efficiently applied to allografts located superficially than to native kidneys which are located retroperitoneally thereby limiting accuracy of this technique. A study by Menzilcioglu et al. reported that even though SE reported higher mean strain index in CKD patients when compared to healthy subjects, it could not differentiate between various stages of CKD [44].

SWI-based techniques have an advantage over SI-based techniques since they do not depend on external compression. However, studies using SWI have reported conflicting results. A study by Wang et al. reported that shear wave velocity measurements did not show any correlation with degree of renal fibrosis [45]. Few studies have reported lower shear wave velocities in patients with CKD than in healthy subjects [46]. It has been observed that there is a negative correlation between shear wave velocity and progression of CKD in kidneys whereas a positive correlation has been observed in liver using the same SWI-based techniques [43]. Apart from these conflicting results, US-based elastography techniques have following limitations: (1) only provides 1D or 2D stiffness of the kidneys; (2) requires extensive training of technicians and is still prone to inter- and intraobserver variability; (3) highly dependent on the body mass index of subjects; and (4) anisotropy of the kidney can impact the results. The US-based transient elastography (Fibroscan™ device) is able to discriminate the different stages of liver fibrosis with a quadratic trend of the curve plotting histologic scores versus elasticity measurements [47]. Among patients with cirrhosis, stiffness thresholds predicting the onset of specific complications (ascites, oesophageal bleeding, hepatocarcinoma, etc.) have been identified. However, as explained with the limiations of US based studies, this technique is limited by its 1D nature in that it does not allow the exploration of the entire liver. MRI has advantages over US since it can image organs located deep in the human body with good image contrast and spatial resolution thereby improving the diagnosis. It also does not involve use of any radiation and therefore can be used to monitor progression of diseases over a period of time. MRE has been successfully used to assess and stage liver fibrosis. The shear stiffness of normal liver was found to be approximately 2.2 kPa by several independent groups, using vibrating frequencies of 60 Hz [1, 3]. MRE has been shown to sucessfully discriminate the different stages of liver fibrosis, with the same quadratic trend of the fibrosis/elasticity curve and a recommended cut-off value derived from a large group of patients [18]. MRE has the advantage of being intrinsically a 2D technique and can be associated to conventional liver imaging at the same time. In the kidney, evaluation of interstitial fibrosis is crucial to the assessment of prognosis and to guide therapy for most kidney diseases. However, how best to measure kidney fibrosis remains

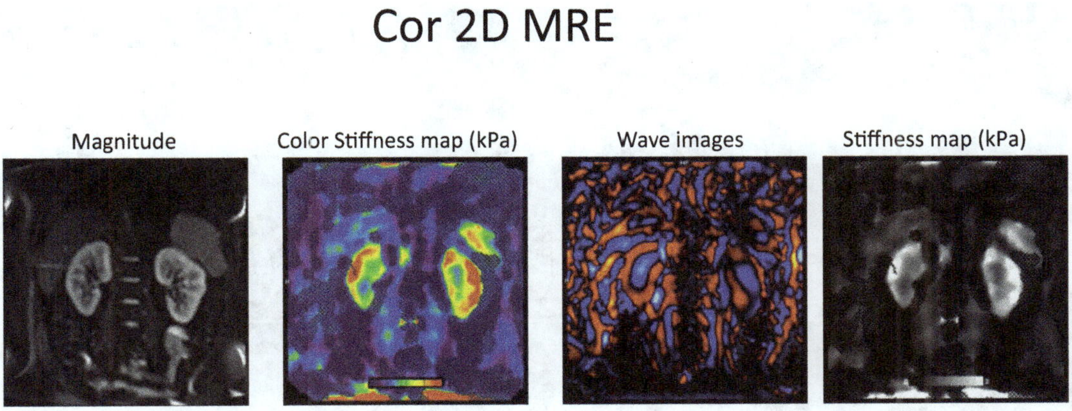

Fig. 5 MRE of the kidney of a healthy volunteer performed at 60 Hz. Magnitude, stiffness map and color-coded wave images of a successful MRE showing excellent illumination of waves through the kidney. The stiffness of the normal kidneys at 60 Hz ranged from 3.5 to 5 kPa

uncertain. An MRE-based technique that measures tissue stiffness, would be a novel application for assessment of renal fibrosis. The resulting microscopic vibrational waves passing through the organ generate shear waves that can be imaged with motion-synchronized MRI. The velocity of wave propagation is dependent on organ stiffness, with stiffer fibrotic tissue leading to more rapidly moving waves with longer wavelength. Exploratory MRE of the kidneys in healthy volunteers has demonstrated that shear waves can be readily generated and imaged in this organ. Unlike the liver and spleen, the patterns of wave propagation in these structures are extremely complex and include significant components propagating at oblique angles relative to an axial plane of section. Given these characteristics, it is necessary to image the pattern of wave propagation in three dimensions and to obtain data from all three polarizations of motion, which requires longer imaging times. This kind of 3D/3-axis MRE acquisition is problematic if the imaging is to be conducted during suspended respiration and using a GRE-based acquisition method. One approach to this is to use respiratory gating, though this can make the total acquisition times quite long. As an alternative, EPI-based techniques can be used to significantly reduce acquisition times. EPI-based MRE sequence have been shown to be capable of acquiring 12 wave images (four phase offsets at each of three motion-encoding directions) with an acquisition time of 8 s per slice. This technique has successfully generated 3D wave data sets with typical voxel dimensions of 4 mm (Figs. 5, 6, and 7). With a 3D extension of the inversion software, including 3D spatial filtering, the preliminary results indicate that it is quite feasible to image tissue stiffness throughout a larger 3D region of interest in the abdomen and has yielded provocative preliminary results in the kidneys that motivate further development in this organ.

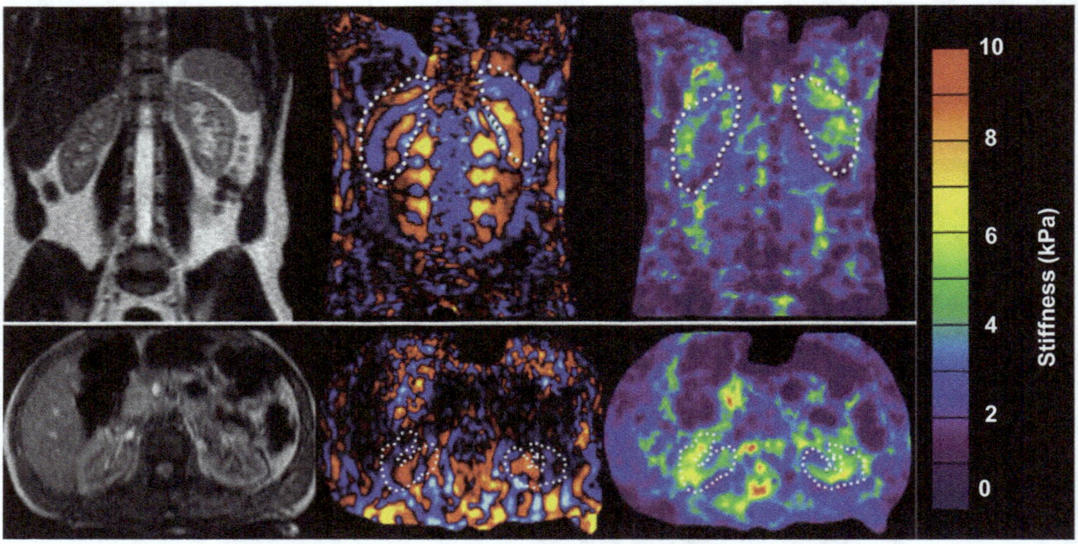

MRE of kidneys performed in two normal healthy volunteers.
MRE performed in coronal and axial planes at 90Hz. The dotted lines on the wave images and stiffness maps outline the kidneys. The stiffness of the normal kidneys ranged from 5 to 7.5 kPa

Fig. 6 MRE performed in coronal and axial planes at 90 Hz. The dotted lines on the wave images and stiffness maps outline the kidneys. The stiffness of the normal kidneys at 90 Hz ranged from 5 to 7.5 kPa (Image courtesy of Dr. Sudhakar Venkatesh, Mayo Clinic, Rochester, Minnesota, USA)

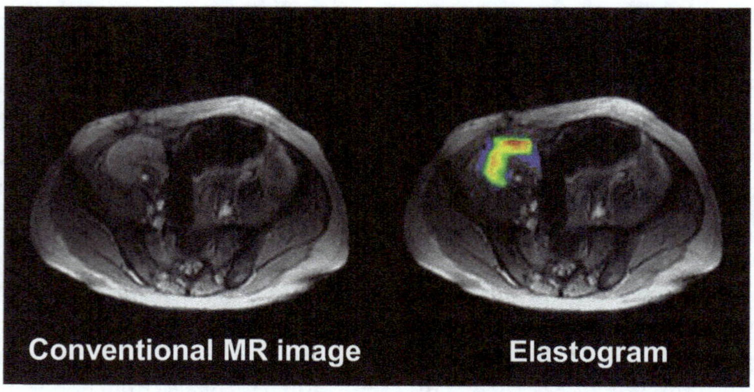

MRE of renal graft in the right iliac fossa 4-months following transplantation.
Stiffness is similar to normal kidneys. The renal function was normal. Biopsy showed no interstitial fibrosis or tubular atrophy.

Fig. 7 MRE of renal graft in the right iliac fossa acquired 4-months following transplantation. Stiffness is similar to normal kidneys. The renal function was normal. Biopsy showed no interstitial fibrosis or tubular atrophy (Image courtesy of Dr. Sudhakar Venkatesh, Mayo Clinic, Rochester, Minnesota, USA)

Pilot studies of MRE have been performed in native kidneys and kidney allografts, attempting to correlate kidney stiffness with either fibrosis burden or kidney function [48]. Although MRE in porcine kidneys showed a correlation between stiffness and fibrosis in the medulla, the results of small pilot human studies have so far been conflicting, and no studies, as yet, have assessed whether stiffness measured by MRE predicts progression of kidney dysfunction [49]. MRE may also be helpful in the evaluation and follow-up of patients undergoing renal transplant [50]. In a study by Orlachio et al., real-time elastography was able to evaluate kidney fibrosis in a noninvasive way and could be used as complementary imaging during follow-up of renal transplant patients [51].

3.5 MRE of the Pancreas

Pancreatic fibrosis is often associated with chronic pancreatitis, pancreatic ductal cancer, or inflammatory pseudotumor [52]. Since pancreatic fibrosis may affect decisions of surgical interventions and prognosis in such pathologies [53], MRE techniques could be exploited for information concerning pancreatic fibrosis reflected by its stiffness. Serai et al. have demonstrated that 3D MRE of the pancreas is feasible in children with and without pancreatic disease, in a small cohort of pediatric patients, referred for clinical imaging with history of acute recurrent pancreatitis (APR) or CP [12]. In this preliminary study, they observed statistically significant lower pancreas stiffness values derived from 3D MRE in children with a history of ARP or CP as compared to healthy control children (1 kPa vs. 1.7 kPa) [12]. The finding of lower pancreas stiffness in ARP/CP than controls is contrary to the findings reported in a small series of adults (mean age 55.6 years) by An et al. [54]. In their study, a mean stiffness value of 1.1 kPa was reported for healthy controls compared to a mean stiffness of 1.5 kPa in five patients with chronic pancreatitis. Further, a study by Wang et al. reported mean stiffness values of 1.5 and 1.9 kPa in adults with mild ($n = 30$) and moderate to severe ($n = 16$) chronic pancreatitis respectively as classified by the Cambridge criteria [55]. Reported stiffness values in patients were higher than the values in healthy patients in the same study.

3.6 Other MRE Body Applications

Since MRE is a new, multistep MR technique, there is potential for improvement, expansion and exploration. Breast tumors are known to be stiffer than normal breast tissue and hence manual palpation is a recommended part of routine screening that helps in the detection of tumors [56]. MRE is being investigated in breast imaging for the detection of breast cancer since this disease is one of the leading causes of death in women and the current diagnostic methods are not satisfactory [57, 58]. Skeletal muscle MRE can be used for studying the physiological response of diseased and pathological muscles [59]. For instance, it has been found that there is a difference in the stiffness of muscles with and without neuromuscular disease [60]. In a recent study on patients with Duchenne muscular dystrophy, the authors concluded that shear wave elastography could be considered a useful noninvasive tool to monitor muscle changes in early stages of the disease [61].

4 Influence of Perfusion on Abdominal Organs

Preliminary results from the studies relating splenic stiffness to hepatic venous pressure gradient (HVPG) suggests that the stiffness of abdominal organs may have two components: a static component reflecting intrinsic structural properties and a dynamic component reflecting extrinsic perfusion changes [62, 63]. To investigate the influence of perfusion on the shear stiffness of abdominal organs, studies of specific conditions of the liver and kidneys are being actively pursued [64].

4.1 Post-prandial Influence on Liver Stiffness

Food intake is known to cause an increase in mesenteric blood flow, which may lead to a postprandial increase in hepatic stiffness that is different in patients with hepatic fibrosis than in normal volunteers [65]. It has been observed that MRE-assessed liver stiffness increases significantly (average increment of 18% with ranges from 5% up to 48%) following a test meal in patients with advanced hepatic fibrosis, whereas fasting and postprandial liver stiffness are similar in the normal state [65]. This finding suggests that there is a dynamic component to the liver stiffness that is dependent on the portal pressure. Therefore, it is very important to have hepatic MRE examinations performed consistently in a fasting state. The postprandial augmentation in hepatic stiffness after a test meal known to increase mesenteric blood flow is likely due to the transiently increased portal pressure in patients with hepatic fibrosis. It is thought that mechanical distortion of the intrahepatic vasculature caused by fibrosis impairs the autoregulatory mechanism for the portal venous pressure, which may cause acceleration of the development of portal systemic varies and stretching of hepatic parenchyma and stellate cells that are instrumental in the progression of hepatic fibrosis. This promising observation provides motivation for further studies to determine the potential value of assessing postprandial hepatic stiffness augmentation for predicting progression of fibrotic disease and the development of portal varices. It may also provide new insights into the natural history and pathophysiology of chronic liver disease.

4.2 Influence of Hydration on Renal Stiffness

Stiffness plays an important role in diagnosing renal fibrosis. However, kidney stiffness is altered by perfusion changes in many kidney diseases. A study by Clark et al. suggests that increasing water intake is recommended for patients with CKD as it helps to preserve renal function [66]. Water intake before a MRE scan can act also as a confounding factor to estimate the stiffness of kidneys. In a recent study, Gandhi et al. observed a negative correlation between difference in stiffness values and changes in bladder volumes before and after water intake [67]. This suggests that at lower bladder volume the kidneys are still filtering the water where perfusion pressure is high leading to an increased stiffness in the kidneys.

4.3 Stenotic Kidney MRE

The kidney is a richly perfused organ receiving 25% of the cardiac output. Renal occlusions, such as renal arterial stenosis, threaten the viability of the kidney by diminishing blood flow leading to irreversible tissue fibrosis and ultimately kidney failure. Preliminary research has been performed to study the impact of renal arterial stenosis on kidney stiffness in a porcine model of acute renal arterial stenosis [68]. MRE measurements showed that the stiffness of the kidney progressively decreased as the renal artery stenosis was increased. The authors reported that the stiffness of the contralateral kidney was observed to increase progressively, which indicates that hemodynamics can significantly affect the mechanical properties of renal parenchyma. Fibrosis is associated with elevated tissue stiffness. However, studies have indicated the rich perfusion of the kidney may affect its distension and, in turn, stiffness [68]. In order to determine the interdependent relationship between perfusion, fibrosis and stiffness, an acute renal arterial stenosis model was established in adult pigs by isolating the renal artery to insert a vascular occluder and an embedded Doppler flow probe. The renal blood flow (RBF) was gradually reduced from the baseline level to total occlusion of 100% with MRE acquisitions performed at each step. The cortex of the acutely stenotic kidney decreased in stiffness as the degree of stenosis was increased to 40% and above. The systemic blood pressure also rose during each decrement in the RBF (from 75 ± 3 to 96 ± 3 mmHg). These preliminary renal MRE results encourage the further evaluation of renal hemodynamics on tissue stiffness, which may be due, in part, to perfusion pressure applied to the organ. These factors may also play a complicating role in detecting the presence of fibrosis due to renal arterial stenosis, and hence may lead to new techniques to assess tissue stiffness. The use of MRE to assess changes in tissue mechanics associated with the dynamic perfusion of tissue may also provide new insights into the natural history and pathophysiology of renal diseases (Table 1).

5 Preclinical MRE

Increasing evidence has demonstrated that, unlike cirrhosis, the early stages of fibrosis are treatable and reversible if appropriate antifibrotic treatment is given [69, 70]. As antifibrotic therapies evolve, a reliable, noninvasive assessment of hepatic fibrosis is needed to manage patients with chronic liver disease. Being able

Table 1
Factors confounding the tissue stiffness measured using MRE

Confounding factor	Direction of effect	Examples scenarios
Iron/T_2*	Loss of SNR	Patients with B-Thalassemia
Inflammation	Positive	Patients with AIH
Congestion	Positive	Patients with Fontan
Magnetic-field (B_0) inhomogeneity	Positive	Bowel gas, poor shim
Steatosis/fat	Negative	Patients with NAFLD, NASH
Renal stenosis	Negative	Patients with renal artery stenosis or perfusion defects
Renal perfusion	Positive	Large hydration volume or higher renal perfusion pressure can alter renal stiffness

A "positive" direction of the effect means that an increase in the confounding factor leads to an increase in measured stiffness and hence an overestimation of the fibrosis, and a "negative" direction of the effect means that decreases the confounding factor lead to a potential under estimation of stiffness

to noninvasively monitor the progression of liver fibrosis helps in understanding the natural history of liver fibrosis in patients with chronic liver disease, determining which patients require antiviral therapy, predicting the approximate time to the development of cirrhosis, and discovering new directions of scientific inquiry. Similarly, being able to early diagnose renal fibrosis or parencyma damage would help in understanding the natural history of renal fibrosis in patients with CKD, determining which patients require which therapy, predicting the approximate time to the development of renal failure, and discovering new directions of scientific inquiry. Therefore, there are ongoing investigations using preclinical models with a reliable, noninvasive method to assess fibrosis, not only to detect and stage the disease itself but also to monitor treatment efficacy and optimize dosing. In recent work by Yin et al. [2] feasibility of MRE was demonstrated on a mouse model of autosomal recessive polycystic kidney disease (ARPKD), which is an inherited disorder of the kidneys and liver caused by mutations in the PKHD1 gene and an important cause of congenital hepatic fibrosis (CHF) in humans. A renal wrapping surgery performed on eight pigs to induce sytemic arterial hypertension, showed that MRE derived aortic stiffness increased with mean arterial pressure [71].

5.1 Considerations Regarding Animal Preparation

- Bowel gas can create susceptibility artifacts in renal imaging; right lateral position helps minimize susceptibility artifacts from bowel gas.
- Respiratory motion can create artifacts and if necessary free breathing methods may be needed to minimize them. Alternately, respiratory triggering could be used, but this may increase the acquisition time [72].
- Studies indicate the choice of anesthesia may have an effect on quantitative MR measurements. This may be partly due to known effects of anesthesia on respiration, temperature, blood pressure, and pO_2.
- Hemodynamic variables may modulate kidney stiffness measured by MRE and may mask the presence of fibrosis [68].
- In liver imaging, elevated stiffness is observed "after meal" due to postprandial effect. Such effects have not yet been reported in measuring kidney stiffness [65].
- While performing renal MRE, renal perfusion status should be taken into account to ensure reproducible detection [73]. Confounding stiffness changes due to excess water intake have been reported [67].
- In the preclinical setting, motion artifacts can usually be minimized using multiple averages.

6 Conclusion

Renal fibrosis causes a change in the anatomy of kidneys wherein there is an excess accumulation of interstitial extracellular matrix and reduction in the number of tubules. Elasticity imaging is an imaging field that has received considerable attention due to its intuitive mechanical contrast based on "palpation" and its great diagnostic potential. Elasticity imaging techniques are based on measuring the response of tissues to an applied excitation and different approaches have been proposed and investigated toward this goal. Elastography encompasses imaging techniques that noninvasively estimate tissue elasticity and the related mechanical properties through the application of external forces. Elasticity reflects the ability of tissue to deform and resume its normal shape under an applied stress and relates to tissue stiffness. Tissue stiffness in turn reflects tissue composition and structure. Fibrosis is an important pathologic and pathogenic feature of each of these conditions, and the assessment of fibrosis is often necessary for prognosis, risk stratification, clinical decision-making, and disease severity monitoring. Due to the cost, need for sedation, and risk associated with biopsy, noninvasive methods such as elastography to assess tissue fibrosis are needed.

US-based methods only provide 1-D stiffness, have lower penetration depth and are highly dependent on body mass index, anisotropy of tissues, transducer force, and intra- and inter-observer variability. Numerous investigations have shown that it is readily possible to perform MRE in abdominal organs for detecting specific diseases, such as hepatic fibrosis and portal hypertension, which increase the stiffness of the liver and spleen. Other preliminary studies have demonstrated that is possible to evaluate the mechanical properties of other abdominal structures, such as the pancreas and kidneys. These results will further motivate future studies incorporating MRE to study the normal and pathological mechanics and physiology of abdominal organs.

MRE has been shown to be capable of detecting alterations in the tissue mechanical properties of kidneys in vivo preclinical and clinical studies. In the kidney, shear wave elastography has been shown to be helpful in early noninvasive detection and management of patients with chronic kidney disease (CKD). Renal MRE is a promising noninvasive technique that might have pathologic and prognostic significance.

Acknowledgments

This publication is based upon work from COST Action PARENCHIMA, supported by European Cooperation in Science and Technology (COST). COST (www.cost.eu) is a funding agency for research and innovation networks. COST Actions help connect research initiatives across Europe and enable scientists to enrich their ideas by sharing them with their peers. This boosts their research, career, and innovation.

PARENCHIMA (renalmri.org) is a community-driven Action in the COST program of the European Union, which unites more than 200 experts in renal MRI from 30 countries with the aim to improve the reproducibility and standardization of renal MRI biomarkers.

References

1. Yin M, Talwalkar JA, Glaser KJ, Manduca A, Grimm RC, Rossman PJ, Fidler JL, Ehman RL (2007) Assessment of hepatic fibrosis with magnetic resonance elastography. Clin Gastroenterol Hepatol 5(10):1207–1213.e1202. https://doi.org/10.1016/j.cgh.2007.06.012
2. Yin M, Woollard J, Wang X, Torres VE, Harris PC, Ward CJ, Glaser KJ, Manduca A, Ehman RL (2007) Quantitative assessment of hepatic fibrosis in an animal model with magnetic resonance elastography. Magn Reson Med 58 (2):346–353. https://doi.org/10.1002/mrm.21286
3. Xanthakos SA, Podberesky DJ, Serai SD, Miles L, King EC, Balistreri WF, Kohli R (2014) Use of magnetic resonance elastography to assess hepatic fibrosis in children with chronic liver disease. J Pediatr 164 (1):186–188. https://doi.org/10.1016/j.jpeds.2013.07.050

4. Muthupillai R, Ehman RL (1996) Magnetic resonance elastography. Nat Med 2 (5):601–603
5. Serai SD, Towbin AJ, Podberesky DJ (2012) Pediatric liver MR elastography. Dig Dis Sci 57 (10):2713–2719. https://doi.org/10.1007/s10620-012-2196-2
6. Fung YC (1993) Biomechanics mechanical properties of living tissues. Springer, New York, NY
7. Papazoglou S, Hirsch S, Braun J, Sack I (2012) Multifrequency inversion in magnetic resonance elastography. Phys Med Biol 57 (8):2329–2346. https://doi.org/10.1088/0031-9155/57/8/2329
8. Serai SD, Dillman JR, Trout AT (2017) Spin-echo echo-planar imaging MR elastography versus gradient-echo MR elastography for assessment of liver stiffness in children and young adults suspected of having liver disease. Radiology 282(3):761–770. https://doi.org/10.1148/radiol.2016160589
9. Calle-Toro JS, Serai SD, Hartung EA, Goldberg DJ, Bolster BD Jr, Darge K, Anupindi SA (2019) Magnetic resonance elastography SE-EPI vs GRE sequences at 3T in a pediatric population with liver disease. Abdom Radiol. https://doi.org/10.1007/s00261-018-1884-6
10. Serai SD, Obuchowski NA, Venkatesh SK, Sirlin CB, Miller FH, Ashton E, Cole PE, Ehman RL (2017) Repeatability of MR elastography of liver: a meta-analysis. Radiology 285 (1):92–100. https://doi.org/10.1148/radiol.2017161398
11. Loomba R, Cui J, Wolfson T, Haufe W, Hooker J, Szeverenyi N, Ang B, Bhatt A, Wang K, Aryafar H, Behling C, Valasek MA, Lin GY, Gamst A, Brenner DA, Yin M, Glaser KJ, Ehman RL, Sirlin CB (2016) Novel 3D magnetic resonance elastography for the noninvasive diagnosis of advanced fibrosis in NAFLD: a prospective study. Am J Gastroenterol 111(7):986–994. https://doi.org/10.1038/ajg.2016.65
12. Serai SD, Abu-El-Haija M, Trout AT (2019) 3D MR elastography of the pancreas in children. Abdom Radiol. https://doi.org/10.1007/s00261-019-01903-w
13. Mohamed AA, Elbedewy TA, El-Serafy M, El-Toukhy N, Ahmed W, Ali El Din Z (2015) Hepatitis C virus: a global view. World J Hepatol 7(26):2676–2680. https://doi.org/10.4254/wjh.v7.i26.2676
14. Ratziu V, Charlotte F, Heurtier A, Gombert S, Giral P, Bruckert E, Grimaldi A, Capron F, Poynard T (2005) Sampling variability of liver biopsy in nonalcoholic fatty liver disease. Gastroenterology 128(7):1898–1906
15. Regev A, Berho M, Jeffers LJ, Milikowski C, Molina EG, Pyrsopoulos NT, Feng ZZ, Reddy KR, Schiff ER (2002) Sampling error and intraobserver variation in liver biopsy in patients with chronic HCV infection. Am J Gastroenterol 97(10):2614–2618. https://doi.org/10.1111/j.1572-0241.2002.06038.x
16. Venkatesh SK, Ehman RL (2014) Magnetic resonance elastography of liver. Magn Reson Imaging Clin N Am 22(3):433–446. https://doi.org/10.1016/j.mric.2014.05.001
17. Trout AT, Serai S, Mahley AD, Wang H, Zhang Y, Zhang B, Dillman JR (2016) Liver stiffness measurements with MR elastography: agreement and repeatability across imaging systems, field strengths, and pulse sequences. Radiology 281(3):793–804. https://doi.org/10.1148/radiol.2016160209
18. Yin M, Glaser KJ, Talwalkar JA, Chen J, Manduca A, Ehman RL (2016) Hepatic MR elastography: clinical performance in a series of 1377 consecutive examinations. Radiology 278(1):114–124. https://doi.org/10.1148/radiol.2015142141
19. Pepin KM, McGee KP (2018) Quantifying tumor stiffness with magnetic resonance elastography: the role of mechanical properties for detection, characterization, and treatment stratification in oncology. Top Magn Reson Imaging 27(5):353–362. https://doi.org/10.1097/rmr.0000000000000181
20. Venkatesh SK, Yin M, Glockner JF, Takahashi N, Araoz PA, Talwalkar JA, Ehman RL (2008) MR elastography of liver tumors: preliminary results. AJR Am J Roentgenol 190 (6):1534–1540. https://doi.org/10.2214/ajr.07.3123
21. Garteiser P, Doblas S, Daire JL, Wagner M, Leitao H, Vilgrain V, Sinkus R, Van Beers BE (2012) MR elastography of liver tumours: value of viscoelastic properties for tumour characterisation. Eur Radiol 22 (10):2169–2177. https://doi.org/10.1007/s00330-012-2474-6
22. Talwalkar JA, Yin M, Venkatesh S, Rossman PJ, Grimm RC, Manduca A, Romano A, Kamath PS, Ehman RL (2009) Feasibility of in vivo MR elastographic splenic stiffness measurements in the assessment of portal hypertension. AJR Am J Roentgenol 193(1):122–127. https://doi.org/10.2214/AJR.07.3504
23. Yin M, Chen J, Glaser KJ, Talwalkar JA, Ehman RL (2009) Abdominal magnetic resonance elastography. Top Magn Reson Imaging 20 (2):79–87. https://doi.org/10.1097/RMR.0b013e3181c4737e
24. Hartung EA, Wen J, Poznick L, Furth SL, Darge K (2019) Ultrasound elastography to

quantify liver disease severity in autosomal recessive polycystic kidney disease. J Pediatrics 209:107–115.e105. https://doi.org/10.1016/j.jpeds.2019.01.055

25. Nangaku M (2004) Mechanisms of tubulointerstitial injury in the kidney: final common pathways to end-stage renal failure. Intern Med 43(1):9–17. https://doi.org/10.2169/internalmedicine.43.9
26. Hodgkins KS, Schnaper HW (2012) Tubulointerstitial injury and the progression of chronic kidney disease. Pediatr Nephrol 27(6):901–909. https://doi.org/10.1007/s00467-011-1992-9
27. Alukal JJ, Thuluvath PJ (2019) Reversal of NASH fibrosis with pharmacotherapy. Hepatol Int 13(5):534–545. https://doi.org/10.1007/s12072-019-09970-3
28. Ismail MH, Pinzani M (2009) Reversal of liver fibrosis. Saudi J Gastroenterol 15(1):72–79. https://doi.org/10.4103/1319-3767.45072
29. Schuppan D, Ashfaq-Khan M, Yang AT, Kim YO (2018) Liver fibrosis: direct antifibrotic agents and targeted therapies. Matrix Biol 68-69:435–451. https://doi.org/10.1016/j.matbio.2018.04.006
30. Tampe D, Zeisberg M (2014) Potential approaches to reverse or repair renal fibrosis. Nat Rev Nephrol 10(4):226–237. https://doi.org/10.1038/nrneph.2014.14
31. Bledsoe G, Shen B, Yao Y, Zhang JJ, Chao L, Chao J (2006) Reversal of renal fibrosis, inflammation, and glomerular hypertrophy by kallikrein gene delivery. Hum Gene Ther 17(5):545–555. https://doi.org/10.1089/hum.2006.17.545
32. Klinkhammer BM, Goldschmeding R, Floege J, Boor P (2017) Treatment of renal fibrosis-turning challenges into opportunities. Adv Chronic Kidney Dis 24(2):117–129. https://doi.org/10.1053/j.ackd.2016.11.002
33. Lee SY, Kim SI, Choi ME (2015) Therapeutic targets for treating fibrotic kidney diseases. Transl Res 165(4):512–530. https://doi.org/10.1016/j.trsl.2014.07.010
34. Menn-Josephy H, Lee CS, Nolin A, Christov M, Rybin DV, Weinberg JM, Henderson J, Bonegio R, Havasi A (2016) Renal interstitial fibrosis: an imperfect predictor of kidney disease progression in some patient cohorts. Am J Nephrol 44(4):289–299. https://doi.org/10.1159/000449511
35. dos Santos EA, Li LP, Ji L, Prasad PV (2007) Early changes with diabetes in renal medullary hemodynamics as evaluated by fiberoptic probes and BOLD magnetic resonance imaging. Investig Radiol 42(3):157–162. https://doi.org/10.1097/01.rli.0000252492.96709.36
36. Li LP, Halter S, Prasad PV (2008) Blood oxygen level-dependent MR imaging of the kidneys. Magn Reson Imaging Clin N Am 16(4):613–625. https://doi.org/10.1016/j.mric.2008.07.008
37. Pruijm M, Mendichovszky IA, Liss P, Van der Niepen P, Textor SC, Lerman LO, Krediet CTP, Caroli A, Burnier M, Prasad PV (2018) Renal blood oxygenation level-dependent magnetic resonance imaging to measure renal tissue oxygenation: a statement paper and systematic review. Nephrol Dial Transplant 33(Suppl_2):ii22–ii28. https://doi.org/10.1093/ndt/gfy243
38. Caroli A, Schneider M, Friedli I, Ljimani A, De Seigneux S, Boor P, Gullapudi L, Kazmi I, Mendichovszky IA, Notohamiprodjo M, Selby NM, Thoeny HC, Grenier N, Vallee JP (2018) Diffusion-weighted magnetic resonance imaging to assess diffuse renal pathology: a systematic review and statement paper. Nephrol Dial Transplant 33(Suppl_2):ii29–ii40. https://doi.org/10.1093/ndt/gfy163
39. Ljimani A, Caroli A, Laustsen C, Francis S, Mendichovszky IA, Bane O, Nery F, Sharma K, Pohlmann A, Dekkers IA, Vallee JP, Derlin K, Notohamiprodjo M, Lim RP, Palmucci S, Serai SD, Periquito J, Wang ZJ, Froeling M, Thoeny HC, Prasad P, Schneider M, Niendorf T, Pullens P, Sourbron S, Sigmund EE (2019) Consensus-based technical recommendations for clinical translation of renal diffusion-weighted MRI. MAGMA. https://doi.org/10.1007/s10334-019-00790-y
40. Mansour SG, Puthumana J, Coca SG, Gentry M, Parikh CR (2017) Biomarkers for the detection of renal fibrosis and prediction of renal outcomes: a systematic review. BMC Nephrol 18(1):72. https://doi.org/10.1186/s12882-017-0490-0
41. Serai SD, Trout AT, Miethke A, Diaz E, Xanthakos SA, Dillman JR (2018) Putting it all together: established and emerging MRI techniques for detecting and measuring liver fibrosis. Pediatr Radiol 48(9):1256–1272. https://doi.org/10.1007/s00247-018-4083-2
42. Serai SD, Trout AT, Sirlin CB (2017) Elastography to assess the stage of liver fibrosis in children: concepts, opportunities, and challenges. Clin Liver Dis 9(1):5–10. https://doi.org/10.1002/cld.607

43. Sigrist RMS, Liau J, Kaffas AE, Chammas MC, Willmann JK (2017) Ultrasound elastography: review of techniques and clinical applications. Theranostics 7(5):1303–1329. https://doi.org/10.7150/thno.18650
44. Menzilcioglu MS, Duymus M, Citil S, Avcu S, Gungor G, Sahin T, Boysan SN, Altunoren O, Sarica A (2015) Strain wave elastography for evaluation of renal parenchyma in chronic kidney disease. Br J Radiol 88(1050):20140714. https://doi.org/10.1259/bjr.20140714
45. Wang L, Xia P, Lv K, Han J, Dai Q, Li XM, Chen LM, Jiang YX (2014) Assessment of renal tissue elasticity by acoustic radiation force impulse quantification with histopathological correlation: preliminary experience in chronic kidney disease. Eur Radiol 24(7):1694–1699. https://doi.org/10.1007/s00330-014-3162-5
46. Bob F, Bota S, Sporea I, Sirli R, Popescu A, Schiller A (2015) Relationship between the estimated glomerular filtration rate and kidney shear wave speed values assessed by acoustic radiation force impulse elastography: a pilot study. J Ultrasound Med 34(4):649–654. https://doi.org/10.7863/ultra.34.4.649
47. Bota S, Herkner H, Sporea I, Salzl P, Sirli R, Neghina AM, Peck-Radosavljevic M (2013) Meta-analysis: ARFI elastography versus transient elastography for the evaluation of liver fibrosis. Liver Int 33(8):1138–1147. https://doi.org/10.1111/liv.12240
48. Lee CU, Glockner JF, Glaser KJ, Yin M, Chen J, Kawashima A, Kim B, Kremers WK, Ehman RL, Gloor JM (2012) MR elastography in renal transplant patients and correlation with renal allograft biopsy: a feasibility study. Acad Radiol 19(7):834–841. https://doi.org/10.1016/j.acra.2012.03.003
49. Zhang X, Zhu X, Ferguson CM, Jiang K, Burningham T, Lerman A, Lerman LO (2018) Magnetic resonance elastography can monitor changes in medullary stiffness in response to treatment in the swine ischemic kidney. MAGMA 31(3):375–382. https://doi.org/10.1007/s10334-017-0671-7
50. Grenier N, Poulain S, Lepreux S, Gennisson JL, Dallaudiere B, Lebras Y, Bavu E, Servais A, Meas-Yedid V, Piccoli M, Bachelet T, Tanter M, Merville P, Couzi L (2012) Quantitative elastography of renal transplants using supersonic shear imaging: a pilot study. Eur Radiol 22(10):2138–2146. https://doi.org/10.1007/s00330-012-2471-9
51. Orlacchio A, Chegai F, Del Giudice C, Anselmo A, Iaria G, Palmieri G, Di Caprera E, Tosti D, Costanzo E, Tisone G, Simonetti G (2014) Kidney transplant: usefulness of real-time elastography (RTE) in the diagnosis of graft interstitial fibrosis. Ultrasound Med Biol 40(11):2564–2572. https://doi.org/10.1016/j.ultrasmedbio.2014.06.002
52. Itokawa F, Itoi T, Sofuni A, Kurihara T, Tsuchiya T, Ishii K, Tsuji S, Ikeuchi N, Umeda J, Tanaka R, Yokoyama N, Moriyasu F, Kasuya K, Nagao T, Kamisawa T, Tsuchida A (2011) EUS elastography combined with the strain ratio of tissue elasticity for diagnosis of solid pancreatic masses. J Gastroenterol 46(6):843–853. https://doi.org/10.1007/s00535-011-0399-5
53. Erkan M, Hausmann S, Michalski CW, Schlitter AM, Fingerle AA, Dobritz M, Friess H, Kleeff J (2012) How fibrosis influences imaging and surgical decisions in pancreatic cancer. Front Physiol 3:389. https://doi.org/10.3389/fphys.2012.00389
54. An H, Shi Y, Guo Q, Liu Y (2016) Test-retest reliability of 3D EPI MR elastography of the pancreas. Clin Radiol 71(10):1068.e1012–1068.e1012. https://doi.org/10.1016/j.crad.2016.03.014
55. Wang M, Gao F, Wang X, Liu Y, Ji R, Cang L, Shi Y (2018) Magnetic resonance elastography and T1 mapping for early diagnosis and classification of chronic pancreatitis. J Magn Reson Imaging. https://doi.org/10.1002/jmri.26008
56. Barton MB, Harris R, Fletcher SW (1999) The rational clinical examination. Does this patient have breast cancer? The screening clinical breast examination: should it be done? How? JAMA 282(13):1270–1280. https://doi.org/10.1001/jama.282.13.1270
57. Lorenzen J, Sinkus R, Lorenzen M, Dargatz M, Leussler C, Roschmann P, Adam G (2002) MR elastography of the breast:preliminary clinical results. Rofo 174(7):830–834. https://doi.org/10.1055/s-2002-32690
58. McKnight AL, Kugel JL, Rossman PJ, Manduca A, Hartmann LC, Ehman RL (2002) MR elastography of breast cancer: preliminary results. AJR Am J Roentgenol 178(6):1411–1417. https://doi.org/10.2214/ajr.178.6.1781411
59. Kim HK, Lindquist DM, Serai SD, Mariappan YK, Wang LL, Merrow AC, McGee KP, Ehman RL, Laor T (2013) Magnetic resonance imaging of pediatric muscular disorders: recent advances and clinical applications. Radiol Clin N Am 51(4):721–742. https://doi.org/10.1016/j.rcl.2013.03.002
60. Basford JR, Jenkyn TR, An KN, Ehman RL, Heers G, Kaufman KR (2002) Evaluation of healthy and diseased muscle with magnetic resonance elastography. Arch Phys Med Rehabil

83(11):1530–1536. https://doi.org/10.1053/apmr.2002.35472

61. Pichiecchio A, Alessandrino F, Bortolotto C, Cerica A, Rosti C, Raciti MV, Rossi M, Berardinelli A, Baranello G, Bastianello S, Calliada F (2018) Muscle ultrasound elastography and MRI in preschool children with Duchenne muscular dystrophy. Neuromuscul Dis 28 (6):476–483. https://doi.org/10.1016/j.nmd.2018.02.007
62. Buechter M, Manka P, Theysohn JM, Reinboldt M, Canbay A, Kahraman A (2018) Spleen stiffness is positively correlated with HVPG and decreases significantly after TIPS implantation. Dig Liver Dis 50(1):54–60. https://doi.org/10.1016/j.dld.2017.09.138
63. Song J, Huang J, Huang H, Liu S, Luo Y (2018) Performance of spleen stiffness measurement in prediction of clinical significant portal hypertension: a meta-analysis. Clin Res Hepatol Gastroenterol 42(3):216–226. https://doi.org/10.1016/j.clinre.2017.11.002
64. Yin M, Kolipaka A, Warner L, Talwalkar JA, Manduca A, Ehman RL (2010) Influence of perfusion on tissue stiffness assessed with MR elastography. Proc Int Soc Magn Reson Med 18:256
65. Yin M, Talwalkar JA, Glaser KJ, Venkatesh SK, Chen J, Manduca A, Ehman RL (2011) Dynamic postprandial hepatic stiffness augmentation assessed with MR elastography in patients with chronic liver disease. AJR Am J Roentgenol 197(1):64–70. https://doi.org/10.2214/AJR.10.5989
66. Clark WF, Sontrop JM, Moist L, Huang SH (2015) Increasing water intake in chronic kidney disease: why? Safe? Possible? Ann Nutr Metab 66(Suppl 3):18–21. https://doi.org/10.1159/000381241
67. Gandhi D, Kalra P, Raterman B, Mo X, Dong H, Kolipaka A (2019) Magnetic resonance elastography-derived stiffness of the kidneys and its correlation with water perfusion. NMR Biomed 33:e4237. https://doi.org/10.1002/nbm.4237
68. Warner L, Yin M, Glaser KJ, Woollard JA, Carrascal CA, Korsmo MJ, Crane JA, Ehman RL, Lerman LO (2011) Noninvasive in vivo assessment of renal tissue elasticity during graded renal ischemia using MR elastography. Investig Radiol 46(8):509–514. https://doi.org/10.1097/RLI.0b013e3182183a95
69. Ramachandran P, Iredale JP (2009) Reversibility of liver fibrosis. Ann Hepatol 8(4):283–291
70. Campana L, Iredale JP (2017) Regression of liver fibrosis. Semin Liver Dis 37(1):1–10. https://doi.org/10.1055/s-0036-1597816
71. Dong H, Mazumder R, Illapani VSP, Mo X, White RD, Kolipaka A (2017) In vivo quantification of aortic stiffness using MR elastography in hypertensive porcine model. Magn Reson Med 78(6):2315–2321. https://doi.org/10.1002/mrm.26601
72. Morin CE, Dillman JR, Serai SD, Trout AT, Tkach JA, Wang H (2018) Comparison of Standard Breath-Held, Free-Breathing, and Compressed Sensing 2D Gradient-Recalled Echo MR Elastography Techniques for Evaluating Liver Stiffness. AJR American journal of roentgenology:1–9. doi:https://doi.org/10.2214/ajr.18.19761
73. Liu X, Li N, Xu T, Sun F, Li R, Gao Q, Chen L, Wen C (2017) Effect of renal perfusion and structural heterogeneity on shear wave elastography of the kidney: an in vivo and ex vivo study. BMC Nephrol 18(1):265. https://doi.org/10.1186/s12882-017-0679-2

7

Renal pH Mapping Using Chemical Exchange Saturation Transfer (CEST) MRI: Experimental Protocol

Kowsalya Devi Pavuluri, Lorena Consolino, Dario Livio Longo, Pietro Irrera, Phillip Zhe Sun, and Michael T. McMahon

Abstract

Chemical exchange saturation transfer (CEST) is recognized as one of the premier methods for measuring pH with this environmental variable expected to be an excellent biomarker for kidney diseases. Here we describe step-by-step CEST MRI experimental protocols for producing pH and perfusion maps for monitoring kidney pH homeostasis in rodents after administering iopamidol as contrast agent. Several CEST techniques, acquisition protocols and ratiometric approaches are described. The impact of length of acquisition time on the quality of the maps is detailed. These methods may be useful for investigating progression in kidney disease in vivo for rodent models.

This chapter is based upon work from the COST Action PARENCHIMA, a community-driven network funded by the European Cooperation in Science and Technology (COST) program of the European Union, which aims to improve the reproducibility and standardization of renal MRI biomarkers. This experimental protocol is complemented by two separate chapters describing the basic concepts and data analysis.

Key words Magnetic resonance imaging (MRI), Kidney, Mice, Rats, Chemical exchange saturation transfer (CEST), pH imaging, Iopamidol, Contrast agent, Responsive contrast agent

1 Introduction

The kidneys are responsible for filtration of plasma in order to remove waste and toxins and for maintaining the acid–base balance of the body through regulation of systemic HCO_3^- concentrations [1]. The kidneys can either reabsorb or generate new HCO_3^- through acid excretion. Renal control of pH could be impacted by a number of factors including whether or not there are abnormalities in perfusion, filtration, amino acid metabolism or if renal tissue edema or inflammation are present. Based on a number of studies relating changes in acid production, secretion or reduced NH_4^+ with pathological conditions [2–8], pH should be a good biomarker for assessing renal function. A number of methods are

Andreas Pohlmann and Thoralf Niendorf (eds.), *Preclinical MRI of the Kidney: Methods and Protocols*, Methods in Molecular Biology, vol. 2216, https://doi.org/10.1007/978-1-0716-0978-1_27,

now established for determining local pH in vivo, including use of pH micro electrodes [9–11], fluorescence imaging [12, 13], ^{1}H, ^{31}P, ^{19}F MRS [14–21] hyperpolarized ^{13}C MRS [22], pH-dependent MR relaxometry [23], and chemical exchange saturation transfer (CEST) MRI [24, 25]. CEST is a novel MRI contrast mechanism allowing detection of low concentrations of contrast agent through the application of saturation radiofrequency (RF) pulses on their labile protons to destroy their magnetization with the resulting signal loss transferred to water through chemical exchange which has now emerged as the premier MRI method for pH imaging [7, 26–32].

Here we describe CEST MRI for monitoring of the local pH variation found in the kidney of rodents in a step-by-step experimental protocol. The rationale for the choosing acquisition parameters is given in generic terms, together with specific parameter examples.

Mapping of contrast agent renal perfusion is described as an optional component of the experiment. Contrast agent perfusion is a functional parameter that is also sensitive to kidney damage. Currently CT, SPECT and gadolinium based MR imaging are available for assessing renal perfusion in patients, each with its own limitations [33]. CEST MRI contrast enables production of high resolution images of perfusion without need of using ionizing radiation making mapping of perfusion a valuable complement to pH imaging [34].

The protocols contained in this chapter were tested on healthy control mice using Iopamidol as the contrast agent to standardize the pH mapping and tested for both an axial slice and a coronal slice for bench marking. These methods may be useful for investigating renal pH and perfusion variations found in vivo for various rodent models with acute kidney injuries or which progress to chronic kidney disease.

This experimental protocol chapter is complemented by two separate chapters describing the basic concepts and data analysis, which are part of this book.

This chapter is part of the book Pohlmann A, Niendorf T (eds) (2020) Preclinical MRI of the Kidney—Methods and Protocols. Springer, New York.

2 Materials

2.1 Animals

This experimental protocol is tailored for immunocompetent (typically C57BL/6 and Balb/C) or immunocompromised (nude, NOD-SCID) mice with a body mass of 15–35 g. Advice for adaptation to rats is given as *Notes* where necessary. All animal studies have to be carried out in compliance with specific legislation covering the use of animals for scientific purposes. Therefore, all experiments must be authorized under national regulations.

2.2 Lab Equipment and Chemicals

1. Mouse tail illuminator/restrainer for catheterizing the tail vein.
2. Saline solution or heparin solution, 1-ml syringe, catheter (e.g., PE 20 polyethylene tubing) of known inner diameter to hold the saline flush and for contrast agent bolus is required.
3. Anesthesia: please refer to the chapter by Kaucsar T et al. "Preparation and Monitoring of Small Animals in Renal MRI" for an in-depth description and discussion of the anesthesia. Typically, 0.5–1.5% isoflurane is used for anesthesia administered to the mice using an anesthetic gas vaporizer (Leica Biosystems, Maryland, USA). For nonrecovery experiments, urethane solution (Sigma-Aldrich, Steinheim, Germany; 20% in distilled water) can provide anesthesia for several hours with comparatively few side effects on renal physiology, which is an important issue. For intramuscular anesthesia, please refer to **Note 1**.
4. Gases: O_2, N_2, and compressed air, as well as a gas-mixing system or general inhalation anesthesia equipment, including an anesthetic vaporizer, a flow meter and an induction chamber.
5. Mouse cradle.
6. pH imaging contrast agent: typically iodinated-based contrast media are employed, as Iopamidol (Isovue® 370, Bracco Imaging SpA, Milano, Italy), Iopromide (300 mg iodine/ml Ultravist®, Bayer Healthcare, Germany) or Iobitridol (Omnipaque®, GE Healthcare, USA). Such clinically available contrast agents have stock concentrations of 0.9–1 M that can be directly used (*see* **Note 2**).
7. Small Animal Ventilator: animals (rats) needs to be ventilated so the CEST MRI acquisition can be gated to minimize the respiratory motion artifacts. We used a TOPO Dual Mode Rodent/Small Animal Ventilator (Kent Scientific, Torrington, CT).
8. Syringe Infusion Pump: an MR-compatible single syringe pump (Harvard Bioscience, Holliston, MA) for contrast agent administration.

2.3 MRI Hardware

The general hardware requirements for renal ^1H MRI on mice and rats are described in the chapter by Ramos Delgado P et al. "Hardware Considerations for Preclinical Magnetic Resonance of the Kidney." The technique described in this chapter has been tailored for MR preclinical systems at magnetic fields higher than 3 T but advice for adaptation to other field strengths is given where necessary (*see* **Note 3**). No special or additional hardware is required, except for the following:

1. A physiological monitoring system that can track the respiration and which is connected to the MR system such that it can be used to synchronize CEST MRI with respiration. Typically, we use the MR-compatible rodent monitoring and gating system (Small Animal Instruments, New York, USA) equipped with an air-pillow to monitor breath rate.

2.4 MRI Sequences

The CEST MRI sequence includes continuous wave (CW) RF saturation followed by fast image readout such as echo planar imaging (EPI), Rapid Imaging with Refocused Echoes (RARE) and/or fast imaging with steady-state precession (FISP) [6, 35–37]. Herein we describe those based on fast refocused multiecho sequences since they provide the higher SNR in acceptable acquisition times and are without geometrical distortions. The same sequence readout is described for B_0 mapping, for full Z-spectrum acquisition and for dynamic acquisition applications.

3 Methods

3.1 MR Protocol Setup

3.1.1 Rapid Acquisition with Refocused Echoes Sequence for External B_0 Mapping Using WASSR

1. Select a 2D Rapid Acquisition with Refocused Echoes sequence in conjunction with a magnetization transfer preparation module that has a frequency offset which can be incremented within a single scan. This is a standard sequence on Bruker MRI systems, called "RARE."
2. Switch on the magnetization transfer module. The magnetization transfer pulse parameters are then adjusted to allow detection of direct water saturation vs. excitation frequency and also the signal-to-noise >50:1 when the saturation pulse is 500 Hz or more away from water. Typically, we employ $N = 11{,}000$ ms rectangular shaped pulse with saturation power (amplitude) of 1–1.5 μT, similar to what was previously described for the WASSR Scheme [38].
3. Sample several frequency offsets around the frequency of bulk water signal (commonly set at 0 ppm, in contrast to the 4.8 ppm as in conventional NMR experiments). Usually the sampled range is between −3 and +3 ppm with different step size, according to the available acquisition time and expected B_0 inhomogeneity. Please *see* **Note 4** for an example of the frequency list used in B_0 mapping.
4. Choose a repetition time (TR) of ~5–6 s for good signal stability and signal-to-noise per time (SNR/t) efficiency. TR will be limited by the length of the saturation pulse, length of echo train and the number of slices to be acquired, and saturation pulse(s)'s field strength.

5. Use the shortest echo time (TE) and echo spacing (ΔTE) possible. One wants to acquire as many lines of k space as possible to minimize motion distortions of the images. For that reason, it is advantageous to have ΔTE well below 10 ms. Larger ΔTE are not advisable because the SNR in the kidney will be so low that these images must be excluded. Acquisition bandwidth should be considered to shorten the ΔTE.
6. Set the rare factor as high as possible to reduce scan time. Same as the CEST acquisition scan (Subheading 3.1.2).
7. Set the acquisition bandwidth (BW) as for the CEST contrast scan (Subheading 3.1.2).
8. Switch on the fat saturation module.
9. Do not use the respiration trigger since this will increase the overall acquisition time.
10. Set the same geometry as for the CEST contrast scan (Subheading 3.1.2).
11. Set the matrix size/acceleration the same as for the CEST contrast scan (Subheading 3.1.2).
12. For an example of a specific parameter set please *see* **Note 5**.

3.1.2 Full Z-Spectrum Acquisition for CEST-pH Mapping

1. Select a 2D Rapid Acquisition with Refocused Echoes sequence with magnetization transfer preparation module. This is a standard sequence on Bruker MRI systems, called "RARE." RARE sequence with centric encoding is used. More details on CEST sequences for Bruker scanners are provided in **Note 6**.
2. Switch on the Magnetization transfer module. The magnetization transfer pulse parameters are then adjusted to allow detection of CEST contrast while keeping the current within limits given by the RF transmit coil and the ^{1}H RF power amplifier. For CEST pH mapping, Z-spectra are acquired by applying a 1.5–6 μT continuous wave (CW) block shaped (bp) presaturation pulse for 2–5 seconds or by applying a pulsed saturation scheme (*see* Subheading 2.4.3.35).
3. Acquire a series of 30–50 frequencies in the range of ±10 ppm for the whole CEST Z-spectrum acquisition. A macro file containing the MR frequencies is manually implemented by the operator in Bruker systems, by creating a list of frequencies covering the positive and negative side of CEST spectra. At the resonating frequencies of mobile protons (4.2/4.3 ppm and 5.5 ppm for Iopamidol and Iopromide, 5.6 ppm for Iobitridol) a denser sampling is usually applied (frequency resolution of 0.1 ppm). Please *see* **Note 7** for an example of the frequency list.

4. Choose the Repetition Time (TR) in the range 4–6 s for good signal stability and signal-to-noise per time (SNR/t) efficiency, also according to the duration of the saturation pulse.
5. Use the shortest TE and echo spacing (ΔTE) possible.
6. Set the Rare factor to 64–96. Typically, a single shot acquisition (Rare Factor equal to Matrix Size) to reduce the acquisition time for each frequency. Partial Fourier acceleration should be considered to reduce the size of the matrix and improve the time efficiency of data acquisition and centric encoding to maximize SNR. Reconstruction to higher matrix size may be also considered to improve spatial resolution.
7. Use a high acquisition bandwidth (BW) to shorten ΔTE, while keeping an eye on the SNR, which decreases with increasing BW.
8. Switch on the fat saturation module. Important to avoid fat signal overlaying with the kidney due to chemical shift.
9. Set off the respiration trigger.
10. Adapt the geometry of the slice(s) so that animal fits into FOV in L-R direction (approx. 30–40 mm, according to the coil inner diameter) and use frequency encoding in H-F direction. Use a slice with the lowest thickness the SNR allows, typically around 1.5–2.0 mm. The thinner the slices the better, as this improves the resolution—which can be readily seen on the raw images.
11. Use the highest in-plane resolution that the SNR allows. A typical matrix size of 64 × 64, 96 × 96, or 128 × 128 is used for CEST images, with in-plane spatial resolution of 468, 312, or 234 μm (for an FOV of 30 mm). This has to be balanced by the need for sufficient SNR in the images. Zero-filling or use of partial Fourier techniques in the phase encoding direction can be helpful to speed up acquisition to minimize motion artifacts and contrast agent concentration changes during the acquisition.
12. For an example of a specific parameter set for mice please *see* **Note 8** or for rats please *see* **Note 9**.

3.1.3 Rapid Acquisition with Refocused Echoes Sequence for CEST pH and Perfusion Measurements

1. Select a 2D rapid acquisition with refocused echoes sequence (RARE) with magnetization transfer preparation module.
2. Switch on the magnetization transfer module. The magnetization transfer pulse parameters are then adjusted to allow detection of CEST contrast while keeping the current within the limits given by the RF transmit coil, the ^{1}H RF power amplifier and the signal-to-noise >50:1 at the frequency of the labile protons of interest on the CEST agent. Typically, we employ signal averaging with $N = 10$, 300 ms rectangular shaped RF

pulses with an amplitude between 3 and 4 μT. The saturation frequency is alternated between 4.2 ppm, 5.5 ppm for collection of signal with saturation on resonance with the two labile protons in iopamidol and for the last ten images −100 ppm for collection of S_0 (signal with no saturation).

3. Choose a repetition time (TR) between 7 and 12 s for good signal stability and signal-to-noise per time (SNR/*t*) efficiency.
4. Use the shortest TE and echo spacing (ΔTE) possible (*see* Subheading 3.1.2).
5. Use a rare factor of 20–32. Typically, 20–32 TEs are sensible and allow acquiring a 32 × 32 matrix slice or 48 × 48 with partial Fourier acceleration in a single shot. Partial Fourier acceleration should be considered to reduce the size of the matrix and improve the time efficiency of data acquisition.
6. Use a high acquisition bandwidth (BW) to shorten ΔTE, while keeping an eye on the SNR, which decreases with increasing BW. For the image with the shortest TE an SNR of at least 60 is recommended.
7. Switch on the fat saturation module. Important to avoid fat signal overlaying with the kidney due to chemical shift.
8. Use an FOV saturation of 4 mm thickness above 9–13 mm from the kidneys for coronal slices. This is not required for axial slices.
9. Set off the respiration trigger.
10. Adapt the geometry of the acquisition slices so that the animal fits into FOV in L-R direction (approx. 30–40 mm according to the coil inner diameter) and use frequency encoding in H-F direction. Use a slice with the lowest thickness the SNR allows, typically around 1.5 mm. The thinner the slices the better, as this improves the resolution—which can be readily seen on the raw images. For adaptation to rats *see* **Note 10**.
11. Use highest in-plane resolution that the SNR allows, typically around 600 × 400 um^2 for axial slices or 200 × 500 μm^2 for coronal slices. This has to be balanced by the need for sufficient SNR in the images. Use zero-filling or partial Fourier techniques in the phase encoding direction to speed up acquisition and to minimize motion artifacts and contrast agent concentration changes during the acquisition. One may use half Fourier in read direction (asymmetric echo) to further shorten the first TE. Reducing the excitation and refocusing pulse lengths to below 1.5 ms can then also help to shorten TE.
12. For an example of a specific parameter set please *see* **Note 11**.

3.2 Setting of the pH Calibration Curve

Prepare multiple vials of Iopamidol phosphate-buffered solution (PBS 1×, 10 mM of inorganic phosphates) or human blood serum solutions, with pH titrated to physiological relevant renal pH values: 5.5, 6.0, 6.5, 7.0, 7.5, 8.0 and place them in a plastic container (e.g., 30–50 ml falcon tube) filled with water. Such a phantom calibration experiment is crucial for in vivo pH quantification at different experimental conditions such as magnetic field strength and CEST irradiation Schemes [39]. A more detailed description for pH calibration curve can be found in the chapter by Kim H et al. "Analysis Protocol for the Quantification of Renal pH Using Chemical Exchange Saturation Transfer (CEST) MRI."

1. Acquire the CEST Z-spectrum by sweeping RF saturation to a series of frequency offsets around the bulk water resonance. Note that the magnitude of the saturation field (B_1) and duration can be adjusted serially to facilitate Z-spectral acquisition. For an example of specific parameters at 7 T please *see* **Note 12**, whereas for an example of specific parameters at 4.7 T please *see* **Note 13** and for the same at 11.7 T please *see* **Note 14**.

3.3 Preparations of the Contrast Agent Injection and of the Catheter

1. Fill the 1-ml syringe with the contrast agent stock solution.
2. Prepare the catheter by filling the PE20 tubing with the contrast agent solution, and with 20–60 μl of a heparin solution (or a saline solution), between the needle (the animal) and the contrast agent solution to prevent clotting before the contrast agent will be injected.
3. According to the length of the catheter (usually 60–100 cm to exit from the magnet bore) the contrast agent solution can be injected directly from the syringe containing the contrast agent or by changing the syringe with one filled with a (heparin-free) saline solution for the postinjection flush.

3.4 Preparation of the Mouse

1. Place the mouse on a mouse tail illuminator restrainer for catheterizing the tail vein. Catheterize the tail vein by placing a 27/29-G needle in the animal.
2. Induce anesthesia via isoflurane in an induction box. Transfer the animal to the scanner (**Note 15**).
3. Set up the temperature monitoring (rectal probe) and respiratory monitoring (balloon on chest) unit. Keep the animal's respiration rate during imaging at 35–80 breaths per min by adjusting the dose of anesthesia (approximately 1–1.5% isoflurane with air and oxygen mixed at a 3:1 ratio administered through a nose cone attached to the animal bed and ophthalmic ointment will be applied to the eyes) (*see* **Note 16**).
4. Perform anatomical imaging as described in the chapter by Pohlmann A et al. "Essential Practical Steps for MRI of the Kidney in Experimental Research."

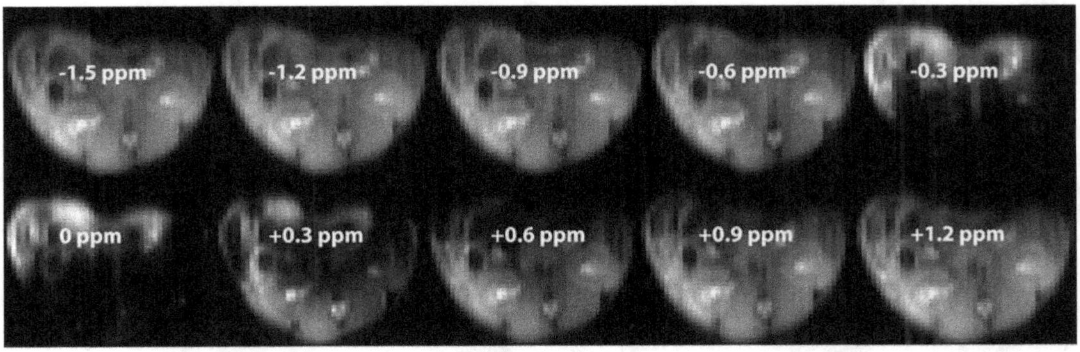

Fig. 1 Series of ten saturation weighted images of a healthy mouse kidney acquired with a 2D CEST-RARE sequence at 11.7 T. Images correspond to saturation frequencies = −1.5, −1.2, −0.9, −0.6, −0.3 ppm (top row) and saturation frequencies = 0, 0.3, 0.6, 0.9, 1.2 ppm (bottom row)

5. Perform localized shimming on the kidney imaging as described in the chapter by Pohlmann A et al. "Essential Practical Steps for MRI of the Kidney in Experimental Research" (*see* **Note 17**).

3.5 B_0 Mapping

3.5.1 External B_0 Mapping

1. Load the B_0 mapping sequence and adapt the slice orientation to provide a coronal or axial view of the two kidneys based on the tripilot/scout and anatomical images collected.
2. Run the B_0 mapping scan using 42 offsets from −1.5 to +1.5 ppm and B_1 = 1.5 μT. Example images are shown in Fig. 1.

3.5.2 Internal B_0 Mapping

1. Acquire a full Z-spectrum with some frequency offsets sampled around 0 ppm to exploit the Z-spectrum for internal measurement of B_0 shifts as described in the chapter by Kim H et al. "Analysis Protocol for the Quantification of Renal pH Using Chemical Exchange Saturation Transfer (CEST) MRI."

3.6 CEST Acquisition for pH Mapping

1. Perform the CEST experiment by acquiring CEST images before, (during) and after injection of the contrast agent. Choose among the different pH mapping procedures by conventional ratiometric approach (Subheading 3.5.1), pH mapping with power ratiometric method (Subheading 3.5.2) or dynamic CEST perfusion and pH mapping (Subheading 3.5.3).

3.6.1 pH Mapping with Conventional Ratiometric Method (Full Z-Spectrum)

1. Load the pH mapping sequence, using the same geometry as used for anatomical and B_0 mapping. Switch off the magnetization module and use this sequence to set the receiver gain.
2. Load the pH mapping sequence, using the same geometry as used for anatomical and B_0 mapping. Set the receiver gain as calculated by the magnetization off sequence (*see* Subheading

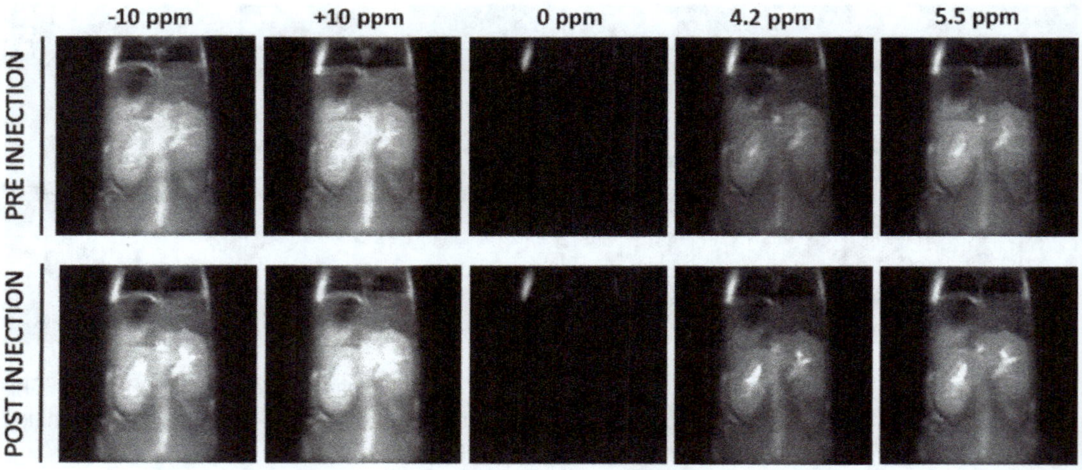

Fig. 2 Series of saturated weighted images of a healthy mouse kidney acquired with a 2D CEST-RARE sequence at 7 T before (up panel) and after (bottom panel) the injection of iopamidol at 1.5 mg I/kg b.w. Images correspond to saturation frequencies of −10, +10, 0, +4.2, and +5.5 ppm

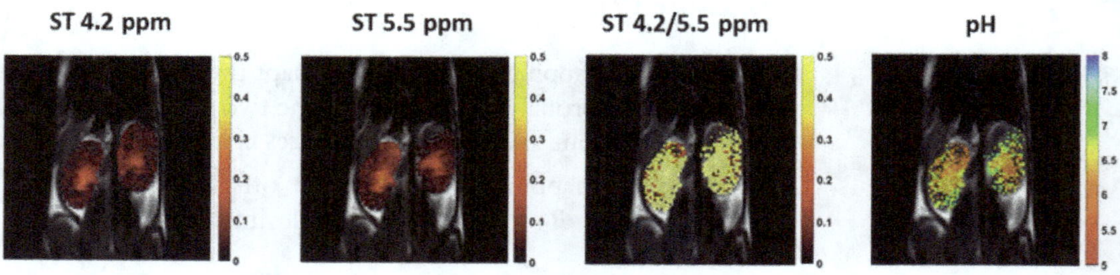

Fig. 3 From left to right: parametric maps of saturation transfer (ST) contrast obtained at 4.2 ppm, at 5.5 ppm, ratiometric 4.2/5.5 map and calculated pH map in kidney regions. The parametric color maps are superimposed on a T_{2w} anatomical image (gray scale)

3.5.1.15). Load the macro file containing the offset frequencies to be saturated and run the sequence for CEST preinjection scanning.

3. Clone the pH mapping scans, at least one time for acquiring one CEST postinjection scan.
4. After the acquisition of the CEST prescan, perform a bolus injection of iodine contrast agent through the tail vein catheter at a dose of 1.0–1.5 iodine/kg b.w. (*see* **Note 18**).
5. Run the postinjection scans.
6. A demonstration of the acquired images at different offsets and of CEST contrast that can be expected for the pH mapping scans are given in Fig. 2 and Fig. 3, respectively.

3.6.2 pH Mapping with Power Ratiometric Method (Full Z-Spectrum)

1. Load the pH mapping sequence, using the same geometry as used for anatomical and B_0 mapping. Switch off the magnetization module and use this sequence to set the receiver gain.
2. Load the pH mapping sequence, using the same geometry as used for anatomical and B_0 mapping. Set the receiver gain as calculated by the magnetization off sequence (*see* Subheading 3.6.1.15). Load the macro file containing the offset frequencies to saturate at a first selected power pulse (1.5 μT) and run the sequence for CEST preinjection scanning.
3. Clone the scan and set the second selected saturation power pulse (6 μT). Run the sequence for CEST preinjection scanning.
4. Clone two times the scans with 1.5 and 6 μT saturation power pulse for acquiring the postinjection scans.
5. Perform a bolus injection of iodine contrast agent with single amide exchanging pool (e.g., iobitridol) through the tail vein catheter at a dose of 1.0–1.5 iodine/kg b.w. (*see* **Note 18**).
6. Run the postinjection scans.

3.6.3 pH and Perfusion Mapping with Two Offset Sampling

1. Load the pH mapping sequence, using the same geometry as used for B_0 mapping and setting up a collection to run for 1 h, 5 min alternating the saturation frequency between 4.2 ppm (labile proton #1 for iopamidol), 5.5 ppm (labile proton #2 for iopamidol), and for the final ten images at −100 ppm (S_0 image) (*see* **Note 19**).
2. Initiate the pH mapping scans.
3. Exactly 5 min after starting the pH mapping scans, perform a bolus injection of contrast agent: inject iopamidol through the tail vein at a dose of 1.0 g iodine/kg using ~100–150 μl.
4. Approximately 1 h after injection, end the pH mapping scan collection.
5. A demonstration of the contrast changes that can be expected for the pH mapping scans are given in Fig. 4.

4 Notes

1. Intramuscular anesthesia can be administered as a mixture of xylazine 5 mg/kg (Rompun, Bayer, Milan, Italy) and tiletamine/zolepan 20 mg/kg (Zoletil 100, Virbac, Milano, Italy).
2. To reduce the viscosity of these solutions, hence the pressure needed to infuse these solutions, syringes can be warmed at 37 °C before the injection. Please avoid the inclusion of air bubbles in the catheter filled with the saline solution or with the contrast agent solution that will be injected into the animals.

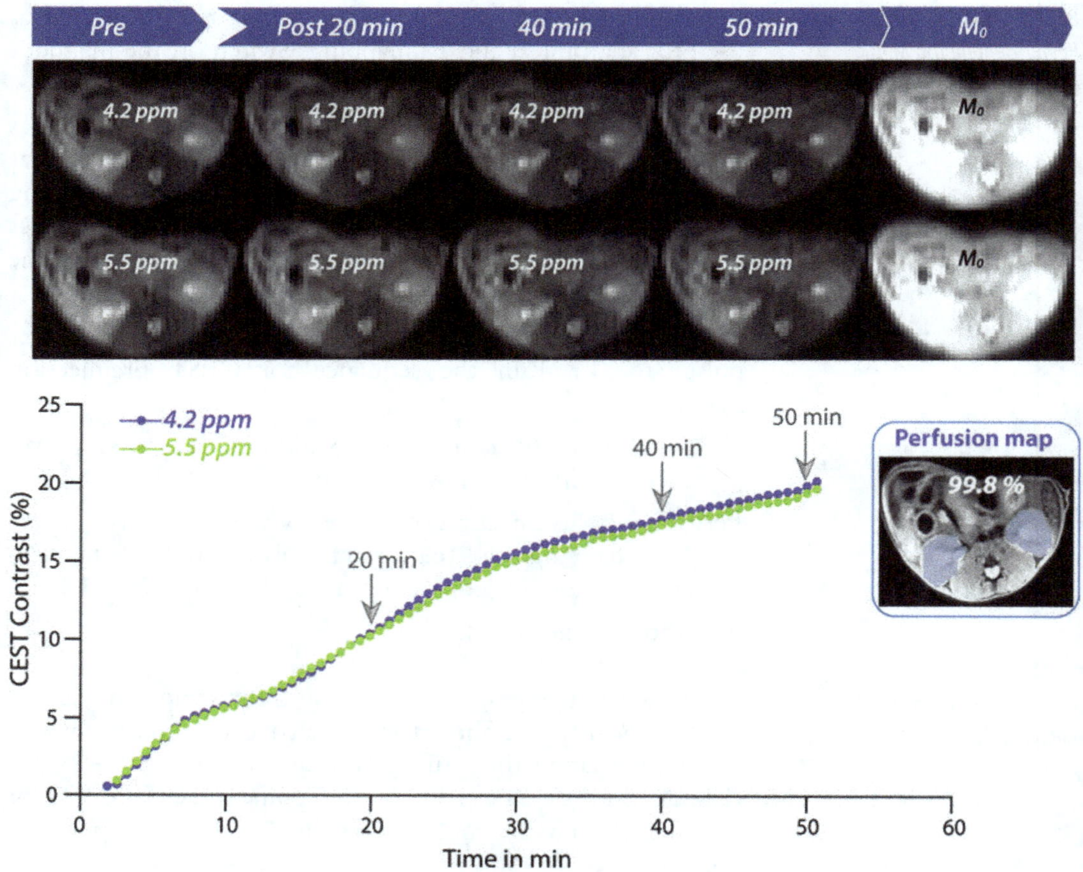

Fig. 4 Demonstration of the contrast changes that can be expected in pH mapping. CEST weighted images (from a 2D RARE acquisition, effective TE = 3.5 ms) of the kidneys throughout a pH measurement experiment, together with a final processed image of perfusion. A moving average filter was applied on the time series data to remove fluctuations in signal due to motion. The percentage of kidney pixels with >20% of maximum contrast were calculated to obtain the perfusion or filtration fraction map

3. CEST pH measurements are basically performed on Bruker MR systems as Biospec 117/20 (11.7 T), Avance 300 (7 T), Pharmascan 70/16 (7 T), or Biospec (3 T) (Bruker, Ettlingen, Germany). Standard 1H transmit/receive coils (birdcage, quadrature) or phased-array coils (4- or 8-channel mouse body phase array receive coil) to improve SNR can be used.
4. WASSR B_0 mapping frequency list (in ppm): −1.5, −1.4, −1.3, −1.2, −1.1, −1.0, −0.9, −0.8, −0.7, −0.6, −0.5, −0.4, −0.3, −0.2, −0.1, 0, 0.1, 0.2, 0.3, 0.4, 0.5, 0.6, 0.7, 0.8, 0.9, 1.0, 1.1, 1.2, 1.3, 1.4, and 1.5.
5. Scan acquisition parameters for B_0 mapping: TR = 5000 ms; magnetization transfer power = 1.5 μT; magnetization transfer module time = 3 s; MT offset mode = Sequential_Offset; effective TE = 3.49 ms; RARE Factor = 32; averages = 1;

centric encoding; slice thickness = 1.5 mm; slice orientation = axial; frequency encoding = head-feet; FOV = 28 × 19 mm; matrix size = 48 × 48 reconstructed to 128 × 128; fat suppression = on.

6. Standard Bruker sequences for the software versions PV5 and PV6 include only a Magnetization Transfer module that allows the saturation of a single frequency offset. As a consequence, full Z-spectrum acquisition can only be acquired by cloning the same scan and modifying for each scan the irradiated frequency offset. Therefore, for in vivo experiments this may lead to acquisition times that are not feasible in reasonable time. Bruker sequences for PV5 and PV6 that have been modified to accept a frequency list for acquiring the full Z-spectrum in a single scan are available upon request to the authors (dario.longo@unito.it; mtmcmaho@gmail.com; pzhesun@emory.edu). Starting from PV360 a new CEST module has been implemented with different readout sequences (RARE, EPI, Spiral) that allows to fix this issue. MR Solutions vendor has already a CEST module that can be applied with an EPI-based readout scheme.
7. Frequency list (in ppm) for a full Z-spectrum acquisition (43 offsets): 0, 0.5, −0.5, 1.0, −1.0, 1.5, −1.5, 2.0, −2.0, 3.0, −3.0, 3.9, −3.9, 4.0, −4.0, 4.1, −4.1, 4.2, −4.2, 4.3, −4.3, 4.4, −4.4, 4.5, −4.5, 5.2, −5.2, 5.3, −5.3, 5.4, −5.4, 5.5, −5.5, 5.6, −5.6, 5.7, −5.7, 5.8, −5.8, 7.5, −7.5, 10.0, and −10.0.
8. Example for a 30 g mouse at 7 T: TR = 6000 ms; magnetization transfer power = 3 μT; magnetization transfer module time = 5 s; MT offset mode = from file; effective TE = 4.14 ms; RARE Factor = 96; averages = 1; centric encoding; slice thickness = 1.5 mm; slice orientation = axial; frequency encoding = head-feet; FOV = 30 mm; matrix size = 96 × 96 reconstructed to 128 × 128; fat suppression = on.
9. Example for a 150 g rat at 4.7 T: Z-spectra are collected with moderate saturation RF power (B_1) levels of 1.0 and 2.0 μT. The in vivo CEST MRI parameters were as the following: RF saturation offsets from −7.0 to 7.0 ppm with intervals of 0.125 ppm, and TR, TS and TE were 6 s, 3 s, and 18 ms, respectively, for an image matrix of 48 × 48.
10. For rats increase the FOV to the body width and keep the matrix size the same or similar. The relative resolution is then identical and the SNR should also be similar, because the larger rat RF coil provides worse SNR (e.g., eight-channel rat body phase array receive coil vs eight-channel mouse body phase array receive coil).

11. Example for a 30 g mouse at 11.7 T: TR = 9000 ms; magnetization transfer power = 4 μT; magnetization transfer pulse number = 10; magnetization transfer inter pulse delay = 10 μs; magnetization transfer pulse length = 300 ms; magnetization transfer module time = 3 s; MT offset mode = from file; effective TE = 3.49 ms; RARE Factor = 32; averages = 1; centric encoding; slice thickness = 1.5 mm; slice orientation = axial; frequency encoding = head-feet; FOV = 28 × 19 mm^2; matrix size = 48 × 48 using partial Fourier of 1.5; fat suppression = on.
12. Phantom CEST acquisition parameters at 7 T: RF saturation offsets from −10.0 to 10.0 ppm with intervals of 0.1–0.2 ppm. TR = 10s, TE = 4.8 ms, saturation = 3 μT × 5 s, matrix size = 64 × 64, FOV = 30 × 30 mm^2 with centric encoding.
13. Phantom CEST acquisition parameters at 4.7 T: RF saturation offsets from −7 to 7 ppm with intervals of 0.25 ppm. TR = 12 s, TE = 39.5 ms, saturation: 1, 1.5, 2, 2.5, 3 and 4 μT × 5 s, matrix size = 64 × 64, FOV =48 × 48 mm with centric encoding.
14. Phantom CEST acquisition parameters at 11.7 T:: 25 mm transmit/receive volume coil; TR = 5000 ms; magnetization transfer power = six different saturation power (B_1) from 1 to 6 μT; magnetization transfer module time = 3 s; MT offset mode = Sequential_Offset; 71 CEST offsets between ±7 ppm plus one at +40 ppm for M_0; effective TE = 3.39 ms; RARE Factor = 16; averages = 1; centric encoding; slice - thickness = 1.0 mm; slice orientation = axial; frequency encoding = head-feet; FOV = 28 × 19 mm^2; matrix size = 64 × 48.
15. Mice can be alternatively anesthetized with intramuscular anesthesia, tail veins heated with hot water/heater equipment at 37 °C and catheter placed in the animal.
16. You must monitor the respiration continuously throughout the entire experiment.
17. B_0 Shimming is particularly important, since macroscopic magnetic field inhomogeneities affect the exact resonance frequency of the labile protons in a voxel, and can impact the pH and perfusion measurements and hinder quantitative intra- and inter-subject comparisons. Shimming should be performed on a voxel enclosing both kidneys using either the default iterative shimming method or the Mapshim technique (recommended).
18. Injections can be manually or automatically performed. For manual injection, keep injection constant within 20–30 s. Automatic injection can be performed with dedicated injection pumps, by setting injection speed of contrast agent at 400 μl/

min. For instance, a 25 g mouse would receive ca 70 μl to achieve a dose of 1 g iodine/kg b.w. with a stock solution of 370 mg iodine/ml.

19. The exact list of frequencies used here can be adjusted based on the B_0 shimming conditions of the kidneys and the saturation power applied. For example, if the B_0 varies by more than say 0.1 ppm, additional frequencies around each labile proton should be added to allow B_0 correction at the expense of SNR due to the reduced redundancy of the data collected.

Acknowledgments

This work was supported by the Maryland Stem Cell Research Foundation MSCRF#2829 and NIH P41EB024495. The Italian Ministry for Education and Research (MIUR) is gratefully acknowledged for yearly FOE funding to the Euro-BioImaging Multi-Modal Molecular Imaging Italian Node (MMMI).

This chapter is based upon work from COST Action PARENCHIMA, supported by European Cooperation in Science and Technology (COST). COST (www.cost.eu) is a funding agency for research and innovation networks. COST Actions help connect research initiatives across Europe and enable scientists to enrich their ideas by sharing them with their peers. This boosts their research, career, and innovation.

PARENCHIMA (renalmri.org) is a community-driven Action in the COST program of the European Union, which unites more than 200 experts in renal MRI from 30 countries with the aim to improve the reproducibility and standardization of renal MRI biomarkers.

References

1. Hamm LL, Nakhoul N, Hering-Smith KS (2015) Acid-base homeostasis. Clin J Am Soc Nephrol 10(12):2232–2242
2. Soleimani M, Rastegar A (2016) Pathophysiology of renal tubular acidosis: core curriculum 2016. Am J Kidney Dis 68(3):488–498. https://doi.org/10.1053/j.ajkd.2016.03.422
3. Gil-Peña H, Mejía N, Santos F (2014) Renal tubular acidosis. J Pediatr 164(4):691–698. https://doi.org/10.1016/j.jpeds.2013.10.085
4. Gillies RJ, Raghunand N, Garcia-Martin ML, Gatenby RA (2004) pH imaging. IEEE Eng Med Biol Mag 23(5):57–64
5. Raghunand N, Howison C, Sherry AD, Zhang S, Gillies RJ (2003) Renal and systemic pH imaging by contrast-enhanced MRI. Magn Reson Med 49(2):249–257
6. Longo DL, Busato A, Lanzardo S, Antico F, Aime S (2013) Imaging the pH evolution of an acute kidney injury model by means of iopamidol, a MRI-CEST pH-responsive contrast agent. Magn Reson Med 70(3):859–864
7. Longo DL, Cutrin JC, Michelotti F, Irrera P, Aime S (2017) Noninvasive evaluation of renal pH homeostasis after ischemia reperfusion injury by CEST-MRI. NMR Biomed 30(7). https://doi.org/10.1002/nbm.372
8. Hashim AI, Zhang XM, Wojtkowiak JW, Martinez GV, Gillies RJ (2011) Imaging pH and metastasis. NMR Biomed 24(6):582–591. https://doi.org/10.1002/nbm.1644

9. Ashby BS (1966) pH studies in human malignant tumours. Lancet 288(7458):312–315
10. Prescott DM, Charles HC, Poulson JM, Page RL, Thrall DE, Vujaskovic Z, Dewhirst MW (2000) The relationship between intracellular and extracellular pH in spontaneous canine tumors. Clin Cancer Res 6(6):2501–2505
11. Wike-Hooley JL, van den Berg AP, van der Zee J, Reinhold HS (1985) Human tumour pH and its variation. Eur J Cancer Clin Oncol 21(7):785789–787791
12. Li C, Xia J, Wei X, Yan H, Si Z, Ju S (2010) pH-activated near-infrared fluorescence nanoprobe imaging tumors by sensing the acidic microenvironment. Adv Funct Mater 20(14):2222–2230
13. Hassan M, Riley J, Chernomordik V, Smith P, Pursley R, Lee SB, Capala J, Amir HG (2007) Fluorescence lifetime imaging system for in vivo studies. Mol Imaging 6 (4):7290.2007.00019
14. García-Martín M-L, Hérigault G, Rémy C, Farion R, Ballesteros P, Coles JA, Cerdán S, Ziegler A (2001) Mapping extracellular pH in rat brain gliomas in vivo by H magnetic resonance spectroscopic imaging: comparison with maps of metabolites. Cancer Res 61 (17):6524–6531
15. Gillies R, Liu Z, Bhujwalla Z (1994) 31P-MRS measurements of extracellular pH of tumors using 3-aminopropylphosphonate. Am J Phys Cell Phys 267(1):C195–C203
16. Gillies RJ, Morse DL (2005) In vivo magnetic resonance spectroscopy in cancer. Annu Rev Biomed Eng 7:287–326
17. Vermathen P, Capizzano AA, Maudsley AA (2000) Administration and 1H MRS detection of histidine in human brain: application to in vivo pH measurement. Magn Reson Med 43(5):665–675
18. Bhujwalla ZM, McCoy C, Glickson J, Gillies R, Stubbs M (1998) Estimations of intra-and extracellular volume and pH by 31P magnetic resonance spectroscopy: effect of therapy on RIF-1 tumours. Br J Cancer 78(5):606
19. Aoki Y, Akagi K, Tanaka Y, Kawai J, Takahashi M (1996) Measurement of intratumor pH by pH indicator used in 19F-magnetic resonance spectroscopy: measurement of extracellular pH decrease caused by hyperthermia combined with hydralazine. Investig Radiol 31 (11):680–689
20. Zhou R, Bansal N, Leeper DB, Glickson JD (2000) Intracellular acidification of human melanoma xenografts by the respiratory inhibitor m-iodobenzylguanidine plus hyperglycemia: a 31P magnetic resonance spectroscopy study. Cancer Res 60(13):3532–3536
21. Ojugo AS, McSheehy PM, McIntyre DJ, McCoy C, Stubbs M, Leach MO, Judson IR, Griffiths JR (1999) Measurement of the extracellular pH of solid tumours in mice by magnetic resonance spectroscopy: a comparison of exogenous 19F and 31P probes. NMR Biomed 12(8):495–504
22. Gallagher FA, Kettunen MI, Day SE, Hu D-E, Ardenkjær-Larsen JH, Jensen PR, Karlsson M, Golman K, Lerche MH, Brindle KM (2008) Magnetic resonance imaging of pH in vivo using hyperpolarized 13C-labelled bicarbonate. Nature 453(7197):940–943
23. Garcia-Martin ML, Martinez GV, Raghunand N, Sherry AD, Zhang S, Gillies RJ (2006) High resolution pHe imaging of rat glioma using pH-dependent relaxivity. Magn Reson Med 55(2):309–315
24. McMahon MT, Gilad AA, Bulte JWM, van Zijl PCM (2017) Chemical exchange saturation transfer imaging: advances and applications, 1st edn. Pan Stanford Publishing, Singapore
25. Longo D, Aime S (2017) Iodinated contrast media as pH-responsive CEST agents. In: McMahon MT, Gilad AA, JBM B, PCM VZ (eds) Chemical exchange saturation transfer imaging. Vol. Advances and applications. Pan Stanford Publishing, Singapore, pp 447–466. https://doi.org/10.1201/9781315364421-20
26. Pavuluri K, McMahon MT (2017) pH imaging using chemical exchange saturation transfer (CEST) MRI. Isr J Chem 57(9):862–879. https://doi.org/10.1002/ijch.201700075
27. Longo DL, Dastrù W, Digilio G, Keupp J, Langereis S, Lanzardo S, Prestigio S, Steinbach O, Terreno E, Uggeri F (2011) Iopamidol as a responsive MRI-chemical exchange saturation transfer contrast agent for pH mapping of kidneys: In vivo studies in mice at 7 T. Magn Reson Med 65(1):202–211
28. Longo DL, Sun PZ, Consolino L, Michelotti FC, Uggeri F, Aime S (2014) A general MRI-CEST ratiometric approach for pH imaging: demonstration of in vivo pH mapping with iobitridol. J Am Chem Soc 136 (41):14333–14336
29. Wu RH, Longo DL, Aime S, Sun PZ (2015) Quantitative description of radiofrequency (RF) power-based ratiometric chemical exchange saturation transfer (CEST) pH imaging. NMR Biomed 28(5):555–565. https://doi.org/10.1002/nbm.3284
30. Yang X, Song X, Ray Banerjee S, Li Y, Byun Y, Liu G, Bhujwalla ZM, Pomper MG, McMahon

MT (2016) Developing imidazoles as CEST MRI pH sensors. Contrast Media Mol Imaging 11(4):304–312

31. McMahon MT, Gilad AA, Zhou J, Sun PZ, Bulte JW, van Zijl P (2006) Quantifying exchange rates in chemical exchange saturation transfer agents using the saturation time and saturation power dependencies of the magnetization transfer effect on the magnetic resonance imaging signal (QUEST and QUESP): pH calibration for poly-L-lysine and a starburst dendrimer. Magn Reson Med 55(4):836–847
32. Anemone A, Consolino L, Arena F, Capozza M, Longo DL (2019) Imaging tumor acidosis: a survey of the available techniques for mapping in vivo tumor pH. Cancer Metastasis Rev. https://doi.org/10.1007/s10555-019-09782-9
33. Grenier N, Cornelis F, Le Bras Y, Rigou G, Boutault JR, Bouzgarrou M (2013) Perfusion imaging in renal diseases. Diagn Interv Imaging 94(12):1313–1322. https://doi.org/10.1016/j.diii.2013.08.018
34. Anemone A, Consolino L, Longo DL (2017) MRI-CEST assessment of tumour perfusion using X-ray iodinated agents: comparison with a conventional Gd-based agent. Eur Radiol 27(5):2170–2179. https://doi.org/10.1007/s00330-016-4552-7
35. Sheth VR, Li Y, Chen LQ, Howison CM, Flask CA, Pagel MD (2012) Measuring in vivo tumor pHe with CEST-FISP MRI. Magn Reson Med 67(3):760–768. https://doi.org/10.1002/mrm.23038
36. Sun PZ, Cheung JS, Wang E, Benner T, Sorensen AG (2011) Fast multislice pH-weighted chemical exchange saturation transfer (CEST) MRI with unevenly segmented RF irradiation. Magn Reson Med 65(2):588–594. https://doi.org/10.1002/mrm.22628
37. Pavuluri K, Manoli I, Pass A, Li Y, Vernon HJ, Venditti CP, McMahon MT (2019) Noninvasive monitoring of chronic kidney disease using pH and perfusion imaging. Sci Adv. https://doi.org/10.1126/sciadv.aaw8357
38. Kim M, Gillen J, Landman BA, Zhou J, van Zijl PC (2009) Water saturation shift referencing (WASSR) for chemical exchange saturation transfer (CEST) experiments. Magn Reson Med 61(6):1441–1450. https://doi.org/10.1002/mrm.21873
39. Sun PZ, Longo DL, Hu W, Xiao G, Wu R (2014) Quantification of iopamidol multi-site chemical exchange properties for ratiometric chemical exchange saturation transfer (CEST) imaging of pH. Phys Med Biol 59(16):4493

8

Monitoring Renal Hemodynamics and Oxygenation by Invasive Probes: Experimental Protocol

Kathleen Cantow, Mechthild Ladwig-Wiegard, Bert Flemming, Andreas Pohlmann, Thoralf Niendorf, and Erdmann Seeliger

Abstract

Renal tissue hypoperfusion and hypoxia are early key elements in the pathophysiology of acute kidney injury of various origins, and may also promote progression from acute injury to chronic kidney disease. Here we describe methods to study control of renal hemodynamics and tissue oxygenation by means of invasive probes in anesthetized rats. Step-by-step protocols are provided for two setups, one for experiments in laboratories for integrative physiology and the other for experiments within small-animal magnetic resonance scanners.

This publication is based upon work from the COST Action PARENCHIMA, a community-driven network funded by the European Cooperation in Science and Technology (COST) program of the European Union, which aims to improve the reproducibility and standardization of renal MRI biomarkers. This experimental protocol chapter is complemented by a separate chapter describing the basic concepts of quantitatively assessing renal perfusion and oxygenation with invasive probes.

Key words Renal hemodynamics and oxygenation, In vivo methods, Rats, Magnetic resonance imaging (MRI)

1 Introduction

Kidney diseases are a global health burden with steadily increasing incidence [1–5]. Animal studies indicate that acute kidney injuries (AKI) of various origins share one common link in the pathophysiological chain of events, ultimately leading to AKI, as well as to progression from AKI to chronic kidney diseases (CKD): imbalance between renal oxygen delivery and oxygen demand [3, 6–13]. Renal tissue hypoperfusion and hypoxia have also been suggested to play a pivotal role in the pathophysiology of other kidney diseases including diabetic nephropathy [14–18].

The majority of the preclinical studies that generated this concept utilized a set of invasive probes to measure renal hemodynamics and oxygenation in anaesthetized rats [12, 14–16, 19–22]. These probes

Andreas Pohlmann and Thoralf Niendorf (eds.), *Preclinical MRI of the Kidney: Methods and Protocols*, Methods in Molecular Biology, vol. 2216, https://doi.org/10.1007/978-1-0716-0978-1_19,

typically include (1) a perivascular flow probe for measurement of total renal blood flow, (2) laser-Doppler-probes for assessment of local tissue perfusion, (3) Clark-type electrodes or fluorescence-quenching optodes for measurements of local tissue partial pressure of oxygen (pO_2), and (4) devices for invasive measurement of arterial blood pressure. These methods are considered the gold standard for the study of renal hemodynamics and oxygenation because the methods—with the exception of the laser-Doppler—provide calibrated quantitative data [23–25]. The methodological principles of these techniques are detailed in the chapter by Cantow K et al. "Quantitative Assessment of Renal Perfusion and Oxygenation by Invasive Probes: Basic Concepts." Besides the study of the pathophysiology of AKI and CKD, these methods have also been used to study (1) mechanisms of control of renal hemodynamics and oxygenation in healthy rats, (2) the effects of various substances on this control, and (3) several putative preventive or therapeutic approaches for AKI and CKD [20–22, 26–30].

It is well known that, due to the considerable capacity of the organism's homeostatic control systems to—at least partially—compensate for disturbances of, or injury to, certain control elements, these alterations are often not easily detectable when studied by measuring baseline data only. Therefore, the control systems must be "challenged" in order to unmask such alterations. This is done by dedicated test interventions (*see* the chapter by Cantow K et al. "Reversible (Patho)Physiologically Relevant Test Interventions: Rationale and Examples") [19, 27, 28, 31].

As all established modalities available in today's experimental and translational research, these techniques have shortcomings and methodological restraints, in particular, the invasiveness that preclude the survival of the animals and therefor the implementation in long-term studies, and, of course, their use in humans. Magnetic resonance imaging (MRI) offers noninvasive techniques to obtain insight into renal perfusion and oxygenation under (patho)-physiological conditions. MRI affords full kidney coverage, soft tissue contrast that helps to differentiate the renal layers, seconds to minutes temporal resolution, support of longitudinal studies, and high anatomical detail [24, 25, 32–34].

However, the validity and efficacy of functional MRI techniques for quantitative characterization of renal tissue perfusion and oxygenation and its changes in various (patho)physiological scenarios remains to be established [24, 33, 35–37]. In particular, the weakness of MRI, its qualitative nature, needs to be addressed by calibration with quantitative methods, that is, the gold standard physiological techniques. Realizing the need of tracking invasive physiological parameters and MR parameters simultaneously for the same kidney, an integrated multimodality approach designated as MR-PHYSIOL was developed by our group [24, 33, 38]. It combines the measurements by the invasive probes described above (hereafter called *PHYSIOL*) with renal functional MRI data acquired by an ultrahigh field small animal scanner. By means of this hybrid setup, the first steps toward calibration of the blood oxygenation-sensitive parameter T_2* (so-called blood oxygenation level-dependent MRI, BOLD-MRI) were done. Dedicated (patho)physiologically relevant test intervention including short periods of suprarenal aortic occlusion, hypoxia, and hyperoxia were applied to modulate renal perfusion and oxygenation, in order to detail the relationship between renal T_2* and tissue oxygenation [24, 33, 39]. Of course, the MR-PHYSIOL setup can be used for calibration of functional MR parameters other than oxygenation-sensitive T_2* as well.

In the following, step-by-step protocols are provided for two setups, one for stand-alone experiments in laboratories for integrative physiology (*PHYSIOL*) and the other for experiments within dedicated small-animal magnetic resonance scanners by use of the hybrid setup (*MR-PHYSIOL*).

This experimental protocol chapter is complemented by a separate chapter describing the basic concepts, which is part of this book.

This chapter is part of the book Pohlmann A, Niendorf T (eds) (2020) Preclinical MRI of the Kidney—Methods and Protocols. Springer, New York.

2 Materials

2.1 Animals

For *PHYSIOL*, male Wistar rats with body mass of 300–400 g are used. For *MR-PHYSIOL*, the spatial constraints dictated by the MR environment require the use of relatively small rats ($\leq$350 g). The rats are allowed ad libitum food (standard maintenance diet) and water and must be housed at standardized conditions (e.g., group housed in Makrolon type IV cages with elevated lids under conventional SPF conditions; for cage enrichment paper towels as nesting material and pieces of wood for gnawing should be provided).

2.2 Surgical Preparation

1. Anesthesia: urethane solution (Sigma-Aldrich, Steinheim, Germany; 20% in distilled water).
2. Temperature controlled operation table.
3. Operation microscope (e.g., Leica MZ6; Leica Microsystems, Wetzlar, Germany) with magnification range between 6.3× and 40×.
4. Set of microsurgical instruments (including dissecting scissors, microsurgical forceps, needle holders) and threads (including Vicryl polyglactin 910, 4/0; Prolene 6/0; Ethicon, Norderstedt, Germany).
5. For blood pressure measurement: (a) a pressure transducer (e.g., DT-XX, Viggo-Spectramed, Swindon, UK) connected

to an amplifier (TAM-A Plugsys, Hugo Sachs Elektronik—Harvard Apparatus, March, Germany); (b) a femoral artery catheter designed and custom-made in our laboratory using Portex Tubing (polythene). For *MR-PHYSIOL* the catheter must be longer than 1 m to allow placing the pressure transducer well outside the bore of the MR scanner. Safety information: Make sure that the positioning of the amplifier meets the safety requirements of the MR environment.

6. For monitoring of total renal blood flow for *PHYSIOL*: a perivascular flow probe (1RB, Transonic Systems, Ithaca, NY, USA), for *MR-PHYSIOL* a perivascular flow probe (MCV2PSB-MRI; Transonic Systems) as depicted in Fig. 1. Please note that the flow probe employed in *MR-PHYSIOL* uses an acoustic reflector made of Macor ceramics instead of a stainless steel or brass reflector to meet the safety and compatibility requirements of MRI. The respective flow probe is connected to a perivascular flow module (TS420; Transonic Systems). Safety information: Make sure that the positioning of the flow module meets the safety requirements of the MR environment.
7. Combined optical laser-Doppler-Flux and pO_2 probes (pO_2 E-Series Sensor; Oxford Optronix, Oxford, UK) for measurements of local tissue oxygenation and local tissue perfusion as

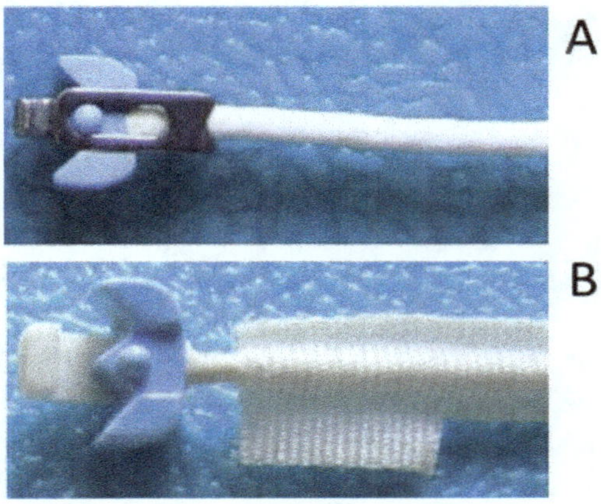

Fig. 1 Probes for monitoring of total renal blood flow. (**a**) Perivascular flow probe (1RB, Transonic Systems, Ithaca, NY, USA) for *PHYSIOL*: the acoustic reflector is made of steel; closing the probe's steel "lock" prevents detachment from the renal artery. (**b**) perivascular flow probe (MV2PSB-MRI; Transonic Systems) for *MR-PHYSIOL*: due to the long extension leads necessary to meet MR safety requirements, this probe has a larger body size. The reflector is made of ceramics (it does not induce MR artifacts), is L-shaped and offers no mechanism to lock the vessel. Therefore, a gauze is attached to the probe's cable, which will be fixed to the retroperitoneal muscles by means of sutures to avoid probe displacement

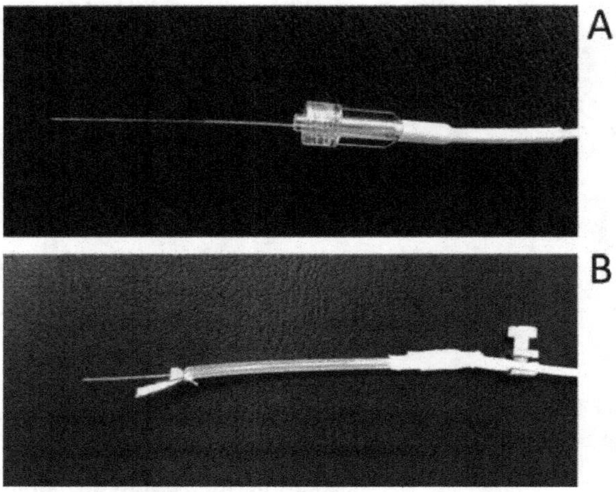

Fig. 2 Probes for monitoring of tissue laser-Doppler-flux and pO_2 (pO_2 E-Series Sensor; Oxford Optronix, Oxford, UK). (**a**) Unmodified probe for *PHYSIOL*. (**b**) Modified probe for *MR-PHYSIOL*: the customary Luer-Lock connector is removed, the fiber glass cores are fixed to the sheathing by means of a clamp. Silicone tubing with its length adjusted to the distance between the caudal and the cranial extremities of the individual kidney enables the exact placement of the cortical probe. A patche of gauze attached to the end of silicone tubing is used to fixed the probe on the kidney surface by Histoacryl glue to prevent displacement

depicted in Fig. 2. The probes are attached to an OxyLite/OxyFlo-apparatus (Oxford Optronics, Oxford, UK). Safety information: For *MR-PHYSIOL* make sure that the positioning of the OxyLite/OxyFlo-apparatus meets the safety requirements of the MR environment.

8. For continuous logging of the signals from the probes for arterial blood pressure, renal blood flow, cortical and medullary pO_2 and flux, their analog outputs must be digitized and recorded. An analog–digital converter (e.g., DT 9800-16SE-BNC, Data Translation GmbH, Bietigheim-Bissingen, Germany) permits connection to the USB port of a PC. A dedicated data acquisition software (HAEMODYN, Hugo Sachs Elektronik—Harvard Apparatus, March, Germany) allows for calibration of the probe signals and their continuous recording.
9. A vascular occluder (*see* Fig. 3): the remotely controlled hydraulic occluder is custom-made; it was designed and manufactured in our laboratory. The occluder consists of an inflatable tube ("head" of the occluder) connected by a catheter to a syringe. The "head" of the occluder is made of a high-grade silicone elastomer tube (Silikonkautschuk, Detakta Isolier-und Messtechnik GmbH & Co KG, Germany). For the connection between the "head" of the occluder and a regulative syringe an inextensible extension catheter (Portex Polythene Tubing; Ref

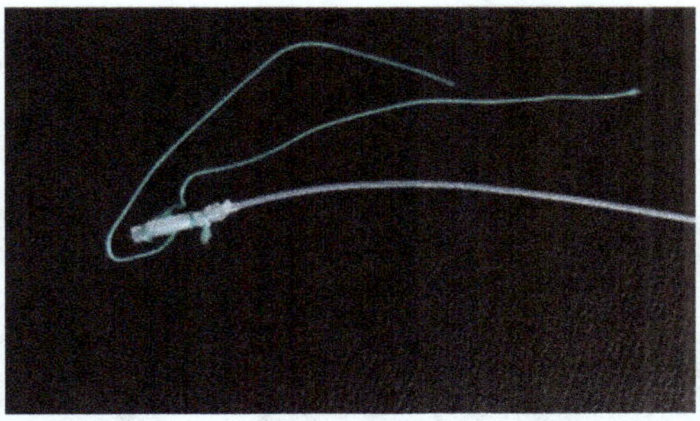

Fig. 3 Custom-made remotely controlled hydraulic vascular occluder as designed and manufactured in our laboratory. An inflatable tube ("head" of the occluder) is connected by an inextensible catheter (about 1 m length for *MR-PHYSIOL*) to a syringe. Inflation of the "head" (which is made of a high-grade silicone elastomer tube) compresses the respective vessel due to its fixation to the vessel by means of the (green) surgical threads

800/110/200; inner diameter 0.58 mm) is used. For *MR-PHYSIOL*, the extension catheter must be longer than 1 m to allow remote control of the occluder from outside the bore of the MR scanner.

10. Vascular catheter(s) for administration of fluids (e.g., isotonic saline) and/or solutions of substances used for selective test interventions (e.g., drugs), and for repeated blood sampling (e.g., for measurements of blood gases and hemoximetry). Catheters for venous and arterial insertion are made in our laboratory using Portex Tubing (polythene).

11. For fixation and stabilization of the probes for *PHYSIOL*: two micromanipulators (e.g., type M-44 and MN-153, Narishige group, Tokyo, Japan) mounted on a rotatable magnetic pedestal (e.g., type M9, World Precision Instruments, Sarasota, FL, USA) as depicted in Fig. 4. The operation table needs a steel surface (e.g., type Micro-g, Technical Manufacturing Corporation, Peabody, MA, USA) to fixate the magnetic pedestals in positions required by the individual placements of the probes within the rat. For *MR-PHYSIOL*: to achieve stabile positions of the probes and to ensure safe transfer of the animal equipped with the probes to the scanner, a custom-made portable animal holder must be used (*see* Fig. 5). It was designed and built in our laboratory using 3D CAD (Autodesk Inventor 2012; Autodesk, San Rafael, CA, USA) and rapid prototyping (BST 1200es; Alphacam GmbH, Schorndorf, Germany). The holder must meet the geometry of the MR setup; it has a half-pipe shape with a section of reduced diameter to allow for the 4-element surface RF coil to be placed beneath. A mark on the holder indicates the center of the RF coil. A bridge-like construction, positioned at the end of the hind paws of the rat, enables fixation of all leads that connect the physiological

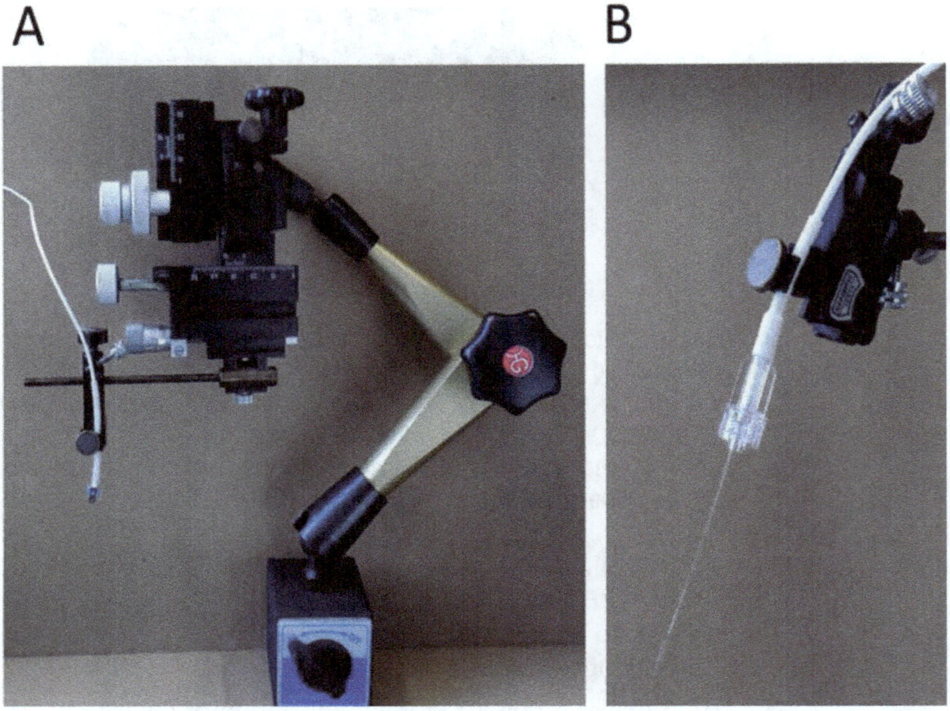

Fig. 4 Micromanipulators used for placement/insertion and fixation of probes for *PHYSIOL*. (**a**) micromanipulator (type M-44 and MN-153, Narishige group, Tokyo, Japan) mounted on a rotatable magnetic pedestal (type M9, World Precision Instruments, Sarasota, FL, USA). A perivascular flow probe (1RB, Transonic Systems, Ithaca, NY, USA) is attached to its "clutch" (type M-44). (**b**) Detail of the "clutch" with a laser-Doppler-flux and pO_2 probe (pO_2 E-Series Sensor; Oxford Optronix, Oxford, UK) attached

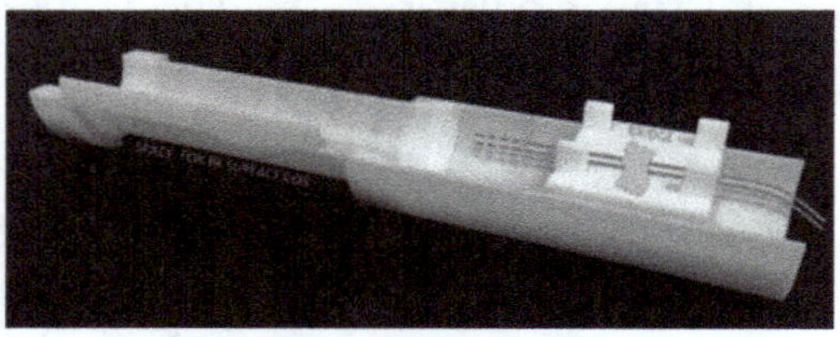

Fig. 5 Portable animal holder for *MR-PHYSIOL*. The holder enables fixation and stabilization of the probes and a safe transfer to the scanner of the animal equipped with the probes. To meet the geometry of the MR setup, it is custom-made by our lab in a half-pipe shape with a section of reduced diameter to allow for the surface RF coil. A bridge-like construction, positioned at the caudal end, enables fixation of all leads that connect the physiological probes with the equipment positioned outside the MR scanner room

probes with the equipment positioned outside the MR scanner room. The portable rigid animal holder in conjunction with the adjustable cable support bridge enables a safe transport of the animal to the MR scanner.

12. A respiratory (anesthetic) mask through which the spontaneously breathing rat is provided with air or other gas mixtures at

a supply rate of about 1000 mL/min. Such a mask can be easily built: take a 20 mL plastic syringe, cut off the tip approximately 15 mm from the bottom of the syringe, yielding a funnel shaped mask. Finally deflash and smooth the cutting edges of the mask using a file. The cone of the syringe can be connected to the gas supplying tube (*see* **Note 1**).

13. Patches of Dacron gauze (Woven Mesh Spacer; Merck Millipore, Billerica, USA).
14. Histoacryl glue (Braun Surgical GmbH, Melsungen, Germany).
15. Medical sticky tape.
16. Silicone elastomer tubes (Silikonkautschuk, Detakta Isolier- und Messtechnik GmbH & Co KG, Germany).

2.3 Magnetic Resonance Imaging (for MR-PHYSIOL)

Magnetic resonance imaging (MRI) requires access to an ultrahigh field MRI system including suitable accessories for the MR acquisition (radio frequency antennas), positioning, warming, and monitoring of physiological parameters, as well as trained personnel for operating the MRI system. The general hardware requirements for renal ^{1}H MRI on rats and mice are described in the chapter by Ramos Delgado P et al. "Hardware Considerations for Preclinical Magnetic Resonance of the Kidney." The methods described in this chapter were tailored for in vivo studies in rats by means of the dedicated MR-PHYSIOL techniques.

Due to the small size of rats in comparison with humans a much higher spatial resolution is required to depict the kidney with adequate detail. This, in turn, demands a high signal-to-noise ratio (SNR), which must be achieved by use of tailored MR equipment.

1. MR system: a dedicated small animal MR system with a magnetic field strength of 7 T and higher is recommended. We use a 9.4 T 20 cm bore system (Biospec 94/20, Bruker Biospin, Ettlingen, Germany) equipped with a gradient system with integrated shim set (B-GA12S2, Bruker Biospin, Ettlingen, Germany; gradient amplitude 440 mT/m, max. Slew rate 3440 T/m/s).
2. Radio frequency (RF) coils: use RF coils (antennas for RF transmission and reception) suitable for abdominal imaging, such as a transmit/receive rat body volume coil (72 mm inner diameter, quadrature; Bruker Biospin, Ettlingen, Germany) or preferably a transmit only *rat body volume coil* (72 mm inner diameter, linear; model T10325V3, Bruker Biospin, Ettlingen, Germany) in combination with a receive only *rat heart RF coil array* (curved, 2 × 2 elements; model T12814V3, Bruker Biospin, Ettlingen, Germany). Use of the latter coil setup is assumed here, as it allows for much higher spatial resolution

due to its superior SNR when compared with the transmit/ receive *volume coil.*

3. Animal holder: an MRI animal holder designed for the size of the rats and the geometry of the RF coils (here model T11739 with 68 mm diameter, Bruker Biospin, Ettlingen, Germany).
4. Device for sustaining the rat's body temperature: use a circulating warm-water based heating system, consisting of a flexible rubber blanket with integrated tubing (part no. T10964, Bruker Biospin, Ettlingen, Germany) connected to a conventional warm water bath (SC100-A10, ThermoFisher, Dreieich, Germany). For alternative coil setups water pipes may be integrated into the animal holder.
5. Monitoring of physiological parameters: for monitoring of respiration and core body temperature throughout the entire MR experiment use a small animal monitoring system (Model 1025, Small Animal Instruments, Inc., Stony Brook, NY, USA), including a rectal temperature probe and pneumatic pillow.

2.4 Test Interventions

1. Gases: O_2, N_2, and compressed air, as well as a gas-mixing system (e.g., Föhr Medical Instruments GmbH, Seeheim-Ober Beerbach, Germany) to achieve required changes in the oxygen fraction of inspired gas mixture (FiO_2). The following gas mixtures are required during the experiment: (a) for hypoxia: 10% O_2–90% N_2; (b) for hyperoxia: 100% O_2; (c) for normoxia: 21% O_2 (air) (*see* **Note 2**).
2. Device for monitoring FiO_2 and $FiCO_2$ in gas mixtures: for example Capnomac AGM-103 (Datex GE, Chalfont St Gils, UK).
3. Vascular occluder as listed under 2.2.9. already.
4. Vascular catheters as listed under 2.2.10. already.
5. Solutions for fluid supplementation (e.g., isotonic saline) and drug administration for dedicated test intervention according to the scientific purpose of the respective study.
6. Equipment for blood sampling via vascular catheters (e.g., capillaries for hemoximetry).
7. Instruments for analyses of blood samples according to the scientific purpose of the respective study, for example, regarding blood gases and hemoximetry (e.g., ABL80 FLEX CO-OX, Radiometer, Copenhagen, Denmark).

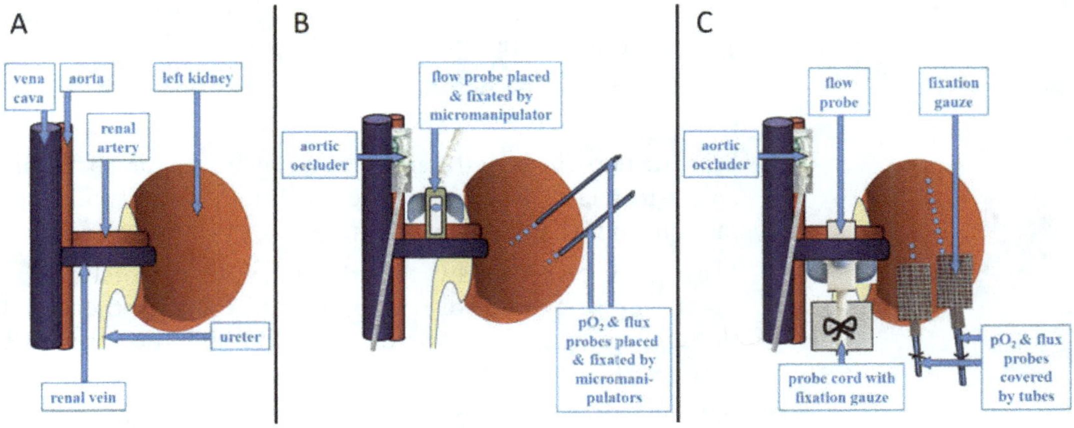

Fig. 6 Schemes depicting (**a**) the rat anatomy relevant for the placing of probes, (**b**) positions and fixations of probes for *PHYSIOL*, and (**c**) positions and fixations of probes for *MR-PHYSIOL*. For details see text

3 Methods

Figure 6 provides schemes of (a) the rat anatomy relevant for the placing of probes, (b) positions and fixations of probes for *PHYSIOL*, and (c) positions and fixations of probes for *MR-PHYSIOL*.

3.1 Surgical Preparation

For *PHYSIOL*, surgery is performed at the same operation table at which the subsequent experiment is executed. For *MR-PHYSIOL*, surgery must be performed outside the MR scanner room (in a neighboring preparation room) for safety reasons.

1. Anesthetize the animal by intraperitoneal injection of urethane (20% solution, 6 mL/kg body mass) (*see* **Note 3**).
2. After reaching the required depth of anesthesia, that is, the state of surgical tolerance (determined by specific physiological signs such as muscle relaxation degree, absence of the paw withdrawal and eye lid reflexes, absence of the swallowing reflex, and whisker movement), carefully shave the coat in the abdominal, inguinal, and ventral neck areas of the rat (hair clipper Elektra II GH2, Aesculap AG, Tuttlingen, Germany).
3. Place the rat in supine position on a warmed-up (39 °C) temperature-controlled operating table and fix the extremities of the animal to the table by means of sticky tapes.
4. Make an incision into the skin of the left inguinal area (approx. 12 mm) along the natural angle of the hind leg by lifting a fold of the skin in order to avoid an injury of the underlying blood vessels.

5. Bluntly dissect the connective tissue until the femoral vein, artery, and nerve are exposed.
6. Gently separate the nerve. Do not cut or damage the nerval tissue.
7. Separate the vein from the artery by using fine tip forceps, while trying to release an approximately 7–8 mm length vein fragment from the surrounding tissue.
8. Place three pieces of 4.0 threads under the femoral artery: situate the *first* thread distal (i.e., toward the leg), the *second* thread proximal (i.e., toward the body) and the *third* one between them.
9. Pull the *first* thread toward the leg and tie a ligature to the distal artery by using a triple knot.
10. Prepare loops with loose surgical knots on the remaining two threads.
11. Pull the *second* thread slightly toward the body so that the blood flow from femoral artery is inhibited.
12. Make a tiny incision in the exposed segment of the femoral artery behind the third thread using fine tip scissors. Fill a catheter with tapered tip with saline.
13. Grasp the catheter with the forceps and gently insert through the incision into the lumen of the femoral artery.
14. Tie the *third* knot slightly, fix catheter and arterial wall with a forceps, relax the tensed *second* thread, and push the catheter with a second forceps slowly deeper ($\approx$10 mm) into the artery in direction of the abdomen.
15. Rinse the catheter carefully with saline, and make sure that it is patent.
16. Tie the prepared loose knot of the *third* and *second* threads.
17. Start the monitoring of arterial blood pressure.
18. For insertion of additional vascular catheters for volume supplementation (e.g., by saline infusion), for test interventions by drugs, and for blood sampling (if warranted by the specific scientific goal of the experiment) surgically prepare the proximal external jugular vein (catheter tip toward vena brachiocephalica) and/or the left common carotid artery (catheter tip toward aorta) similar to **steps 5–16** detailed for the femoral artery catheter implantation.
19. Open the abdominal cavity by a midventral incision (4–5 cm) into the skin. Then open the abdominal cavity by an incision along the linea alba, thereby preventing damage to the abdominal organs. Carefully displace the bowel to the right side of the abdomen to expose the aorta and the left kidney. Carefully detach the aorta directly cranial of the renal arteries from the

surrounding tissues without damaging the very tender lymphatic vessels of that area.

20. Fix the hydraulic occluder around the aorta cranial of the renal arteries in a manner, that the occluder is well attached to the aorta without impairing the blood flow while being deflated (*see* **Note 4**).
21. Carefully separate the left renal artery from the renal vein using fine tip forceps. Try to expose an approximately 6–7 mm long fragment. Do not cut or damage the nerves.
22. For *MR-PHYSIOL*, transfer the animal onto the portable animal holder such that the kidney is aligned with the mark on the holder that indicates the center of the RF coil.
23. Start the HAEMODYN software (*see* Subheading 3.3).
24. Place the Transonic flow probe around the left renal artery and start monitoring RBF. It is important that the head of the flow probe is filled with fluid. For *PHYSIOL*, attach the cable of the probe on the "clutch" of a micromanipulator (*see* Fig. 4a). Position and fixate the probe (Type 1RB) by means of the micromanipulator in the appropriate position of the artery (*see* Fig. 6b). For *MR-PHYSIOL*, the placement of the probe upon the artery must be done without the benefit of a micromanipulator. A gauze is attached to the probe cable (Type MV2PSB-MRI) as shown in Fig. 1b. To avoid displacements of the probe, the gauze is fixed to the retroperitoneal muscles by sutures (*see* Fig. 6c) (*see* **Note 5**).
25. For *PHYSIOL*, attach the cortical and medullary laser-flux-pO_2 probes, respectively, at one of the two "clutches" (*see* Fig. 4b) of a micromanipulator. With the help of the micromanipulator, the probes are placed into the renal cortex (depth about 1–1.5 mm below the capsule) and the medulla (3–4 mm below the capsule), respectively, as shown in Fig. 6b (*see* **Note 6**).
26. For *MR-PHYSIOL*, remove the customary Luer-Lock connectors of the laser-flux-pO2 probes and carefully fix the fiber glass cores to the sheathing using a clamp. Provide the probe with a customary silicone tubing; its length must be adjusted to the distance between the caudal and the cranial extremities of the left kidney. Attach tailored patches of gauze to the end of silicone tubing (*see* Fig. 2b). Measure the distance between the caudal and the cranial extremities of the left kidney by a caliper gauge. Based on this measurement, the cortical laser-flux-pO2-probe must be carefully prepared so that the distance between insertion point and the tip exactly matches the individual kidney's diameter minus 1.5 mm.

27. For *MR-PHYSIOL*, advance the cortical laser-flux-pO_2-probe meticulously from the caudal extremity of the kidney along the caudocranial axis (*see* Fig. 6c). To prevent craniocaudal displacement, the patch of gauze fixed to the silicone tubing of the probe (*see* Fig. 2b) must be stuck to the capsule of kidney's ventral surface by a thin layer of Histoacryl glue.
28. For *MR-PHYSIOL*, prepare the medullary laser-flux-pO_2-probe so that the distance between insertion point and the tip exactly matches the distance 3–4 mm. Carefully advance the medullary laser-flux-pO_2-probe from the caudal extremity of the kidney along the caudocranial axis. Stick the patch of gauze fixed to the silicone tubing of the probe to the capsule of kidney's ventral surface by Histoacryl glue (*see* Fig. 6c).
29. For *MR-PHYSIOL*, carefully fix the two probes' tubing to the retroperitoneal muscles by sutures in order to prevent displacement (*see* Fig. 6c).
30. Fill the abdominal cavity with warm saline (37 °C). For *PHYSIOL*, intermittent exchange of this fluid throughout the experiment is done via the open abdominal wall. As the abdomen will be closed for *MR-PHYSIOL* (see below), for replenishment of abdominal saline a catheter must be placed into the abdominal cavity. Furthermore, for *MR-PHYSIOL*, a fiber-optical temperature probe is placed in close proximity to the left kidney, in order to monitor the temperature of the kidney throughout the experiment.
31. Connect the probes with OxyLite/OxyFlo-apparatus and start the monitoring of tissue pO_2 and laser-Doppler-flux.
32. For *MR-PHYSIOL*, mark the localization of the investigated kidney's upper and lower pole from the outside on the abdominal skin using a pen. Check that the kidney (pen markings on skin) is still aligned with the mark on the portable animal holder that indicates the center of the RF coil—if necessary carefully correct the animal's position. This is essential for optimal positioning of the rat in the MRI scanner (i.e., optimal position of the rat's kidney relative to the MR coil).
33. For *MR-PHYSIOL*, place the special bridge of the portable animal holder right behind the rat's hind paws and fix all the technical extensions (temperature probe, Transonic probe, laser-flux-pO_2-probes, aortic occluder line and abdominal flushing catheter) to the bridge (*see* Fig. 5). Close the abdominal cavity of the rat by continuous suture while passing all extensions through the caudal cutting edge of the median abdominal incision. The extensions of the laser-flux-pO_2-probes must be led through the abdominal wall using a small incision in the left inguinal region.

34. Place a respiratory mask loosely around the muzzle of the spontaneously breathing rat. Open air supply to a rate of 1000 mL/min.
35. Restart the HAEMODYN software (to start a new data file) and check the quality of all physiological signals, that is, arterial pressure (measured caudal the aortic occlude and therefore equivalent to renal artery pressure, RAP), renal blood flow (RBF), cortical and medullary laser-Doppler-flux, and cortical and medullary pO_2.

3.2 Setting Up Animal for MR-PHYSIOL Examination

1. Transfer the animal into the MR scanner room using the portable animal holder (*see* **Note 7**). Position portable animal holder with the rat on the MR scanner's animal bed.
2. Switch on the small animal monitoring system. Place the pneumatic pillow on the abdomen, and cover the animal with the warming blanket. Watch the respiration trace on the monitor of the small animal monitoring system and adjust pillow position until the respiratory motion is captured well (*see* **Note 8**). Set the trigger options of the small animal monitoring system such that the trigger gate opens for the duration of the expiratory phase.
3. Position the animal bed in the MR scanner such that the kidney of interest is located at the isocenter of the magnet.
4. Perform anatomical imaging as described in the chapter by Pohlmann A et al. "Essential Practical Steps for MRI of the Kidney in Experimental Research."
5. Perform localized shimming on the kidney imaging as described in the chapter by Pohlmann A et al. "Essential Practical Steps for MRI of the Kidney in Experimental Research."

3.3 Experimental Procedures

A number of dedicated test procedures and the rationale behind the usage of the respective procedure is detailed in the chapter by Cantow K et al. "Reversible (Patho)Physiologically Relevant Test Interventions: Rationale and Examples." If adequate for the specific purpose of the study, reversible procedures (such as short periods of hypoxia, hyperoxia, and suprarenal aortic occlusion) are preferred, to keep the number of animals as small as possible as required by the 3R principle (*see* the chapter by Hosszu A et al. "Animal Models of Renal Pathophysiology and Disease"). Following each reversible intervention, appropriate time is given for complete recovery. The exact duration of the reversible intervention is dictated by the duration and number of MR measurements. Because MRI can interfere with parameters acquired by invasive probes (as has been observed for laser-Doppler flux), short intervals without MR measurements must be implemented. In the following, an exemplary protocol is given for an *MR-PHYSIOL* experiment. It must be noted, that for these experiments, the closest coordination among the operator(s) of the MR scanner, the person(s) who perform the test interventions and those who run the electronic data storage (including setting markers for events such as start and end of an intervention) is of the essence.

1. On the PC that acquires the physiological data set a "START" marker in the HAEMODYN software to monitor and store a first set of baseline data.
2. On the MR system run the protocol(s) of your choice (T_1-, T_2-, T_2*-mapping, DWI, etc.) to acquire a set of baseline data. Duplicate these scans for repeated measurements during/between/after the test interventions and ensure that all parameters remain identical, including the shim and receiver gain.
3. *Start of hypoxia*. Change the gas flowing through the respiratory mask to 10% O_2–90% N_2.
4. Set markers and acquire both physiological and MR data during the hypoxic challenge.
5. *End of hypoxia*. Change the gas flowing through the respiratory mask back to air (21% O_2).
6. Set markers and acquire both physiological and MR data during the recovery.
7. *Start of hyperoxia*. Change the gas flowing through the respiratory mask to 100% O_2.
8. Set markers and acquire both physiological and MR data during the hyperoxic challenge.
9. *End of hyperoxia*. Change the gas flowing through the respiratory mask back to air (21% O_2).
10. Set markers and acquire both physiological and MR data during the recovery.
11. *Start of occlusion*. Inflate the remotely controlled suprarenal aortic occluder.
12. Set markers and acquire both physiological and MR data during the occlusion (*see* **Note 9**).
13. *End of occlusion*. Rapidly deflate the occluder.
14. Set markers and acquire both physiological and MR data during the recovery.

3.4 End of Experiment

1. Carefully remove the respiratory mask from the animal's muzzle.
2. Cut all sutures; remove the fluid from the abdominal cavity using a pipette.
3. Control and note the overall condition of the kidney after experiment (e.g., surface coloring and its homogeneity).

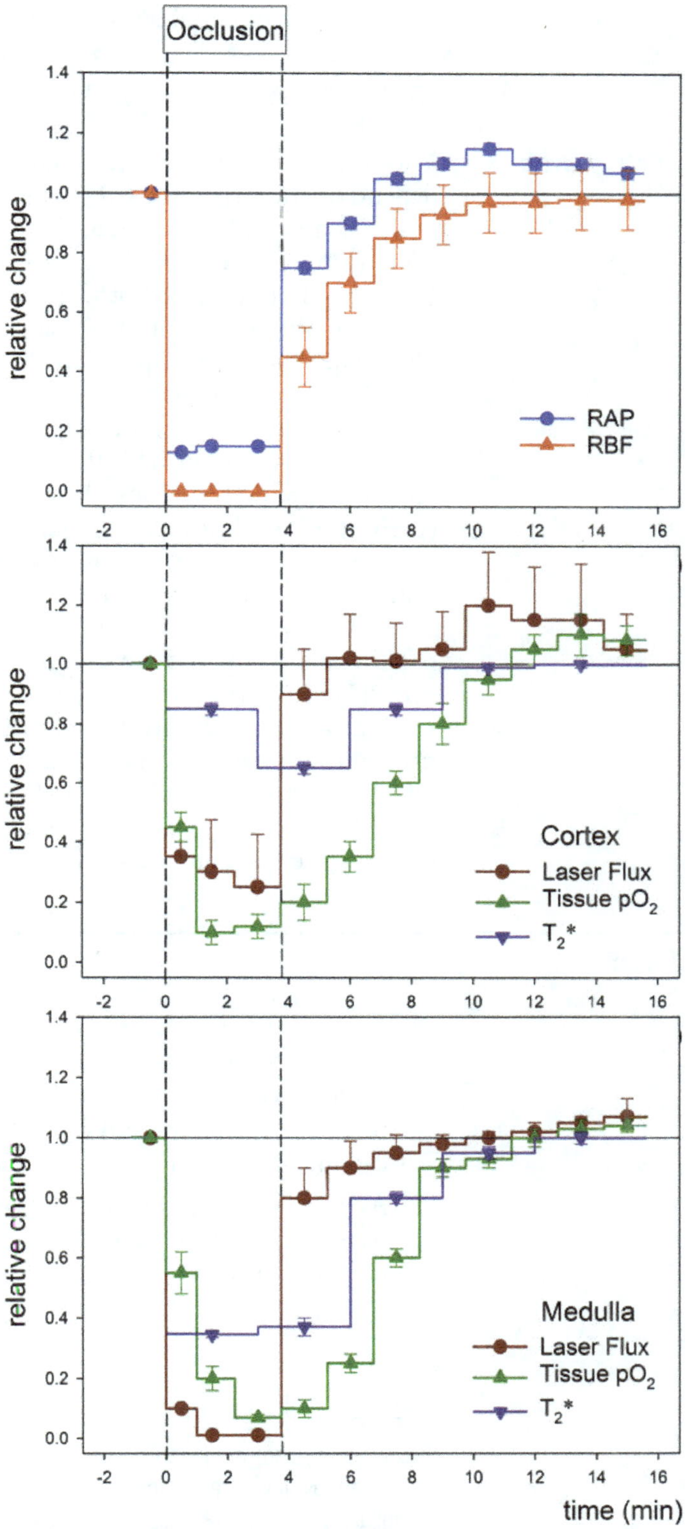

Fig. 7 Example of data obtained with *MR-PHYSIOL* in anesthetized rats (adapted from Ref. 39). Time courses of renal arterial pressure (RAP), total renal blood flow (RBF), cortical and medullary tissue perfusion (Laser Flux), cortical and

4. Carefully untie all sutures and knots; remove all probes and catheters, as well as the occluder.
5. Exsanguinate the animal by cutting the abdominal aorta.

3.5 Data Analysis

The analyses of MRI data acquired for *MR-PHYSIOL* experiments depend on the respective MR protocol and are detailed in dedicated analysis chapters for each MR method, which are part of the book Pohlmann A, Niendorf T (eds) (2020) Preclinical MRI of the Kidney—Methods and Protocols, Springer, New York.

Temporal alignment of MR and PHYSIOL data is achieved by identifying the starting point of the experiment within both data sets. For a direct comparison of the *MR-PHYSIOL* parameters only PHYSIOL data acquired during the relevant MRI acquisitions can be used. While the PHYSIOL parameters are measured with subsecond temporal resolution the acquisition of the MR parameters (derived from a MR image) requires much more time (e.g., about 60 s for a typical T_2^* mapping). PHYSIOL and MR parameters can only be compared based on the (low) temporal resolution of the MRI. For this purpose the average value of each physiological parameter over the acquisition time of each MRI scan is calculated. For PHYSIOL data that are influenced by MR acquisition (such as Laser flux signals) the averages over the times without MR acquisition must be taken. Finally, group analyses of the results (e.g., relative changes of MR and PHYSIOL data; *see* **Note 10**) are done, as shown by exemplary data obtained by *MR-PHYSIOL* during a short suprarenal aortic occlusion and recovery in Fig. 7.

4 Notes

1. Instead of a respiratory (anesthetic) mask, a tracheal cannula can be used, as it is custom-made in our lab using designed and made in our laboratory using polythene tubing. The ventral region of the throat and the trachea are opened surgically, the cannula is inserted and fixated by suture.
2. As another dedicated test of control of hemodynamics and oxygenation, hypercapnia can be used with an inspiratory fraction of CO_2 of 5% in air.

Fig. 7 (continued) medullary tissue partial pressure of oxygen (Tissue pO_2) as monitored by invasive methods (PHYSIOL) simultaneously with cortical and medullary T_2^* data (MR) acquired by a 9.4 T small animal MR scanner during suprarenal aortic occlusion and recovery. Date are given as relative changes (mean $\pm$ SEM) versus baseline (immediately before the occlusion)

3. Urethane supports anesthesia throughout the surgical preparation and the MRI examination (for several hours) and leaves cardiovascular and respiratory reflexes largely undisturbed.
4. (a) In order to prevent additional pressure on the aorta (and therefore development of an unintended kidney ischemia) the positioning and fixation of the aortic occluder must be performed under careful monitoring of the overall condition of the kidney (e.g., surface coloring and its homogeneity); (b) since the occluder consists of silicone and polyethylene and is positioned about 15 mm away from the kidney, it does not cause artefacts in MRI that affect the kidney.
5. (a) The signal of the probe used for *PHYSIOL* is too weak due to the long extension leads. For *MR-PHYSIOL* a probe with a larger body size and a reflector made of ceramics instead of metal must be used (*see* Fig. 1). Its reflector does not induce MR artifacts, is L-shaped and offers no mechanism to lock the vessel, which presents a significant challenge for the implantation if the probe. (b) The bulk of the intestine bears the risk to cause additional pressure that can dislocate the probe and cause probe pressure on the aorta, the renal artery and vein, or the kidney itself. (c) Since Transonic measurements rely on ultrasound an appropriate coupling into tissue is of high relevance. To this end the abdominal cavity must be filled with saline solution (37 °C) and no air bubbles must remain between probe and vessel. An additional catheter was placed in the abdominal cavity to replenish saline leakage in time course of the experiment.
6. Before inserting the tip of the respective probe, a small incision about the diameter of the probe is made into the renal capsule by means of the tip of a hypodermic needle to facilitate insertion of the rather dull tip probe.
7. Special attention during transfer must be paid to the tube/cable extensions (aortic occluder, abdominal flushing, and all probes). Make sure to keep tubes or cable close to the animal bed so they cannot get caught anywhere on the way into the magnet!
8. The peak-to-peak amplitude of the respiratory trace should span about 2/3 of the vertical axis on the display. Any gross movement (for instance during repositioning the pillow) will lead to large peaks and force the monitoring system to adapt the signal amplification, so that temporarily the signal will become much smaller on the display. Keep an eye on the magnification, which is given left next to the display, this will drop to a low value such as 15×—wait until it recovered back to a value around 100× before further adjusting it.

9. If unsuccessful, repeat the occlusion and inflate the occluder with higher hydraulic pressure and make sure that the fluid reservoir for the inflation is sufficiently filled. Always check that the inflation is sufficient to bring total renal blood flow (RBF) rapidly toward zero.
10. It is usually more practical and useful to compare relative changes in the parameters rather than absolute changes. To do this divide all parameter values by that of the last baseline value (e.g., *see* Fig. 7).

Acknowledgments

The authors wish to thank Ariane Anger, Andrea Gerhardt, Stefanie Münchberg, Yvonne Balke, and Victoria Prochnov for expert technical assistance.

This work was funded in part (Kathleen Cantow, Thoralf Niendorf, Andreas Pohlmann and Erdmann Seeliger) by the German Research Foundation (Gefoerdert durch die Deutsche Forschungsgemeinschaft (DFG), Project number / Projektnummer 394046635, SFB 1365, RENOPROTECTION).

This publication is based upon work from COST Action PARENCHIMA, supported by European Cooperation in Science and Technology (COST). COST (www.cost.eu) is a funding agency for research and innovation networks. COST Actions help connect research initiatives across Europe and enable scientists to enrich their ideas by sharing them with their peers. This boosts their research, career, and innovation.

PARENCHIMA (renalmri.org) is a community-driven Action in the COST program of the European Union, which unites more than 200 experts in renal MRI from 30 countries with the aim to improve the reproducibility and standardization of renal MRI biomarkers.

References

1. Fortrie G, de Geus HRH, Betjes MGH (2019) The aftermath of acute kidney injury: a narrative review of long-term mortality and renal function. Crit Care 23(1):24. https://doi.org/10.1186/s13054-019-2314-z
2. Selby NM, Taal MW (2019) Long-term outcomes after AKI-a major unmet clinical need. Kidney Int 95(1):21–23. https://doi.org/10.1016/j.kint.2018.09.005
3. Zuk A, Bonventre JV (2019) Recent advances in acute kidney injury and its consequences and impact on chronic kidney disease. Curr Opin Nephrol Hypertens. https://doi.org/10.1097/mnh.0000000000000504
4. Levin A, Tonelli M, Bonventre J, Coresh J, Donner JA, Fogo AB, Fox CS, Gansevoort RT, Heerspink HJL, Jardine M, Kasiske B, Kottgen A, Kretzler M, Levey AS, Luyckx VA, Mehta R, Moe O, Obrador G, Pannu N, Parikh CR, Perkovic V, Pollock C, Stenvinkel P, Tuttle KR, Wheeler DC, Eckardt KU (2017) Global kidney health 2017 and beyond: a roadmap for closing gaps in care, research, and policy. Lancet 390(10105):1888–1917. https://doi.org/10.1016/s0140-6736(17)30788-2
5. Bello AK, Levin A, Tonelli M, Okpechi IG, Feehally J, Harris D, Jindal K, Salako BL, Rateb A, Osman MA, Qarni B, Saad S,

Lunney M, Wiebe N, Ye F, Johnson DW (2017) Assessment of global kidney health care status. JAMA 317(18):1864–1881. https://doi.org/10.1001/jama.2017.4046

6. Brezis M, Rosen S (1995) Hypoxia of the renal medulla—its implications for disease. N Engl J Med 332:647–655
7. Fähling M, Seeliger E, Patzak A, Persson PB (2017) Understanding and preventing contrast-induced acute kidney injury. Nat Rev Nephrol 13(3):169–180
8. Evans RG, Ince C, Joles JA, Smith DW, May CN, O'Connor PM, Gardiner BS (2013) Haemodynamic influences on kidney oxygenation: the clinical implications of integrative physiology. Clin Exp Pharmacol Physiol 40:106–122
9. Evans RG, Ow CP, Bie P (2015) The chronic hypoxia hypothesis: the search for the smoking gun goes on. Am J Physiol Renal Physiol 308 (2):F101–F102
10. Shu S, Wang Y, Zheng M, Liu Z, Cai J, Tang C, Dong Z (2019) Hypoxia and hypoxia-inducible factors in kidney injury and repair. Cell 8(3). https://doi.org/10.3390/cells8030207
11. Hultstrom M, Becirovic-Agic M, Jonsson S (2018) Comparison of acute kidney injury of different etiology reveals in-common mechanisms of tissue damage. Physiol Genomics 50 (3):127–141. https://doi.org/10.1152/physiolgenomics.00037.2017
12. Calzavacca P, Evans RG, Bailey M, Bellomo R, May CN (2015) Cortical and medullary tissue perfusion and oxygenation in experimental septic acute kidney injury. Crit Care Med 43 (10):e431–e439
13. Ma S, Evans RG, Iguchi N, Tare M, Parkington HC, Bellomo R, May CN, Lankadeva YR (2019) Sepsis-induced acute kidney injury: a disease of the microcirculation. Microcirculation 26(2):e12483. https://doi.org/10.1111/micc.12483
14. Palm F, Carlsson PO, Hansell P, Hellberg O, Nygren A, Liss P (2003) Altered response in renal blood flow and oxygen tension to contrast media in diabetic rats. Acta Radiol 44 (3):347–353
15. Palm F, Cederberg J, Hansell P, Liss P, Carlsson PO (2003) Reactive oxygen species cause diabetes-induced decrease in renal oxygen tension. Diabetologia 46(8):1153–1160
16. dos Santos EA, Li LP, Ji L, Prasad PV (2007) Early changes with diabetes in renal medullary hemodynamics as evaluated by fiberoptic probes and BOLD magnetic resonance imaging. Investig Radiol 42(3):157–162. https://doi.org/10.1097/01.rli.0000252492.96709.36
17. Calvin AD, Misra S, Pflueger A (2010) Contrast-induced acute kidney injury and diabetic nephropathy. Nat Rev Nephrol 6 (11):679–688
18. Hansell P, Welch WJ, Blantz RC, Palm F (2013) Determinants of kidney oxygen consumption and their relationship to tissue oxygen tension in diabetes and hypertension. Clin Exp Pharmacol Physiol 40(2):123–137
19. Seeliger E, Flemming B, Wronski T, Ladwig M, Arakelyan K, Godes M, Mockel M, Persson PB (2007) Viscosity of contrast media perturbs renal hemodynamics. J Am Soc Nephrol 18 (11):2912–2920
20. Hoff U, Lukitsch I, Chaykovska L, Ladwig M, Arnold C, Manthati VL, Fuller TF, Schneider W, Gollasch M, Muller DN, Flemming B, Seeliger E, Luft FC, Falck JR, Dragun D, Schunck WH (2011) Inhibition of 20-HETE synthesis and action protects the kidney from ischemia/reperfusion injury. Kidney Int 79(1):57–65
21. Cantow K, Flemming B, Ladwig-Wiegard M, Persson PB, Seeliger E (2017) Low dose nitrite improves reoxygenation following renal ischemia in rats. Sci Rep 7(1):14597–15058
22. Seeliger E, Cantow K, Arakelyan K, Ladwig M, Persson PB, Flemming B (2014) Low-dose nitrite alleviates early effects of an X-ray contrast medium on renal hemodynamics and oxygenation in rats. Investig Radiol 49(2):70–77
23. Evans RG, Gardiner BS, Smith DW, O'Connor PM (2008) Methods for studying the physiology of kidney oxygenation. Clin Exp Pharmacol Physiol 35(12):1405–1412
24. Pohlmann A, Cantow K, Hentschel J, Arakelyan K, Ladwig M, Flemming B, Hoff U, Persson PB, Seeliger E, Niendorf T (2013) Linking non-invasive parametric MRI with invasive physiological measurements (MR-PHYSIOL): towards a hybrid and integrated approach for investigation of acute kidney injury in rats. Acta Physiol (Oxf) 207 (4):673–689
25. Hirakawa Y, Tanaka T, Nangaku M (2017) Renal hypoxia in CKD; pathophysiology and detecting methods. Front Physiol 8:99. https://doi.org/10.3389/fphys.2017.00099
26. Seeliger E, Wronski T, Ladwig M, Dobrowolski L, Vogel T, Godes M, Persson PB, Flemming B (2009) The renin-angiotensin system and the third mechanism of renal blood flow autoregulation. Am J Physiol Renal Physiol 296(6):F1334–F1345

27. Flemming B, Seeliger E, Wronski T, Steer K, Arenz N, Persson PB (2000) Oxygen and renal hemodynamics in the conscious rat. J Am Soc Nephrol 11(1):18–24
28. Ferrara F, Cantow K, Flemming B, Skalweit A, Ladwig M, Fähling M, Seeliger E (2017) Effects of liraglutide on control of renal hemodynamics and oxygenation in diabetic rats. Acta Physiol (Oxf) 219(Suppl 711):38
29. Cantow K, Pohlmann A, Flemming B, Ferrara F, Waiczies S, Grosenick D, Niendorf T, Seeliger E (2016) Acute effects of ferumoxytol on regulation of renal hemodynamics and oxygenation. Sci Rep 6:29965. https://doi.org/10.1038/srep29965
30. Emans TW, Janssen BJ, Pinkham MI, Ow CP, Evans RG, Joles JA, Malpas SC, Krediet CT, Koeners MP (2016) Exogenous and endogenous angiotensin-II decrease renal cortical oxygen tension in conscious rats by limiting renal blood flow. J Physiol 594(21):6287–6300. https://doi.org/10.1113/jp270731
31. Grosenick D, Cantow K, Arakelyan K, Wabnitz H, Flemming B, Skalweit A, Ladwig M, Macdonald R, Niendorf T, Seeliger E (2015) Detailing renal hemodynamics and oxygenation in rats by a combined near-infrared spectroscopy and invasive probe approach. Biomed Opt Express 6(2):309–323
32. Li LP, Halter S, Prasad PV (2008) Blood oxygen level-dependent MR imaging of the kidneys. Magn Reson Imaging Clin N Am 16 (4):613–625. viii
33. Niendorf T, Pohlmann A, Arakelyan K, Flemming B, Cantow K, Hentschel J, Grosenick D, Ladwig M, Reimann H, Klix S, Waiczies S, Seeliger E (2015) How bold is blood oxygenation level-dependent (BOLD) magnetic resonance imaging of the kidney? Opportunities, challenges and future directions. Acta Physiol (Oxf) 213(1):19–38
34. Grenier N, Merville P, Combe C (2016) Radiologic imaging of the renal parenchyma structure and function. Nat Rev Nephrol 12 (6):348–359
35. Niendorf T, Flemming B, Evans RG, Seeliger E (2016) What do BOLD MR imaging changes in donors' remaining kidneys tell us? Radiology 281(2):653–655
36. Brix S, Cantow K, Flemming B, Pohlmann A, Niendorf T, Seeliger E (2018) Interpretation of functional renal MRI findings: where physiology and imaging sciences need to talk across domains. J Magn Reson Imaging 47 (4):1140–1141. https://doi.org/10.1002/jmri.25829
37. Evans RG, Leong CL, Anderson WP, O'Connor PM (2007) Don't be so BOLD: potential limitations in the use of BOLD MRI for studies of renal oxygenation. Kidney Int 71 (12):1327–1328
38. Cantow K, Arakelyan K, Seeliger E, Niendorf T, Pohlmann A (2016) Assessment of renal hemodynamics and oxygenation by simultaneous magnetic resonance imaging (MRI) and quantitative invasive physiological measurements. Methods Mol Biol 1397:129–154. https://doi.org/10.1007/978-1-4939-3353-2_11
39. Pohlmann A, Arakelyan K, Hentschel J, Cantow K, Flemming B, Ladwig M, Waiczies S, Seeliger E, Niendorf T (2014) Detailing the relation between renal T2* and renal tissue pO2 using an integrated approach of parametric magnetic resonance imaging and invasive physiological measurements. Investig Radiol 49(8):547–560

9

Assessment of Renal Volume with MRI: Experimental Protocol

Andreas Müller and Martin Meier

Abstract

Renal length and volume are important parameters in the clinical assessment of patients with diabetes mellitus, kidney transplants, or renal artery stenosis. Kidney size is used in primary diagnostics to differentiate between acute (rather swollen kidneys) and chronic (rather small kidney) pathophysiology. Total kidney volume is also an established biomarker in studies for the treatment of autosomal dominant polycystic kidney disease (ADPKD). There are several factors influencing kidney size, and there is still a debate on the value of the measured kidney size in terms of renal function or cardiovascular risk. The renal volume is most often calculated by measuring the three axes of the kidney, on the assumption that the organ resembles an ellipsoid. By default, the longitudinal and transverse diameters of the kidney are measured. In animal models renal length and volume[1] are also important parameters in the assessment of organ rejection after transplantation and in determination of kidney failure due to renal artery stenosis, recurrent urinary tract infections, or diabetes mellitus. In general total kidney volume (TKV) is a valuable parameter for predicting prognosis and monitoring disease progression in animal models of human diseases like polycystic kidney disease (PKD) or acute kidney injury (AKI) and chronic kidney disease (CKD).

This chapter is based upon work from the COST Action PARENCHIMA, a community-driven network funded by the European Cooperation in Science and Technology (COST) program of the European Union, which aims to improve the reproducibility and standardization of renal MRI biomarkers. This analysis protocol is complemented by two separate chapters describing the basic concept and experimental procedure.

Key words Magnetic resonance imaging (MRI), Kidney, Mice, Rats, T_2, T_1, Volume

1 Introduction

Kidney size is used in primary diagnostics to differentiate between acute (rather swollen kidneys) and chronic (rather small kidney) pathophysiologies. Renal length and volume are important parameters in the clinical assessment of patients with diabetes mellitus, kidney transplants, or renal artery stenosis. Total kidney volume (TKV) is also qualified as a biomarker in studies for treatment of autosomal dominant polycystic kidney disease (ADPKD). According to the nonbinding recommendations of the FDA this

Andreas Pohlmann and Thoralf Niendorf (eds.), *Preclinical MRI of the Kidney: Methods and Protocols*, Methods in Molecular Biology, vol. 2216, https://doi.org/10.1007/978-1-0716-0978-1_21,

biomarker can be used by drug developers for the qualified context of use in submissions of investigational new drug applications, new drug applications, and biologics license applications (www.fda.gov/media/93105/download). There are many factors governing kidney size and volume.

In patients, renal volume is probably one of the most important predictive parameters for the loss of renal function. Therefore, a determination of kidney size is recommended for patients at risk. For example in ADPKD patients <30 years with a combined renal volume >1500 mL and an estimated glomerular filtration rate (eGFR) <90 mL/min are at high risk even with otherwise normal renal function. Such patients will need renal replacement therapy within 20 years. In ADPKD patients renal volume measurements have been studied extensively and provide a method for patient stratification, monitoring of disease progression and therapeutic efficacy [1–3].

Also, therapeutic decisions are frequently based on the size of the kidney, and for example routinely assessed in follow-up of patients with renal stenosis or for assessment of renal transplant candidates [4, 5]. Therefore it is important to employ a measuring method that provides accurate and precise results in vivo.

In animal models renal length and volume are also important parameters in the assessment of organ rejection after transplantation and in determination of kidney failure due to renal artery stenosis, recurrent urinary tract infections, or diabetes mellitus. In general total kidney volume (TKV) is a valuable parameter for predicting prognosis and monitoring disease progression in models of polycystic kidney disease (PKD). Still, so far, no gold standard exists for renal volumetry in vivo.

The renal volume is most often calculated by measuring the three axes of the kidney, on the assumption that the organ resembles an ellipsoid. By default, the longitudinal and transverse diameters of the kidney are measured. The kidney volume is calculated according to the following approximation formula (in humans these kidney volume data correlate well with the body length and age) (*see* Fig. 1):

$$\text{volume} = \text{length} \times \text{width} \times \text{average depth} \times 0.5.$$

Conventional anatomic MRI offers easy access to high quality image data. Kidney volume is reliably reproduced, and measurements can be performed with minimal bias and low inter- and intraoperator variability [6]. In the voxel-count method accurate calculation is facilitated by acquisition of multiple consecutive images sectioning the kidney. After identification of the organ boundaries, summation of all voxel volumes lying within the organ boundaries provides the total renal volume. While such an approach is highly accurate, it is also time-consuming. Transferring TKV measurement into everyday practice requires imaging techniques and protocols that are widely available while easy to employ

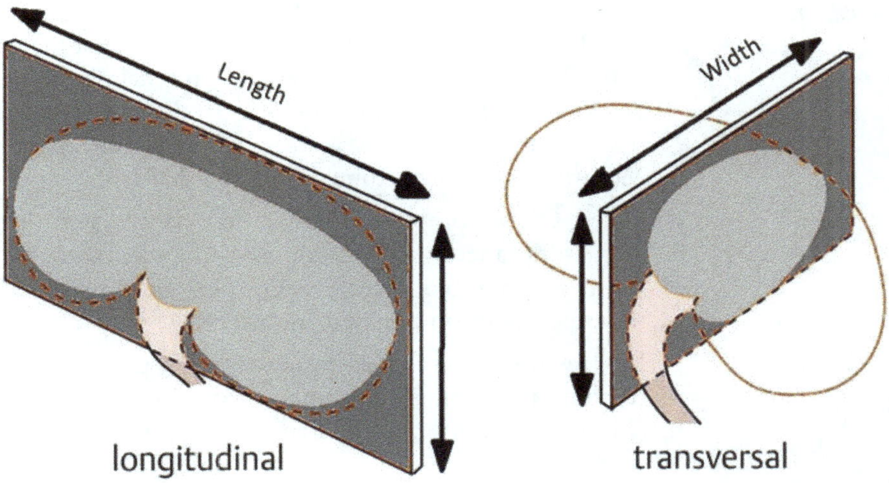

Fig. 1 Depicting standard measurement of length and width for ellipsoidal volume approximation of a kidney

and fast. Furthermore methods for interpretation of results are needed that are feasible and easy to apply. For this purpose open source image analysis tools are available that facilitate fast and easy determination of TKV.

For anatomical MRI of the kidney T_2 weighted MRI sequences are the modality of choice. They provide excellent contrast between different tissues and for the different compartments of the kidney itself. Standard spin-echo T_2 weighted imaging sequences are time-consuming due to the long repetition times TR. However, they still offer best image quality with respect to reproducibility and inter slice variability. Additionally such sequences can be modified easily to perform multiecho imaging, resulting in a set of images with different weighting that even can be used to calculate T_2 maps. In this tutorial we demonstrate the applicability of a 2D T_2 weighted multi echo MRI for accurate determination of kidney volume and compare different standardized TKV measurement techniques using MRI scanners developed for clinical routine imaging or dedicated to (preclinical) small animal imaging.

This chapter is part of the book Pohlmann A, Niendorf T (eds) (2020) Preclinical MRI of the Kidney—Methods and Protocols. Springer, New York.

2 Materials

2.1 Animals

These experimental protocols are tailored for mice (C57BL/6J) with a body mass of 20–30 g. Advice for adaptation to rat (Wistar, Sprague-Dawley or Lewis) is given in Subheading 4 where necessary.

2.2 Lab Equipment

1. Anesthesia: For standard experiments isoflurane inhalation (CP-Pharma, Baxter) provides robust anesthesia for up to 2 h with comparatively little side-effects on renal physiology. For a detailed description and discussion of the anesthesia please refer to the chapter by Kaucsar T et al. "Preparation and Monitoring of Small Animals in Renal MRI."
2. Gases: O_2 or compressed air, as delivering system for evaporated isoflurane. Besides air for use with pulse oximetry systems for monitoring blood oxygenation, O_2 gas is preferred during the experiment on diseased animals.
3. Devices for physiological monitoring ECG, temperature and respiration, to trigger the image acquisition: for example SAI (Model 1030, SAII, Stony Brook, NY, US).

2.3 MRI Hardware

The general hardware requirements for renal ^{1}H MRI on mice and rats are described in the chapter by Ramos Delgado P et al. "Hardware Considerations for Preclinical Magnetic Resonance of the Kidney" (open-access). The technique described in this chapter was tailored for a 9.4 T MR system (Biospec 94/20, Bruker Biospin, Ettlingen, Germany) but advice for adaptation to other field strengths and systems (e.g., 4.7 T Varian and 3 T Siemens Skyra human MR scanner using a wrist RF coil (for signal reception) or knee RF coil (transmit-receive)) is given where necessary.

With preclinical MRI systems volume RF coils covering the entire mouse or rat bodies can be used for signal transmission and reception. However, if needed signal-to-noise ratio (SNR) can be elevated by using dedicated surface receive RF coils (i.e., mouse heart four-element surface RF coil or rat heart four-element surface RF coil) in combination with linear polarized transmit only volume RF coils.

No other special or additional hardware is required.

2.4 MRI Protocols

For anatomical MRI of the kidney T_2-weighted MRI sequences are the modality of choice. Accelerated imaging techniques are available on all MRI systems. On Bruker systems they are identified by acronyms "RARE" or "turboRARE" (for *r*apid *a*cquisition *r*elaxation *e*nhanced). On Philips and Siemens scanners such sequences usually are denoted "FSE" or "TSE" (for *f*ast *s*pin *e*cho or *t*urbo *s*pin *e*cho).

2.5 Image Analysis Tools

MRI data can be analyzed easily by manual planimetry or by calculating TKV from length and width measurements with different standardized equations[2] (the "Traditional Ellipsoid," the "Mayo Ellipsoid," and the "Mid-slice Method"). For this we recommend employing the open source imaging tools ImageJ or IcY:

1. ImageJ (https://imagej.nih.gov/ij/) and the Versatile Wand Tool (https://imagej.nih.gov/ij/plugins/versatile-wand-tool/index.html).
2. IcY (http://icy.bioimageanalysis.org/).

For providing the ex vivo gold standard, kidney volumes can be additionally measured post mortem, using the fluid displacement method.

3 Methods

Renal volumes can be calculated in several ways, using the ellipsoid formula or the voxel-count method. For the ellipsoid formula calculation, the length is determined on the sagittal scans. The width and thickness will be measured at the hilum on the transverse scans. Width can also be measured at the largest transverse diameter. Both volume-hilum and volume-maximum will be calculated. Volume measurements using the ellipsoid formula can easily be done in less than 2 min. In most clinical studies, the ellipsoid method is commonly applied for renal volume assessment. With this method, it is assumed that the kidney resembles an ellipsoid structure. This leads to systematic underestimation of the renal volume. In fact the kidney is not a true ellipsoid structure.

With the voxel-count method, the volumes of all voxels within the boundary of the kidney are summated, thus giving the true total volume of the kidney so that obtaining inaccurate results is highly unlikely. For the voxel-count method, the kidney has to be segmented manually. Segmentations can be done by tracing the boundaries of the kidney on each slice. The total renal volume will then be calculated by summation of all voxel volumes lying within the boundaries of the kidney. Partial volume effects, which occur if voxels contain both kidney and surrounding tissue, could lead to overestimation of the kidney volume, if such voxels are included within the boundaries of the kidney. To avoid such an overestimation, the segmentation line can be drawn halfway along the change in signal intensity between the kidney and surrounding tissues. Semiautomatic segmentation techniques, such as region-growing, can save time. However, such methods are not really practical to use for most available software. Neighboring tissues with very similar signal intensity still have to be separated manually. Fat within the kidneys might perturb the segmentation of the boundaries due to fat-water chemical shift artifacts when using region-growing segmentation technique, leading to an underestimation of the total volume. Semiautomatic segmentation techniques are also challenging to perform on images obtained with accelerated T_2 weighted MRI sequences. While accelerated T_2 weighted imaging yields good results when organ morphology is considered, signal to noise ratio fluctuations between the individual slices due to spatial changes in the noise amplification intrinsic to parallel imaging techniques cannot be entirely prevented. For this reason, selection of threshold values and propagation has to be done individually for each slice and is a source for investigator bias and experimental error. Newer segmentation techniques, like automatic contour detection, might be an option in future software implementations.

Calculating renal volume from both coronal and sagittal scans can help eliminating differences due to aberrations in slice positioning.

Furthermore there is a simplified Mid-Slice Technique for MRI. In this technique, the renal volume is calculated from the area of a single middle slice image of the kidney multiplied by the number of slices. The kidney volumes correlate well with stereology and have high reproducibility comparable with manual planimetry. However, when calculating single kidney volumes, both the mid-slice technique and the ellipsoid formula are less accurate than stereology and manual or semiautomatic planimetry. Although significantly faster than manual tracing for calculating kidney volume, this technique is slower than the standard ellipsoid method. Volume estimates are based on a multiplier linked to the hypothesis that the shape of the kidney is ellipsoidal.

All these approaches rely on geometrical assumptions, that might not be true.

3.1 MR Protocol Setup

3.1.1 Multislice Multiecho Sequence for T_2 Imaging

1. Load the 2D multislice multiecho sequence (MSME). (preferred *see* **Note 1**)
2. Set the shortest echo time (TE) and echo spacing (ΔTE) possible, under the condition that fat and water are in phase (*see* **Note 2**). The last TE should be close to the largest expected $T_2^{(*)}$ in the kidney multiplied by 1.5 (*see* **Note 3**). The aim is to acquire at least five echo images. Consider increasing the acquisition bandwidth and using half Fourier acceleration to shorten the first TE and ΔTE (*see* **Note 4**).
3. Choose the shortest possible repetition time (TR) for good signal-to-noise per time (SNR/t) efficiency. TR will be limited by the length of the echo train and the number of slices you acquire.
4. Adapt the flip angle (FA) to the TR and T_1 in order to achieve the best possible SNR. Use the Ernst angle $\alpha_E = \arccos(\exp(-TR/T_1))$ as a good starting value. Then try a few smaller and larger FAs and determine the optimal FA experimentally by comparing the measured SNRs.
5. Set a high acquisition bandwidth (BW) to shorten ΔTE, while keeping an eye on the SNR, which decreases with the square

root of BW. Low SNR may be balanced out with averaging (*see* **Note 5**).

6. Enable fat saturation. On ultrahigh field systems this works well to avoid fat signal overlaying the kidney due to chemical shift. At lower field strengths it might work less efficient.
7. Enable the respiration trigger (per phase step or per slice). This is essential to reduce motion artifacts (*see* also **Note 6**), reduce motion blurring and unwanted intensities variations among the images acquired with different TEs.
8. Choose as phase-encoding direction the L-R direction and adapt the geometry so that the FOV in this direction includes the entire animal (approx. 40 mm).
9. Use frequency encoding in head-feet (rostral-caudal) direction to avoid severe aliasing. Adjust the FOV to your needs keeping in mind that in this direction the FOV can be smaller than the animal and a smaller FOV permits a smaller acquisition matrix, and in turn a shorter echo-spacing.
10. Use an appropriate slice thickness, typically around 1.0 mm.
11. Use high in-plane resolution that the SNR allows, typically between 100 and 200 μm. Zero-filling in phase encoding direction can be helpful to speed up acquisition. One may use half Fourier in read direction (asymmetric echo) to further shorten the first TE, if very short T_2* (<5 ms) can occur. Reducing the excitation pulse length to below 1 ms would then also help to shorten TE.
12. A spin echo sequence (MSME) with an echo time of >20 ms is very sensitive for instabilities of your system. If the system is not stable for any reason, this can often be observed directly at the time signal.
13. For examples of specific parameter sets please *see* **Notes 9–13**.

3.2 In Vivo MR Imaging

After obtaining scout images in the *x*, *y*, and *z* planes, T_2-weighted MRI should be performed in sagittal and coronal orientation.

When selecting a certain type of MRI sequence and its parameters, an optimum should be established between spatial resolution, signal-to-noise ratio, and scan duration. Accuracy of the volume measurements can be enhanced by reducing slice thickness and/or choosing an additional section orientation transverse to the major axis of the kidney, mostly in axial orientation.

While theoretically beneficial for discrimination of kidney size differences, measurements in multiple orthogonal planes across the kidney prolong examination times and increase the time required for segmentation, thus hampering both clinical and preclinical practice. This holds also true for application of sophisticated high resolution T_2 weighted 3D imaging techniques instead of standard (multislice) 2D T_2 weighted MRI covering the entire kidney. Especially in preclinical studies of diseased animals, it is often more appropriate to use solely a single slice orientation 2D MRI approach to gather standardized images in minimum time (i.e., to reduce length of anesthesia). If reduction of imaging time is of particular importance, accelerated imaging techniques are recommended. Such sequences should be available on all MRI systems. On Bruker systems they are identified by acronyms "RARE" or "turboRARE" (for rapid acquisition relaxation enhanced). On Siemens scanners such sequences usually are denoted "FSE" or "TSE" (for fast spin echo or turbo spin echo). In these measurement techniques acceleration is facilitated mainly by recording of multiple lines of k-space, that is, performing multiple phase-encoding steps on the echo train.

3.2.1 Scanner Adjustments and Anatomical Imaging

1. Acquire a fast pilot scan to obtain images in the three orthogonal planes *x*, *y*, and *z*.
2. Acquire anatomical images in several oblique orientations to facilitate planning a coronal slice orientation with regard to the long axis of the kidney, as described in the chapter by Pohlmann A et al. "Essential Practical Steps for MRI of the Kidney in Experimental Research."
3. Perform localized shimming on the kidney as described in the chapter by Pohlmann A et al. "Essential Practical Steps for MRI of the Kidney in Experimental Research."

3.2.2 Morphometric MR Imaging

1. Load the MSME sequence, adapt the slice orientation to provide a coronal or axial view with respect to the kidney (in scanner coordinates this is double-oblique). (caveat *see* **Note 8**)
2. In the monitoring unit set the trigger delay so that the trigger starts at the beginning of the expiratory plateau (no chest or diaphragm motion) and the duration such that it covers the entire expiratory phase, that is, until just before inhalation starts (1/2 to 2/3 of breath-to-breath interval) (*see* **Note 7**).
3. Adapt TR to be a little shorter (about 100 ms) than the average respiration interval that is displayed on the physiological monitoring unit.
4. Run the MSME scan. Example images are shown in Figs. 2, 3, and 4.

A demonstration of the volume changes that can be expected in pathophysiological scenarios is given in Fig. 4.

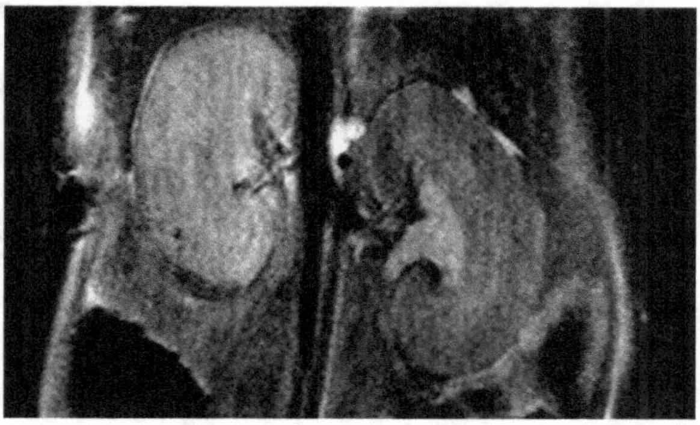

Fig. 2 T_2 weighted image of mouse kidneys in coronal view. For the quantification of kidney volume, respiratory triggered, fat-saturated T2-weighted turbo spin echo (TSE) sequences were acquired in axial and coronal planes, covering both kidneys. The coronal plane was adjusted to the long axis of both kidneys. Scan parameters were: TR/TE = 1500/33 ms, averages = 2, matrix = 256x256, field of view = 35x35 mm2, slice thickness = 1 mm

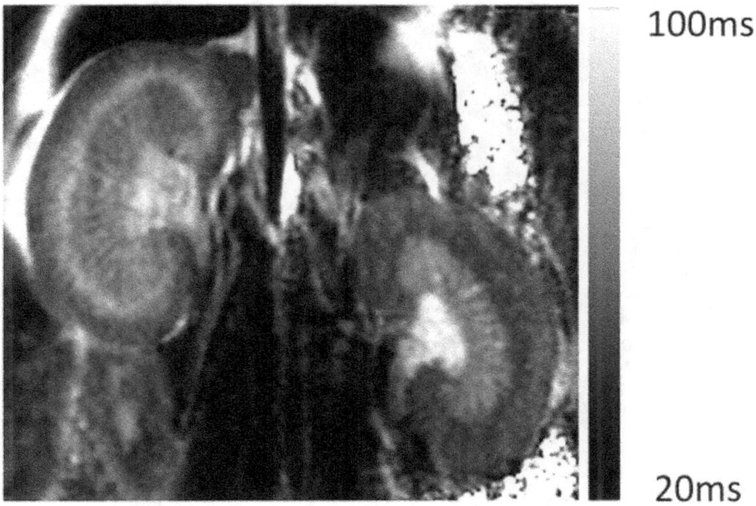

Fig. 3 T_2 map of mouse kidneys with AKI (left). Note the different T_2 values in cortex and medulla between left and right kidney

4 Notes

1. A 3D version of the turboRARE sequence is also available, which allows thinner slices with better SNR, but tends to be too slow for most in vivo applications.
2. The fat signal has a slightly different Larmor frequency (fat-water shift: Δf = 3.5 ppm × Larmor frequency or

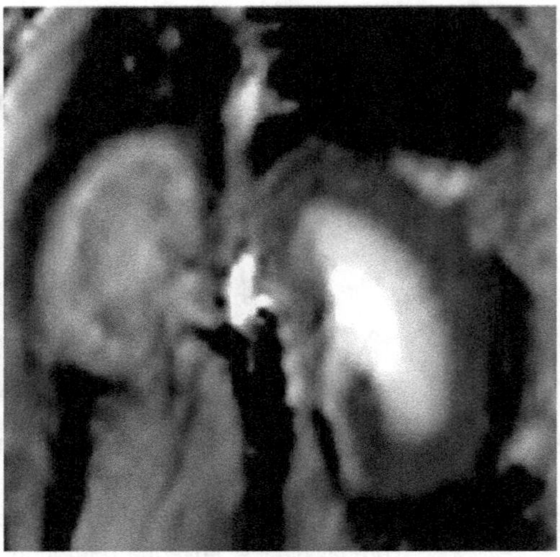

Fig. 4 MSME permits easy detection of size differences in kidneys after acute kidney failure

146 Hz/T, for example: $\Delta f = 220$ Hz at 1.5 T) than the water signal. The faster precession of the fat protons means that with increasing time the fat and water signal fractions within a voxel are sometimes in phase (signals add up) and sometime out of phase (signals subtract). This can lead to an unwanted fat-water shift induced signal intensity modulation along the exponential signal decay curve. This is mostly relevant for diseased kidneys with increased fat content (e.g., diabetes), but we recommend to generally take this into account, that is, also for healthy kidneys. The TEs at which fat and water are in phase depend on the field strength: TE [ms] $= n \times (6.7069/B_0[T])$.

3. When establishing the MR technique you need to define an SNR acceptance threshold for the image with the shortest TE. The aim is to have at least three (better five or more) number of echoes with an SNR > 5. This threshold will depend on the expected $T_2^{(*)}$ values, which in turn depends on parameters like the magnetic field strength, shim quality, and tissue properties (pathology). Example: For a rat imaged at 9.4 T using a four-element rat heart array receive surface RF coil together with a volume RF resonator for excitation in combination with interventions leading to strong hypoxia, an SNR > 60 was needed.
4. For rats increase the FOV to the body width and keep the matrix size the same. The relative resolution is then identical and the SNR should also be similar, because the smaller mouse RF coil provides better SNR.

5. A good starting point is to use the same relative resolution as for rats. For this, reduce the FOV to the mouse body width and keep the matrix size the same.
6. If no specific animal holder is used, it is preferable to position the animals in left or right decubitus position to keep the bowels away from the kidneys to mitigate susceptibility artifacts.
7. You must monitor the respiration continuously throughout the entire experiment and if necessary adapt the TR accordingly.
8. Acquiring more echoes with smaller echo spacing will be beneficial because it improves the fitting when calculating a T_2 map (*see* Fig.3), but keep in mind the specific absorption rate (SAR) associated with sending many 180° RF pulses in a short time could heat up the tissue. This will usually not be detectable via a rectal temperature probe, but measurements with a temperature probe placed in the abdomen next to the kidney showed that significant temperature increases are possible with a multispin echo sequence.
9. Ellipsoid based calculation: Example parameters for a 300 g rat at 9.4 T (Bruker small animal system): TR = [respiration interval] -100 ms; receiver bandwidth = 50 kHz; number of echoes = 12; first echo = 10.0 ms; echo spacing 10.0 ms; TE = 10, 20, 30, 40, 50, 60, 70, 80, 90, 100, 110, 120 ms; averages = 1; slice orientation = coronal to kidney; frequency encoding = head-feet; FOV = (38.2 × 48.5) mm; matrix size = 169 × 115 zero-filled to 169 × 215; resolution = (0.226 × 0.421) mm; 1 slice with 1.4 mm thickness; fat suppression = on; respiration trigger = per slice; acquisition time = 55–75 s (with triggering under urethane anesthesia).
10. *Ellipsoid based calculation: Example parameters for a 30 g mouse at 4.7 T (Agilent small animal system)*: TR = [respiration interval] − 100 ms; receiver bandwidth = 50 kHz; number of echoes = 12; first echo = 10.0 ms; echo spacing 10.0 ms; TE = 10, ..., 120 ms; averages = 1; slice orientation = coronal to kidney; frequency encoding = head-feet; FOV = (30 × 30) mm; matrix size = 128 × 128; resolution = (0.230 × 0.230) mm; 1 slice with 1.0 mm thickness; fat suppression = on; respiration trigger = on; acquisition time = 3.5–9.0 min (with triggering under isoflurane anesthesia).
11. *Ellipsoid based calculation: Example parameters for a 300 g rat at 3.0 T (Siemens Skyra^{fit}, a clinical system)*: Animal position: Right decubitus; Coil: Knee; TR = [respiration interval] − 500 ms; receiver bandwidth = 399 Hz/pixel; number of echoes = 12; first echo = 10.0 ms; echo spacing 10.0 ms; TE = 10, ..., 120 ms; averages = 2; slice orientation = axial;

frequency encoding = left-right; FOV = (120x60) mm; matrix size = 256 × 128; resolution = (0.470 × 0.470) mm; 1 slice with 2.0 mm thickness; fat suppression = on; respiration trigger = off; acquisition time ~ 2 min. If no specific animal holder is used, it is preferable to position the animals in left of right decubitus position to keep the bowels away from the kidneys to mitigate susceptibility artifacts.

12. *Planimetry based calculation: Example parameters for a 300 g rat at 9.4 T (Bruker small animal system)*: TR = 1700 ms; receiver bandwidth = 50 kHz; number of echoes = 12; first echo = 10.0 ms; echo spacing 10.0 ms; TE = 10, 20, 30, 40, 50, 60, 70, 80, 90, 100, 110, 120 ms; averages = 1; slice orientation = coronal to kidney; frequency encoding = head-feet; FOV = (38.2 × 48.5) mm; matrix size = 169 × 115 zero-filled to 169 × 215; resolution = (0.226 × 0.421) mm; 13 slices at 1 mm thickness; fat suppression = on; respiration trigger = per slice; acquisition time = 220–300 s (with triggering under isoflurane anesthesia).

    The following images should be acquired: coronal and transverse T2-weighted fast spin-echo sequence (TSE) and coronal T1-weighted TSE.

    The following images should be acquired: coronal and transverse T2-weighted fast spin-echo sequence (TSE) and coronal T1-weighted TSE.

    The parameters for coronal position TSE can be as follows: slice thickness, 2.0 mm; slice interval, 0.2 mm.

    For T_1 weighted turbo spin-echo (TSE): repetition time (TR), 650 ms; echo time (TE), 10 ms; field of view (FOV), 120 mm × 120 mm; band width, 250 Hz/Px; matrix, 256 × 256; and number of excitations (NEX), 4.0;

    For T_2 weighted TSE you can use: TR, 3460 ms; TE, 35 ms; FOV, 120 mm × 120 mm; band width, 250 Hz/Px; matrix, 256 × 256; and NEX, 4.0.

    The parameters for the transverse position T_2 TSE can be as follows: slice thickness, 2.0 mm; slice interval, 0.2 mm; TR, 650 ms; TE, 10 ms; FOV, 120 mm × 120 mm; band width, 250 Hz/Px; matrix, 256 × 256; and NEX, 4.0.

    Shimming is particularly important, since macroscopic magnetic field inhomogeneities shorten T_2*, but provide no tissue specific information—rather they overshadow the microscopic T_2* effects of interest and hinder quantitative intra- and intersubject comparisons. Shimming should be performed on a voxel enclosing only the kidney using either the default iterative shimming method or based on previously recorded field maps (recommended).

13. If the height adjusted total kidney volume (HtTKV) must be calculated it can be done by measuring the kidneys in three

axes. To calculate HtTKV a structural MRI or at least CT scan is required. The height of the patient is also required for the calculation. The total kidney volume (TKV) is determined using an ellipsoid equation. This is clinically validated for patients with polycystic disease, with bilateral and diffuse small to medium sized cysts. The ellipsoid equation requires only three measurements from both kidneys:

- Kidney length.
- Kidney width.
- Kidney depth.

If you are viewing images on PACs or any DICOM-Viewer it is easiest to calculate the HtTKV with all planes of the kidney visible at the same time. To do this, you mostly have to select "MPR" under the available "View Options" in the specific menu.With this you can view the kidney in the coronal, sagittal, and axial planes. The maximum length of the kidney should be measured in the sagittal plane.

The width and depth can be measured in the axial plane in a slice that shows the greatest kidney width and depth.Repeat this for both kidneys. Once you have all six measurements and the patient's height, you can calculate HtTKV or use one of the available online calculators for kidney volume.

Acknowledgments

This chapter is based upon work from COST Action PARENCHIMA, supported by European Cooperation in Science and Technology (COST). COST (www.cost.eu) is a funding agency for research and innovation networks. COST Actions help connect research initiatives across Europe and enable scientists to enrich their ideas by sharing them with their peers. This boosts their research, career, and innovation.

PARENCHIMA (renalmri.org) is a community-driven Action in the COST program of the European Union, which unites more than 200 experts in renal MRI from 30 countries with the aim to improve the reproducibility and standardization of renal MRI biomarkers.

References

1. King BF, Reed JE, Bergstralh EJ, et al (2000) Quantification and longitudinal trends of kidney, renal cyst, and renal parenchyma volumes in autosomal dominant polycystic kidney disease. 11:1505–1511
2. Sise C, Kusaka M, Wetzel LH et al (2000) Volumetric determination of progression in autosomal dominant polycystic kidney disease by computed tomography. Kidney Int 58:2492–2501
3. Grantham JJ, Torres VE (2016) The importance of total kidney volume in evaluating progression of polycystic kidney disease. Nat Rev Nephrol 12:667–677

4. Hederström E, Forsberg L (1985) Kidney size in children assessed by ultrasonography and urography. Acta Radiol Diagn (Stockh) 26:85–91
5. Ferrer FA, McKenna PH, Bauer MB et al (1997) Accuracy of renal ultrasound measurements for predicting actual kidney size. J Urol 157:2278–2281
6. Sharma K, Caroli A, Quach LV et al (2017) Kidney volume measurement methods for clinical studies on autosomal dominant polycystic kidney disease. PLoS One 12:e0178488

10

Sodium (^{23}Na) MRI of the Kidney: Basic Concept

James T. Grist, Esben Søvsø Hansen, Frank G. Zöllner, and Christoffer Laustsen

Abstract

The handling of sodium by the renal system is a key indicator of renal function. Alterations in the corticomedullary distribution of sodium are considered important indicators of pathology in renal diseases. The derangement of sodium handling can be noninvasively imaged using sodium magnetic resonance imaging (^{23}Na MRI), with data analysis allowing for the assessment of the corticomedullary sodium gradient. Here we introduce sodium imaging, describe the existing methods, and give an overview of preclinical sodium imaging applications to illustrate the utility and applicability of this technique for measuring renal sodium handling.

This chapter is based upon work from the COST Action PARENCHIMA, a community-driven network funded by the European Cooperation in Science and Technology (COST) program of the European Union, which aims to improve the reproducibility and standardization of renal MRI biomarkers. This introduction chapter is complemented by two separate chapters describing the experimental procedure and data analysis.

Key words Magnetic resonance imaging (MRI), Kidney, Mice, Rats, ^{23}Na, Sodium

1 Introduction

In this chapter, we describe renal sodium imaging, as acquired with magnetic resonance imaging (MRI). An introduction to the many methods that can be used to acquire sodium (23Na) signal is presented, as well as the postprocessing required to quantitatively describe the signal in terms of relaxation or concentration. Example applications of sodium renal imaging are discussed—ranging from the action of diuretic drugs to early sodium handling alterations in acute kidney injury. This introduction is complemented by two separate chapters describing the experimental procedure and data analysis, which are part of this book.

This chapter is part of the book Pohlmann A, Niendorf T (eds) (2020) Preclinical MRI of the Kidney—Methods and Protocols. Springer, New York.

Andreas Pohlmann and Thoralf Niendorf (eds.), *Preclinical MRI of the Kidney: Methods and Protocols*, Methods in Molecular Biology, vol. 2216, https://doi.org/10.1007/978-1-0716-0978-1_15, © The Author(s) 2021

2 Measurement Concept

2.1 Basic Concept of Sodium Imaging

Sodium imaging can provide quantitative measures of the ^{23}Na concentration in tissue [1]. It utilizes the signal from the sodium nucleus, found in both the intra- and extracellular compartments, to acquire images of the ^{23}Na biodistribution. Due to the low natural abundance of biological sodium, in comparison to water, as well as a rapid quadrupolar relaxation and lower gyromagnetic ratio (spin $= \frac{3}{2}$, $\gamma = 11.262\,\frac{\text{MHz}}{\text{T}}$), approximately ¼ of protons, the signal available is much lower than that of conventional ^{1}H MRI [2]. The fast quadrupolar relaxation recovers some of the disadvantages of imaging ^{23}Na, as very short repetition times (TR) can be used, albeit the ultrafast T_2^* relaxation imposing constraints on the imaging technique used. Commonly, the total (meaning from both the intra- and extracellular compartments) sodium signal is acquired through the use of surface or RF volume coils, at high magnetic field strengths (3–9.4 T) using gradient echo-based imaging technique [3–6]. It is possible to suppress some of the extracellular signal, to give an "intracellular weighted" image, with advanced techniques such as inversion signal nulling or triple quantum filtering (TQF) [7, 8]. An estimate of the difference in the intra- and extracellular compartment sizes is feasible through the use of T_2^* mapping [9]. It is noted that no current use of TQF or inversion recovery signal nulling have been undertaken in renal studies; however, there are a number of publications in neurological work [8, 10, 11].

2.2 Sodium Imaging Methods

There are a number of imaging methods available for mapping the biodistribution of sodium in the renal system. The sodium signal detected in a simple imaging experiment is a combination of intra- and extracellular compartments, termed the "total" sodium signal. The three main methods used to differentiate the intra- and extracellular sodium signals are triple quantum filtering, inversion recovery fluid attenuation (IR), and T_2^* mapping.

2.2.1 Sodium MRI Hardware

For signal reception, the MR scanners need to be equipped by RF transmitters and receive RF coils tuned to the resonance frequency of the sodium nuclei at the respective magnetic field strength. Today, such extensions are supported by some vendors of preclinical systems. In the following, hardware developments for quantitative ^{23}Na-MRI in preclinical are briefly outlined.

For the first time, Barberi et al. introduced the transmit-only receive-only (TORO) system, the so-called dual radiofrequency (RF) resonator, which is based on the idea of separated transmit and receive RF elements [12]. In contrast to the standard RF resonators in transceiver (TXRX) mode (e.g., surface coil or birdcage), the dual RF resonator allows for both a homogeneous transmit B_1^+ field and a highly sensitive receive B_1^- field [12, 13].

Kalacycian et al. developed a homogeneous transmit-only volume resonator and a highly sensitive RO surface resonator for renal ^{23}Na-MRI for 3 T or 9.4 T MRI scanners [14]. For this setup the sensitivity correction needs to be performed only for the receive profile. Furthermore, the dual resonator allows for increased ^{23}Na-MR signal sensitivity due to the localized signal detection using RO surface coils. For the dedicated task of bilateral kidney imaging, a dual resonator system (TORO) including a two-element phased array at 9.4 T and a receiver saddle shaped RF resonator at 3 T was implemented [13]. These systems were tailored for measuring the absolute renal TSC in rat kidney models with high spatiotemporal resolution, and high concentration measurement accuracy.

2.2.2 Total Sodium Imaging

Total sodium imaging is typically performed using a gradient echo-based technique. To ensure that the conversion from the imaging signal to the sodium concentration is accurate, a repetition time of approximately 2.5 times the T_1 of tissue sodium (approximately 25 ms at 3 T, and longer at higher field strengths) is essential. Further optimization of the sequence readout can be undertaken to capture the fast T_2^* relaxation of the sodium nucleus. For example, an ultrashort echo time (UTE) approach such as radial or twisted projection imaging is preferred over conventional Cartesian strategies. Due to the inherent low SNR of sodium acquisitions, it is common to average a number of sodium scans from the same subject; however, this may lead to long scan times.

An example of total sodium imaging pulse sequence, and renal images, are provided in Figs. 1a and 2.

2.2.3 Triple Quantum Filtering (TQF)

Due to the $\frac{3}{2}$ spin of the sodium nucleus, a biexponential T_2^* is exhibited by the isotope. A single excitation with a 90-degree hard pulse causes a transition of spins between the outer spin states ($\frac{3}{2}$ to $\frac{1}{2}$ and $-\frac{1}{2}$ to $-\frac{3}{2}$) as well as the inner states ($\frac{1}{2}$ to $-\frac{1}{2}$). The outer spin states exhibit a faster T_2^* decay than the inner. Using phase-cycled radiofrequency pulses it is possible to isolate the signal of slow-moving spins in the intracellular compartment, while removing the extracellular contribution [15].

There are a number of limitations to TQF though. The challenges include long scan times and high energy deposition required due to a large SNR penalty of the TQF technique. Furthermore, inhomogeneity in main magnetic field distribution can lead to spurious results, with corrections in reconstruction required to counter the B_0-nonuniformity effects [10]. An example triple quantum filtering sodium imaging pulse sequence is shown in Fig. 1b.

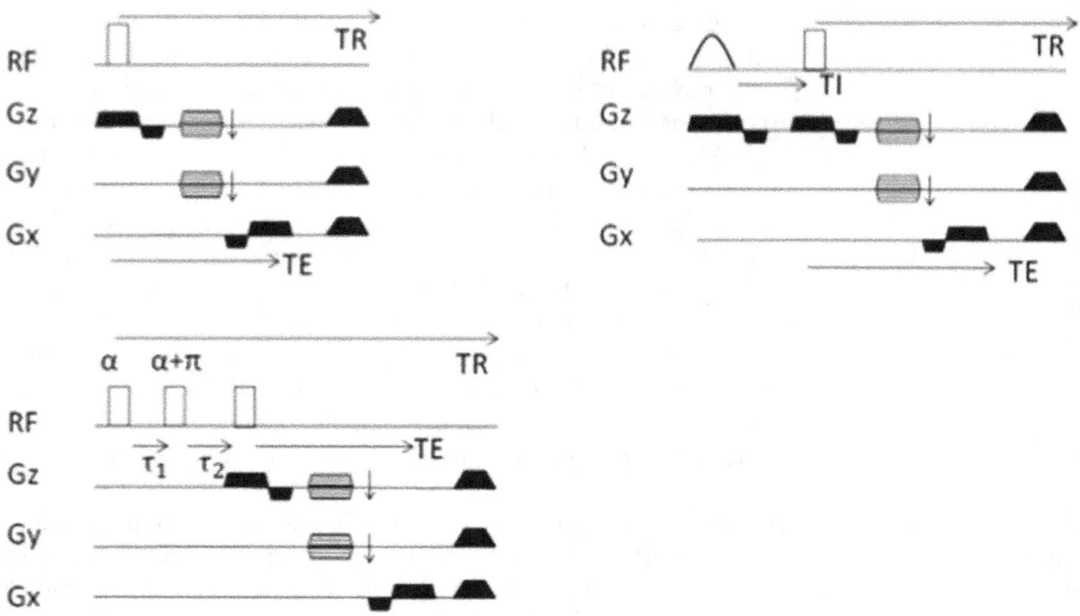

Fig. 1 Sodium imaging pulse sequences. (**a**) Total sodium imaging sequence using a 3D GRE readout. TR = Repetition time, TE = Echo time. (**b**) Triple Quantum Filtered sodium imaging pulse sequence using a 3D GRE readout. α = phase of pulse 1, T1 = Mixing time 1, T2 = Mixing time 2. (**c**) Inversion prepared sodium imaging pulse sequence. TI = Inversion preparation time (determined experimentally)

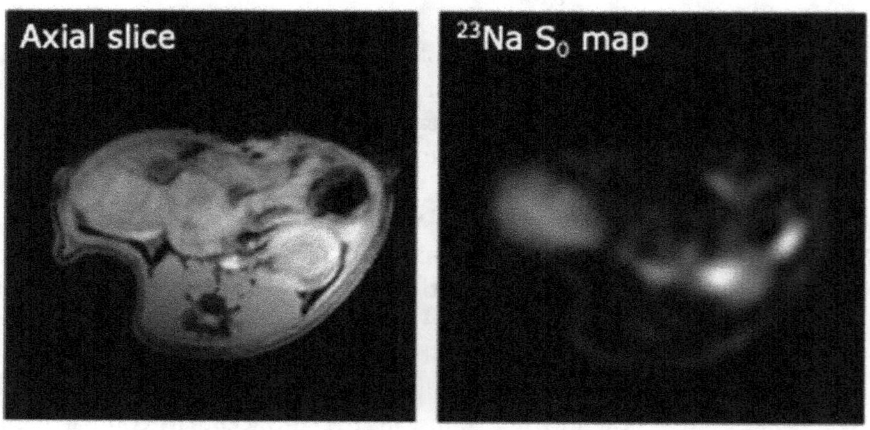

Fig. 2 Example rodent renal ^{1}H (left) and sodium (right) imaging acquired at 9.4 T

2.2.4 Inversion Recovery

Utilizing the difference in T_1 between bound and unbound sodium, it is possible to null the signal contribution fluid compartment using an inversion pulse, whilst retaining the bound signal, as described through Eqs. 1 and 2 [7].

$$S(\mathrm{TI}) = S_0\left(1 - \exp\left(-\frac{\mathrm{TI}}{T_1}\right)\right) \quad (1)$$

$$\mathrm{TI}_{\mathrm{null}} = \ln(2)\, T_1^{\mathrm{Fluid}} \quad (2)$$

where TI is the inversion time, T_1 is the relaxation constant of free sodium, S_0 is the initial sodium NMR signal, and S(TI) is the signal at TI. An example of an inversion recovery sodium imaging technique is illustrated in Fig. 1c.

2.2.5 T2* Mapping

T_2^* mapping is performed with either a multiecho based gradient echo sequence, or many individual scans with an incremented echo time (TE). It is currently thought that the shorter T_2^* component (1-5 ms at 3 T) is derived from the intracellular compartment, and the longer (10–30 ms at 3 T) from the extracellular compartment [9, 16]. T2* mapping therefore could be sensitive to changes in the intracellular–extracellular renal sodium balance.

A multiecho or incremented echo series can be used to derive both the pool sizes and T_2^* time constant for each compartment through Eq. **3**.

$$S(\mathrm{TE}) = \left(a\exp\left(-\frac{\mathrm{TE}}{T^*_{2,\mathrm{Short}}}\right) + b\exp\left(-\frac{\mathrm{TE}}{T^*_{2,\mathrm{Long}}}\right)\right) \tag{3}$$

where S(TE) is the signal at a given echo time, a and b are the intra- and extracellular pool sizes, respectively, and $T^*_{2,\mathrm{Short}}$ and $T^*_{2,\mathrm{Long}}$ are the biexponential relaxation constants.

2.3 Imaging Readout

Due to the rapid decay of the sodium signal, fast gradient echo-based imaging methods are commonly employed for data acquisition. A large number of encoding schemes are present in the literature, encompassing Cartesian and non-Cartesian imaging [17]. Below is a summary of most frequently applied methods.

2.3.1 3D Cartesian Imaging

The majority of preclinical imaging has been undertaken with 3D gradient echo Cartesian imaging, whereby a volume of k-space is sampled using trapezoidal readout gradients. Due to the ease of implementation on a preclinical system, this has been the sequence of choice for a number studies in rodents [3–5]. However, as Cartesian imaging requires encoding in k_y and k_z directions prior to data acquisition, the minimum echo time available for imaging is substantially longer than in other methods available for use in future studies.

2.3.2 Ultrashort Echo Time (UTE) Imaging

In order to shorten the echo time of acquisition, thereby increasing the total signal available for sampling, non-Cartesian imaging trajectories can be employed. Non-Cartesian trajectories are less commonly used in imaging, and require special design of magnetic field gradient waveforms and a more sophisticated reconstruction process. However, with a very short minimum echo time, 3D non-Cartesian trajectories are better suited for probing the fast-relaxing sodium signal. Where a 3D Cartesian sequence requires localisation in k_y and k_z prior to data acquisition, a 3D non-Cartesian acquisition starts each excitation at the center of k-space, and data are simultaneously acquired in k_x, k_y, and k_z. To ensure short TE in UTE imaging a hard RF pulse is commonly used to excite all spins in the imaging volume. A number of trajectories used for non-Cartesian data readout are available from literature, for example radial imaging, twisted projection imaging (TPI), density adapted radial (DAR) imaging, and 3D CONES, briefly described in the following.

Twisted projection imaging (TPI) was first described by Fernando Boada in 1997, as an extension to 2D TWIRL imaging [18]. The technique utilizes a hybrid radial-spiral sampling of k-space, allowing for acceleration in comparison to radial imaging with an underdamping factor defined during trajectory construction. TPI requires high gradient slew rates for image acquisition, due to the sharp transition between the radial and spiral potions of the trajectory. Further optimizations to the trajectory can be made by optimizing maximum gradient amplitudes throughout scan time [19].

Density adapted radial (DAR) trajectories are described in work by Nagel, whereby concentric rings of k-space are acquired with a radial readout. DAR allows for under sampling of k-space, shortening acquisition times in comparison to radial imaging [20].

The 3D cones approach was initially described for UTE proton imaging and has found applications in sodium acquisitions [21, 22]. Due to the high *k*-space efficiency of the trajectory, it is possible to acquire a full imaging volume in a very short time, leading to rapid high resolution imaging [23]. However, due to the high k-space efficiency, the SNR of each volume is lower than a radial acquisition; therefore, it is common practice to perform a number of spatial averages in a single acquisition.

2.4 Reconstruction

There are three main methods for reconstruction of sodium imaging data, depending on the acquisition scheme used. If Cartesian data is acquired, a Fourier transform is applied in all dimensions (x, y,z,t). If non-Cartesian acquisitions are employed more complex reconstruction strategies such as gridding or nonuniform fast Fourier transforms are used. Compensation for the oversampling of the center of k-space is performed in non-Cartesian imaging using precalculated density compensation functions (*see* **Note 1**).

2.5 Sodium Phantoms

External calibration phantoms are used to convert sodium imaging data to quantitative maps, with voxels fitted to a calibration curve formed from measurements of signal from known concentration phantoms as well as from regions of noise in the image.

Phantoms are generally made from agarose doped with sodium chloride, to ensure a T_1 and T_2 that mimic that of tissue. However, other designs are also possible. Phantoms are placed within the imaging field of view before the start of the experiment to ensure that signal is acquired from both tissue and calibration standards in the same exam.

2.6 Segmentation

Segmentation of the kidney is commonly achieved through region of interests initially drawn on proton anatomical imaging and transferred to the sodium images. Other methods have been proposed for the segmentation of the renal system, in particular to measure the corticomedullary sodium gradient, focusing on defining layers of the kidney from an initial whole kidney region [24].

3 Overview of Applications

3.1 Total sodium Imaging for Assessing Alterations in the Corticomedullary sodium Gradient

The corticomedullary sodium gradient has been studied with sodium imaging in a number of healthy and pathological scenarios [3–5, 25–29]. Broadly, the current preclinical literature focuses either on the action of diuretic drugs upon the sodium gradient, or upon acute tubular necrosis. The action of furosemide has been estimated by acquiring longitudinal imaging before and after the introduction of the acute diuretic. Furosemide acts as a loop diuretic, halting reabsorption of sodium through the loop of Henley, leading to acute diuresis. Results from studies have shown the capability of sodium MRI to detect the acute renal sodium alterations induced by furosemide, revealing a flattening of the corticomedullary sodium gradient within minutes of administration [3, 4, 26].

Studies focusing upon the early formation of acute kidney injury through tubular necrosis have revealed alterations in the sodium gradient, with a decreased gradient in the damaged kidney [5].

3.2 Potential Future Applications of sodium Imaging

Although the literature is limited to the current applications of renal sodium imaging, there is a large scope for further preclinical studies demonstrating the power of this technique to probe disease formation. In particular, the formation of acute kidney disease and chronic kidney disease remain prime targets for further ^{23}Na MRI studies.

3.3 Acute Kidney Disease

Acute kidney disease is heralded by a sudden loss of renal function, and impaired reabsorption of electrolytes such as urea and sodium [30]. Indeed, this is a key clinical problem, with a number of patients diagnosed upon admission with AKI and leads to high mortality rates. AKI can occur over a number of hours or days, and is heralded by an decrease of the glomerular filtration rate, leading to retention of nitrogenous waste [31]. Due to the increase in waste retention, common methods for diagnosis are serum-based measures of creatinine clearance and blood nitrogen [31]. Further to the increase in the retention of waste, sodium reabsorption is impaired in AKI. An initial sodium imaging study showed a flattening of the corticomedullary sodium gradient [32]. A particular challenge in diagnosis and management of AKI is the direct estimation of renal health and function pre- and post-therapy, with many imaging methods either requiring the introduction of potentially hazardous contrast agents, or unable to provide physiological information [33]. Here sodium imaging may provide a more specific measure of renal health. The initial imaging study, mentioned above, offers a potential for further studies assessing therapeutic response [32]. Assessing the angle of the corticomedullary sodium gradient may also provide insights in to the degree of the insult that the disrupted kidney is facing.

3.4 Chronic Kidney Disease

Chronic kidney disease (CKD) is characterized by a gradual loss of kidney function over time, leading to a decrease in the intrarenal transport of metabolites such as urea and sodium [34, 35]. A challenge in this disease is, as with AKI, both monitoring disease progression and estimating therapeutic response. Sodium imaging has the potential to evaluate renal function via the corticomedullary sodium gradient, to differentiate the earliest changes in the metabolic and functional mismatch that occur in the renal system prior to the development of kidney disease [28, 32, 36]. The use of a combined multimodal anatomical and functional imaging approach with methods such as sodium, arterial spin labeling, BOLD, dynamic contrast enhanced imaging, and diffusion weighted imaging may provide a more complete picture of the alterations in renal function in relation to chronic kidney disease [24, 36–42].

4 Notes

1. Example gridding and density compensation calculation functions used for the reconstruction of data acquired with non-Cartesian trajectories can be found at https://www.ismrm.org/mri_unbound/sequence.htm.

Acknowledgments

The authors would like to thank Andreas Pohlmann and Thoralf Niendorf for assistance in preparing this chapter (Max-Delbrück Center for Molecular Medicine in the Helmholtz Association, Berlin, Germany.

This chapter is based upon work from COST Action PARENCHIMA, supported by European Cooperation in Science and Technology (COST). COST (www.cost.eu) is a funding agency for research and innovation networks. COST Actions help connect research initiatives across Europe and enable scientists to enrich their ideas by sharing them with their peers. This boosts their research, career, and innovation.

PARENCHIMA (renalmri.org) is a community-driven Action in the COST program of the European Union, which unites more than 200 experts in renal MRI from 30 countries with the aim to improve the reproducibility and standardization of renal MRI biomarkers.

References

1. Christensen JD, Barrère BJ, Boada FE et al (1996) Quantitative tissue sodium concentration mapping of normal rat brain. Magn Reson Med 36:83–89
2. Zöllner FG, Konstandin S, Lommen J et al (2016) Quantitative sodium MRI of kidney. NMR Biomed 29:197–205
3. Maril N, Margalit R, Mispelter J, Degani H (2004) Functional sodium magnetic resonance imaging of the intact rat kidney. Kidney Int 65:927–935
4. Maril N, Margalit R, Mispelter J, Degani H (2005) Sodium magnetic resonance imaging of diuresis: spatial and kinetic response. Magn Reson Med 53:545–552
5. Maril N, Margalit R, Rosen S et al (2006) Detection of evolving acute tubular necrosis with renal 23Na MRI: studies in rats. Kidney Int 69:765–768
6. Zöllner FG, Kalayciyan R, Chacón-Caldera J et al (2014) Pre-clinical functional magnetic resonance imaging part I: the kidney. Z Med Phys 24:286–306
7. Stobbe R, Beaulieu C (2005) In vivo sodium magnetic resonance imaging of the human brain using soft inversion recovery fluid attenuation. Magn Reson Med 54:1305–1310
8. Benkhedah N, Bachert P, Semmler W, Nagel AM (2012) Three-dimensional biexponential weighted (23) Na imaging of the human brain with higher SNR and shorter acquisition time. Magn Reson Med 765:754–765
9. Riemer F, Solanky BS, Wheeler-Kingshott CAM, Golay X (2018) Bi-exponential ^{23} Na T_2 * component analysis in the human brain. NMR Biomed 31(5):e3899
10. Tsang A, Stobbe RW, Beaulieu C (2013) Evaluation of B0-inhomogeneity correction for triple-quantum-filtered sodium MRI of the human brain at 4.7 T. J Magn Reson 230:134–144
11. Hancu I, Boada FE, Shen GX (1999) Three-dimensional triple-quantum-filtered 23Na imaging of in vivo human brain. Magn Reson Med 42:1146–1154
12. Ackerman JJH, Grove TH, Wong GG et al (1980) Mapping of metabolites in whole animals by 31P NMR using surface coils. Nature 283:2–5
13. Mueller OM, Hayes CE, Eash M et al (2006) An efficient, highly homogeneous radiofrequency coil for whole-body NMR imaging at 1.5 T. J Magn Reson 63:622–628
14. Kalayciyan R, Malzacher M, Neudecker S, Gretz N SL (2013) 23Na/1H in-vivo renal MRI of rodent kidney at 3T by using a double-tuned transceiver resonator system. In: International Society for Magnetic Resonance in Medicine. Salt-Lake City, p 4355
15. Hancu I, Boada FE, Shen GX (1999) Three-dimensional triple-quantum – filtered 23 Na imaging of in vivo human brain. Magn Reson Med 42(6):1146–1154
16. Qian Y, Panigrahy A, Laymon CM et al (2014) Short-T2 imaging for quantifying concentration of sodium ((23) Na) of bi-exponential T2 relaxation. Magn Reson Med 00:00–00
17. Konstandin S, Nagel AM (2014) Measurement techniques for magnetic resonance imaging of fast relaxing nuclei. MAGMA 27:5–19
18. Boada FE, Gillen JS, Shen GX et al (1997) Fast three dimensional sodium imaging. Magn Reson Med 37:706–715
19. Angelica MD, Fong Y (2008) Quantitative sodium imaging with a flexible twisted projection pulse sequence. Magn Reson Med 141:520–529
20. Nagel AM, Laun FB, Weber M-A et al (2009) Sodium MRI using a density-adapted 3D radial acquisition technique. Magn Reson Med 62:1565–1573
21. Riemer F, Solanky BS, Stehning C et al (2014) Sodium (23Na) ultra-short echo time imaging in the human brain using a 3D-Cones trajectory. MAGMA 27:35–46
22. Gurney PT, Hargreaves BA, Nishimura DG (2006) Design and analysis of a practical 3D cones trajectory. Magn Reson Med 55:575–582
23. Grist JT, Riemer F, McLean MA et al (2018) Imaging intralesional heterogeneity of sodium concentration in multiple sclerosis: initial evidence from 23Na-MRI. J Neurol Sci 387:111–114
24. Milani B, Ansaloni A, Sousa-Guimaraes S et al (2016) Reduction of cortical oxygenation in chronic kidney disease: evidence obtained with a new analysis method of blood oxygenation level-dependent magnetic resonance imaging. Nephrol Dial Transplant 32 (12):2097–2105
25. Maril N, Rosen Y, Reynolds GH et al (2006) Sodium MRI of the human kidney at 3 tesla. Magn Reson Med 56:1229–1234
26. Neuberger T, Gulani V, Webb A (2007) Sodium renal imaging in mice at high magnetic fields. Magn Reson Med 58:1067–1071
27. Haneder S, Juras V, Michaely HJ et al (2014) In vivo sodium (23Na) imaging of the human

kidneys at 7 T: preliminary results. Eur Radiol 24:494–501

28. Qi H, Nørlinger TS, Nielsen PM et al (2016) Early diabetic kidney maintains the corticomedullary urea and sodium gradient. Physiol Rep 4:1–6
29. Giovannetti G, Pingitore A, Positano V et al (2014) Improving sodium magnetic resonance in humans by design of a dedicated 23Na surface coil. Measurement 50:285–292
30. Hansell P, Welch WJ, Blantz RC, Palm F (2013) Determinants of kidney oxygen consumption and their relationship to tissue oxygen tension in diabetes and hypertension. Clin Exp Pharmacol Physiol 40:123–137
31. Basile DP, Anderson MD, Sutton TA (2012) Pathophysiology of acute kidney injury. Compr Physiol 2:1303–1353
32. Nielsen PM, Szocska Hansen ES, Nørlinger TS et al (2016) Renal ischemia and reperfusion assessment with three-dimensional hyperpolarized13C,15N2-urea. Magn Reson Med 76:1524–1530
33. Perazella MA (2015) Gadolinium-contrast toxicity in patients with kidney disease: nephrotoxicity and nephrogenic systemic fibrosis. Curr Drug Saf 3:67–75
34. McFarland JG (1999) Perioperative blood transfusions: indications and options. Chest 115:113S–121S
35. Thomas R, Kanso A, Sedor JR (2008) Chronic kidney disease and its complications. Prim Care 35:329–344
36. Bertelsen LB, Nielsen PM, Qi H et al (2017) Diabetes induced renal urea transport alterations assessed with 3D hyperpolarized13C,15N-urea. Magn Reson Med 77:1650–1655
37. Cox EF, Buchanan CE, Bradley CR et al (2017) Multiparametric renal magnetic resonance imaging: validation, interventions, and alterations in chronic kidney disease. Front Physiol 8:1–15
38. Piskunowicz M, Hofmann L, Zuercher E et al (2015) A new technique with high reproducibility to estimate renal oxygenation using BOLD-MRI in chronic kidney disease. Magn Reson Imaging 33:253–261
39. Pruijm M, Milani B, Burnier M (2017) Blood oxygenation level-dependent mri to assess renal oxygenation in renal diseases: progresses and challenges. Front Physiol 7:1–7
40. Nielsen PM, Eldirdiri A, Bertelsen LB et al (2017) Fumarase activity: an in vivo and in vitro biomarker for acute kidney injury. Sci Rep 7:40812
41. Zimmer F, Zöllner FG, Hoeger S et al (2013) Quantitative renal perfusion measurements in a rat model of acute kidney injury at 3T: testing inter- and intramethodical significance of ASL and DCE-MRI. PLoS One 8:e53849
42. Zhou HY, Chen TW, Zhang XM (2016) Functional magnetic resonance imaging in acute kidney injury: present status. Biomed Res Int 2016:2027370

11

Experimental Protocols for MRI Mapping of Renal T_1

Philippe Garteiser, Octavia Bane, Sabrina Doblas, Iris Friedli, Stefanie Hectors, Gwenaël Pagé, Bernard E. Van Beers, and John C. Waterton

Abstract

The water proton longitudinal relaxation time, T_1, is a common and useful MR parameter in nephrology research. Here we provide three step-by-step T_1-mapping protocols suitable for different types of nephrology research. Firstly, we provide a single-slice 2D saturation recovery protocol suitable for studies of global pathology, where whole-kidney coverage is unnecessary. Secondly, we provide an inversion recovery type imaging protocol that may be optimized for specific kidney disease applications. Finally, we also provide imaging protocol for small animal kidney imaging in a clinical scanner.

This chapter is based upon work from the COST Action PARENCHIMA, a community-driven network funded by the European Cooperation in Science and Technology (COST) program of the European Union, which aims to improve the reproducibility and standardization of renal MRI biomarkers. This analysis protocol chapter is complemented by two separate chapters describing the basic concept and experimental procedure.

Key words Magnetic resonance imaging (MRI), Kidney, Mice, Rats, Longitudinal relaxation time (T_1), Spin-lattice relaxation time (T_1)

1 Introduction

The water proton longitudinal (or spin-lattice) relaxation time, T_1 (s), is a MR parameter commonly used in biomedical imaging. Unlike machine-dependent metrics such as "signal intensity in T_1-weighted MRI," T_1 measures a real physical process (i.e., the return to Boltzmann equilibrium of water proton longitudinal magnetisation) measured in absolute units (s) and, for any given magnetic field strength, independent of the machine used. Renal pathology often results in abnormal T_1 either globally (e.g., in renal failure) or focally (e.g., in renal cancer). Moreover, disease-induced changes in T_1 can often be assigned, at least qualitatively, to pathological changes such as fibrosis, inflammation, and oedema [1]. A second motivation to measure T_1 is in so-called dynamic experiments. In

Andreas Pohlmann and Thoralf Niendorf (eds.), *Preclinical MRI of the Kidney: Methods and Protocols*, Methods in Molecular Biology, vol. 2216, https://doi.org/10.1007/978-1-0716-0978-1_22,

this case the object under investigation in the MRI scanner for a short period (e.g., 10 min) while T_1 is measured repetitively, during some intervention to perturb T_1 (e.g., contrast agent administration). After administration of a contrast agent such as manganese, a gadolinium chelate, or dioxygen, changes in T_1 are linearly related to the contrast agent concentration, which could not reliably be determined from signal intensity changes alone.

Here we describe MRI protocols for mapping and monitoring T_1 in the kidney of small rodents in a step-by-step experimental protocol. The rationale for choosing different acquisition parameters depending to the aims of the study is discussed, together with specific parameter examples. T_1 measurements for dynamic studies are discussed in the chapter by Irrera P et al. "Dynamic Contrast Enhanced (DCE) MRI-Derived Renal Perfusion and Filtration: Experimental Protocol."

1.1 Motivation for Measuring T_1 in Animal Kidneys

Imaging provides many useful metrics in animal models of kidney physiology and pathophysiology. These include "extensive" or size variables, such as renal volume (ml) or thickness (mm) of renal cortex, and "intensive" or tissue characterisation variables, such as the longitudinal relaxation time, T_1 (s). Some investigators prefer to report the longitudinal relaxation rate R_1, the reciprocal of T_1, because from a metrology perspective R_1 is a "ratio variable" while T_1 is merely an "interval variable" [2]. In this work we use T_1. "Intensive" variables can be mapped, the maps themselves being a type of image. Such image metrics used in animal studies are valuable in translational research, as they are directly comparable with the imaging markers [3–5] used in studies of human subjects.

1.2 Study Design Concepts

Great care is needed in the choice of method to map T_1. No single method is optimal for all in vivo studies. The most accurate methods (e.g., inversion recovery with long TR and short TE readout) are neither fast nor efficient. In vivo studies involve complex tradeoffs between accuracy, speed, spatial resolution, field of view, need for fat suppression, sensitivity to inflow, sensitivity to motion artifact, biexponential T_1 decay, and other confounding tissue magnetisation behaviours such as transverse relaxation and magnetisation transfer. Moreover, even after a specific method is chosen, errors can be very sensitive to pulse sequence parameters such as delays, flip angles, spoiling and refocussing strategies, mis-set RF pulses and so on. For the renal investigator the first question in designing a study to measure T_1 must always be: *what is the aim of the study*?

1. For studies of global pathology, very high spatial and temporal resolution may be unnecessary provided that the cortex, the zones of the medulla, and the papilla can be resolved. In such studies a 2D image with voxel size of around 0.25 mm (in mice, e.g., [6–8]) or around 0.5 mm (in rats, e.g., [9–12]) may be adequate. It is often desirable to acquire T_1 with low

uncertainty so that small early pathological changes can be detected, and also to acquire accurate T_1 values that are reproducible between centers so that findings are generalizable. A saturation recovery sequence with ten or more inversion times, a 2D RARE readout, moderate spatial resolution, and a two- or three-parameter fit, should provide T_1 values which are not biased by B_1^+ errors. Alternately an inversion recovery sequence with a 2D echo-planar readout [6, 8] may be used although this is less time-efficient. The accuracy of the T_1 acquisition and analysis method should be verified using phantoms of known T_1 [2].

2. Studies of focal pathology may require high spatial resolution in 3D appropriate to the disease under investigation. Low uncertainty, high accuracy, and high reproducibility are also likely to be important so that scan times may be relatively long. 3D variable flip angle sequences are convenient, although they are quite vulnerable to B_1^+ errors. In these cases, phantom studies are highly desirable to mitigate B_1^+ errors, although phantom studies do not mitigate the motion artifact error to which these sequences are also highly vulnerable.
3. Longitudinal studies, during the development and/or treatment of disease have similar demands on spatial and temporal resolution, although if the study endpoint is the change in T_1, requirements for accuracy may be relaxed: in a significance test of post vs pre, or treated vs untreated, systematic errors from biased T_1 measurement may partly cancel out.
4. Dynamic studies have similar demands on spatial resolution (e.g., high 3D resolution for focal disease) together with very good temporal resolution to allow dynamic changes to be quantitated. In consequence accuracy may be compromised, but since the study endpoint relies on T_1 change during the dynamic run, bias may partly cancel out. Propagation of errors in these cases can be exceedingly complex and requires careful simulation.

1.3 Data Quality

It is highly desirable to verify the accuracy and repeatability of T_1 using phantoms [2], before experimental animals are exposed to study procedures. The design of MR phantoms can be challenging, and while validated traceable phantoms have been developed by metrologists for clinical MR [13–15], these are usually too large for use in rodent MR scanners. Design considerations should include biological, chemical, and physical stability, temperature independence, convenience, and cost. The phantom should cover both the expected T_1 range and the spatial range, since it may be advantageous to position the kidneys offset relative to the magnet's isocenter [16]. Nickel-doped agarose gels [17–19] are particularly convenient as simple liquid flood phantoms may introduce artifacts from unfamiliar MR phenomena such as radiation damping, convection, excessive T_2 or self-diffusion, standing waves, or abrupt boundaries.

This chapter is part of the book Pohlmann A, Niendorf T (eds) (2020) Preclinical MRI of the Kidney—Methods and Protocols. Springer, New York.

2 General Considerations

2.1 Magnetic Field Strengths

Animal kidney MRI has been performed at a wide range of magnetic field strengths (B_0) between at least 0.4 T [20] and 16.4 T [21]. T_1 increases with B_0 [22]. Hence it is important to consider B_0 as an important factor in experiment design, although in practice B_0 may not be an adjustable parameter since many facilities only have a single MRI machine operated at a single magnetic field strength available. Higher magnetic field strengths are not always preferable, as the scan times required to properly sample the recovery of longitudinal magnetization will be somewhat longer, and problems from motion artifact, chemical shift artifact or susceptibility variation may increase. For an investigator who wishes to use rodent renal T_1 changes to study, say, the development of fibrosis or inflammation, the relevant metric is T_1 contrast-to-noise ratio per unit time, which does not necessarily improve as field strength increases: a high-field ($\geq$9.4 T) magnet may be no better than a conventional 3-7 T magnet. On the other hand, for an investigator who measures the uptake of a relaxive substance such as dioxygen, manganese, or gadolinium chelate, a high-field magnet provides a lower baseline R_1, making the induced changes ΔR_1 more evident.

2.2 Physiologic Motion

Acquisition parameters should ensure that interference from physiologic motion on the signal is kept to a minimum. Indeed, although kidneys are positioned quite low in the abdomen, they are still subject to mild respiratory motion artifacts. It is possible to acquire continuously under shallow breathing, taking advantage of the slow speed of breathing in anesthetized animals [23]. With such datasets, some of this motion can be corrected for during image processing with appropriate coregistration strategies or by intentionally skipping frames presenting a high degree of respiratory motion from the analysis. However, because this strategy potentially removes important datapoints or because it introduces physiological noise into the quantitative estimation, it is still recommended to implement motion compensation strategies at the acquisition level. In particular, respiratory motion compensation takes advantage of a respiratory signal (acquired externally or with MR signals such as navigators) to only allow acquisition during the long periods of breathing motion arrest that are typical of anesthetized animals. An example of such a setup applied to a clinical scanner, is depicted in Fig. 1. Special care is needed to ensure such triggering approaches are compatible with T_1 mapping protocols. In such protocols, sequence timing dictates the effective repetition time, upon which the accuracy of the T_1 computation is

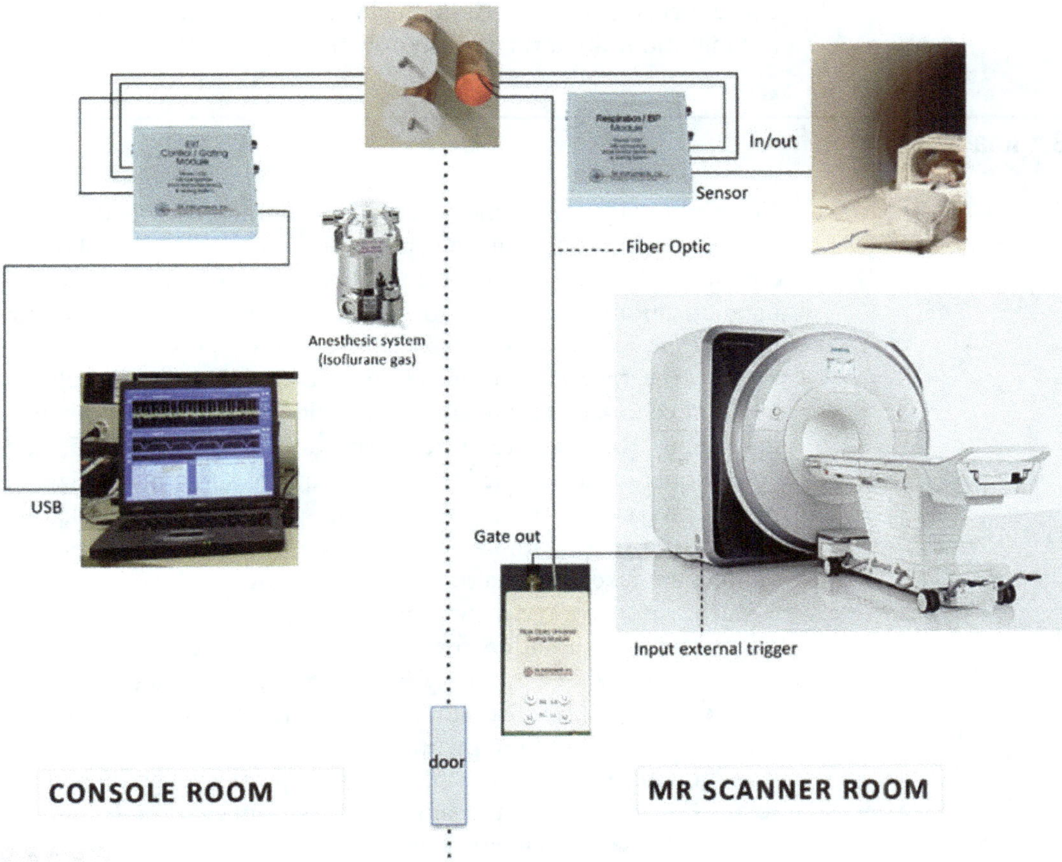

Fig. 1 Scheme of the experimental setup for a respiratory-gated implementation with monitoring small animal system SA Instruments, Inc., Stony Brook, NY11790 USA

based. It is sometimes preferred to position the trigger on the inversion (or saturation) RF pulse rather than on the slice selection or other imaging loops [16] so that the timing of image acquisition relative to inversion is guaranteed. The only timing affected in this strategy is the delay between saturation or inversion slices. In inversion recovery protocols this delay is already very long, (often more than 10 s), so any additional delay incurred will not significantly affect T_1 accuracy, while in saturation recovery the saturation pulse destroys the longitudinal magnetization so that preceding delays are unable to affect T_1 accuracy.

An alternative approach for respiratory motion compensation is retrospective gating or self-gating, which is compatible with gradient echo methods such as Variable Flip Angle (VFA). In this case, data are acquired continuously but an additional "navigator" signal allows data displaced by respiration to be sorted or discarded. This is marketed under the brand-name "IntraGate" (Bruker Biospin, Ettlingen, Germany).

Because kidneys are anatomically close to the bowels, some authors favor imaging sessions done after fasting periods [10]. Fasting should only be done after considering the physiologic consequences, and from the animal welfare perspective should be of the minimum duration consistent with the imaging aims.

3 Imaging Techniques

Conventionally, for T_1 measurement, signal intensity is probed at different time points during exponential decay back to Boltzmann equilibrium following inversion or saturation of the longitudinal magnetization: inversion recovery or saturation recovery. Saturation can be achieved using a specific saturation pulse, or simply by varying the repetition time TR of a conventional spin echo or gradient echo acquisition which also incidentally saturates the magnetization. To reduce the total acquisition time, the Look Locker (LL) sequence can be used. With LL sequences, the magnetization is also prepared with an inversion or saturation pulse [24], but instead of a single sample of the recovery curve per TR, multiple samples are taken using a train of low flip angle pulses [25].

The inversion recovery sequence is the reference method to calculate T_1 but it suffers from long acquisition times. Therefore, the use of Look-Locker inversion recovery is advantageous, but is limited to single 2D slice acquisition: if multiple slices are needed, they must be acquired sequentially.

The alternative approach involves repeating a gradient echo acquisition at varying flip angles (VFA) while keeping TR and other sequence parameters constant: since the signal depends sinusoidally on flip angle but decays exponentially with T_1, the T_1 can be calculated from the Ernst equation (chapter by Garteiser P et al. "Analysis Protocols for MRI Mapping of Renal T_1"). Three-dimensional acquisition (3D) can be performed with VFA, but since VFA is sensitive to B_1^+ inhomogeneity, the B_1^+ field should be mapped to allow correction (chapter by Garteiser P et al. "Analysis Protocols for MRI Mapping of Renal T_1"). Although 3D VFA is familiar in clinical imaging, it is not commonly employed in rodent kidney studies, and we have not provided a protocol here.

3.1 RARE-VTR

3.1.1 Protocol Description

Rapid acquisition with relaxation enhancement at variable TR (RARE-VTR) is a type of saturation recovery sequence. Data are acquired as 2D slices, so this sequence is ideal when a single slice provides an adequate sample of the kidney, for example in the case of homogeneous global pathology. If volumetric data are required then a stack of slices must be acquired sequentially, which is time-consuming.

The RARE-VTR protocol is based on the multiecho RARE protocol, with a slice-selective 90° rf pulse followed by a train of slice-selective 180° refocusing pulses separated by an inter-echo time TE (Fig. 2). Each 180° pulse induces a refocused echo comprising spin-echo and stimulated echo contributions, which is

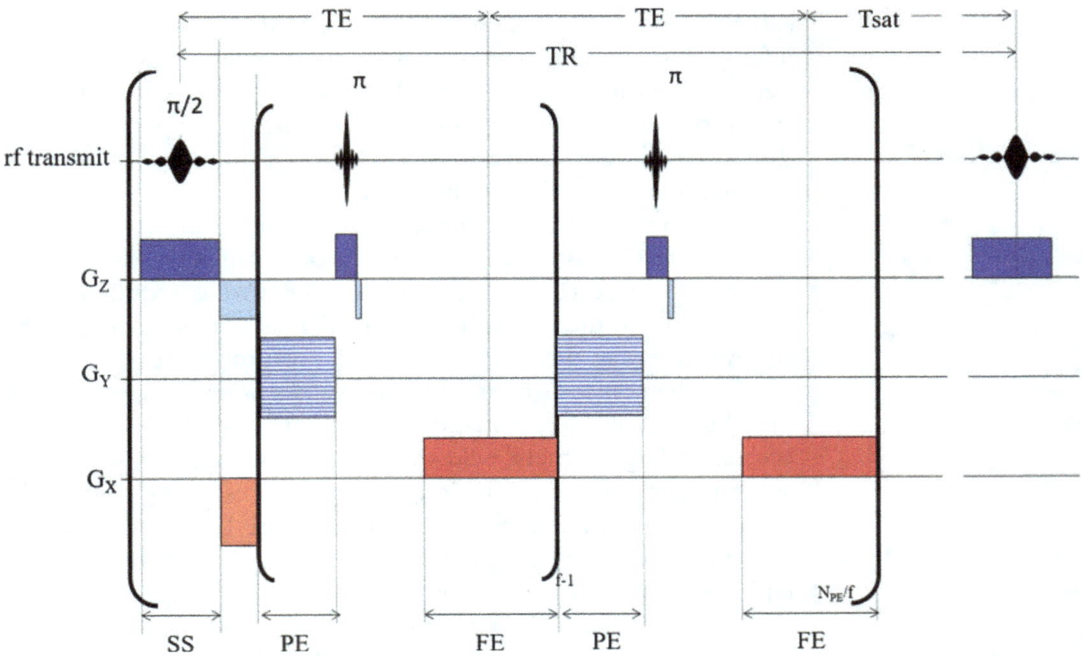

Fig. 2 Simplified timing diagram for 2D saturation recovery sequence with RARE readout. A series of 180° pulses creates *f* echoes at TE, 2 × TE, 3 × TE, and so on, where *f* is the RARE factor, typically $f = 8$. During the phase encoding (PE) step, spatial location is encoded by incrementing the *Y* gradient N_Y times so that each echo is encoded with a different phase, thereby accelerating the k-space coverage. During the frequency encoding (FE) readout periods, the spatial location is encoded in the frequency content of the digitized signal from the echo. If the pulses are perfect and if neglecting the longitudinal regrowth occurring during the echo train, all the magnetization is effectively kept in the transverse plane until the last echo (Phase cycling and spoiling not shown)

digitized, and each echo experiences a different phase encode gradient. Following the last echo there is a delay following which the sequence is repeated with a repetition time TR. The number of 180° pulses is called the echo train length (ETL) or RARE factor: a typical value is 8. TR is then varied to sample the magnetization recovery. A saturation recovery time T_{sat} is defined as TR − (ETL × TE). Thus if an investigator requires a 128^2 matrix, the entire acquisition duration would be ΣTR × 128/ETL, where ΣTR is the sum of all the TR values used to sample the longitudinal magnetization recovery. Recommended acquisition parameters are given in section 4 below.

Because of the presence of refocusing RF pulses, this protocol is relatively insensitive to B_0 imperfections and susceptibility artifacts. For 2D single-slice T_1 mapping it is quite time-efficient, but acquisition of a multislice stack requires rather long acquisition times.

3.1.2 Repetition Times

The set of repetition times that are sampled needs careful consideration. The TR values should be rationally selected during preliminary studies with the animal model under investigation. In saturation recovery experiments, the signal starts at $S_0 \sim 0$ at short TRs (TR $\ll T_1$) and increases with approximately linear S_∞/T_1 dependence on TR. At longer TRs (TR $\approx T_1$), the signal enters a transition regime where the increase in signal per unit TR diminishes. Finally at large TRs (TR $\gg T_1$), the signal asymptotically approaches S_∞. Hence, proper TR sampling strategy should be adopted to cover both regimes and the transition in between.

In determining the set of repetition times to use, the first question may be to select the highest TR that is required. This choice is mainly dictated by the expected T_1 in the tissue of interest, the available scan time and the planned postprocessing strategy.

For the first constraint, literature values or preliminary studies may help in the determination of the expected tissue T_1 at the corresponding magnetic field strength. The longest TR should be substantially larger than the longest expected tissue T_1. Typical T_1 values for cortex and medulla are in the range 1–2 s and for urine around 3 s. There is no generally accepted consensus, but authors typically have the maximal TR be 3–5 times the longest expected T_1, typically 8–12 s. If the investigator finds this makes the overall study duration too long then spatial resolution can be reduced, particularly when small focal changes are not of interest. Alternatively a maximal TR of two times the longest expected T_1 could be considered, but in this case it is recommended to perform careful simulations to ensure the propagated errors are at an acceptable level. A special case arises in contrast agent injection studies. Here, the distribution of the agent into the tissue of interest is quantified by looking at the absolute change in R_1 after vs before injection. Hence, care should be taken to consider that the T_1 value may be significantly shorter after injection. It may be necessary to adopt a different maximal TR for the pre- and postinjection scans. Contrast agents decrease T_1, hence the possible decrease in longest TR that is afforded has the additional consequence of shortening the scan duration. This is potentially advantageous, especially when the dynamics of contrast agent distribution needs to be interrogated and is slow (on the order of minutes). In this case it becomes feasible to monitor the contrast agent distribution dynamically by repetitively acquiring T_1 maps. Temporal resolutions of under 2 min can reasonably be achieved by trading off, for example, spatial resolution. This strategy is compatible with some contrast agent dynamics such as in manganese-enhanced MRI [21].

The choice of the longest TR should be done in harmony with the particular postprocessing solution that is planned. Indeed, the dataset obtained with the longest applied TR may be used to provide an estimate for the total equilibrium signal S_∞. In that case, the mathematical problem to be solved is reduced since S_∞ can be inserted in the fitting equation, thereby removing a degree of freedom and making the fit more robust. This comes at the cost of the necessity to acquire a scan at very long TR to ensure the signal is close enough to equilibrium values. When such an estimate of S_∞ is available, it may no longer be necessary to sample other TRs longer than the tissue T_1, concentrating instead on TR values at and below the tissue T_1 [21].

Once the largest TR to acquire has been selected, the number of TRs should be determined. The set of TR values should span the range of expected T_1. Depending on the fitting equation that is used, a larger number of repetition times may be required to provide sufficient overdetermination for the fitting procedure. In other words, there should be significantly more TRs sampled than there are free parameters in the fitted equation. In an ideal situation with negligible experimental noise, it may be sufficient to select only a number of TR values equal to the number of free parameters in the fit. However, with experimental noise, this rapidly becomes insufficient and introduces bias into the results. Hence, when signal to noise ratio is limited, it is recommended to acquire a larger number of TR values. This comes at the cost of increased scan time, since each TR is generally acquired sequentially. In saturation recovery sequences, the fitting equation only has a limited number of parameters (i.e., S_∞, R_1, and maybe S_0 and/or an error term); hence, as few as four TR values are acceptable providing sufficient signal to noise is available and sampling is appropriately selected.

In disease models the pathology evolves slowly over days or weeks, the scan duration becomes less important, and it is possible to increase the number of TR values to 6, 8, or even 12, although from an ethical perspective the duration of the procedures should always be as short as possible. The choice of TR values can even be done a priori using Cramer-Rao lower-bound methodology. This technique optimizes the distribution of the sampled variable (in that case TR), for a given number of samples, an expected noise distribution and a signal model. It was used already with some success for cardiac T_1 mapping, where it was found that at constant number of acquired averages, increasing the SNR by averaging a carefully selected subset of TR values could prove beneficial relative to a set of uniformly distributed TR values [26]. A similar approach can be proposed to optimize the repetition times to use in kidney T_1 mapping.

In typical MRI scanners, the specific TR values can be set manually with a TR table having a user-specified number of TR entries. Manufacturers also often provide utilities that assist the user in prescribing the TR series. These utilities query from the user only a minimal value, a maximal value and a number of steps, or a minimal value, a number of steps and an estimate of the tissue T_1. These input values are then used to generate the series of TR values to use during the acquisition.

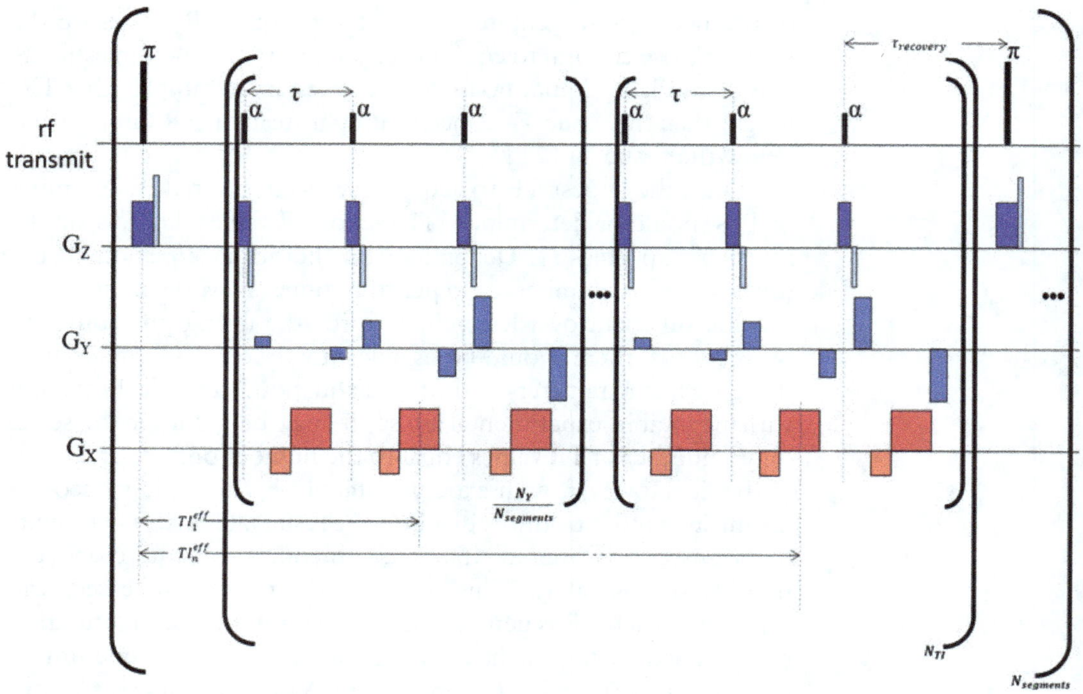

Fig. 3 Schematic view of the look-locker inversion recovery pulse sequence (fast low flip angle spoiled gradient echoes variant with spoiler gradient pulses omitted for simplicity). τ repetition time, N_y prescribed number of k-space lines, $N_{segments}$ number of k space segments (acceleration factor), *TI* inversion recovery time. Effective recovery times are considered at the centerline of each imaging segment. $\tau_{recovery}$: delay added to enable full recovery of the longitudinal magnetization before the subsequent inversion pulse is applied. In other variants, the fast low angle shots can be replaced by steady state free precession modules or EPI modules (Accessory gradient lobes are not shown for clarity)

3.2 Recovery Techniques: Look-Locker and Derivatives

3.2.1 Protocol Description

Look-Locker (LL) is a variant of inversion recovery or saturation recovery sequence. Data are acquired as 2D slices, and if volumetric data are required, a stack of slices must be acquired sequentially. LL involves sampling the magnetization using rapid, small angle imaging readouts while it recovers from the inversion or a saturation RF pulse (Fig. 3). The temporal spacing between imaging readouts provides a rapid way to sample the longitudinal regrowth. Indeed, each imaging shot will occur at a different time during regrowth, hence many different recovery times can be sampled during a single recovery event. Full longitudinal regrowth takes longer after an inversion RF pulse than after a saturation RF pulse, however, adopting an inversion RF pulse increases the dynamic range of the sampled signal. Thus the choice between saturation or inversion for the preparation of magnetization in a recovery sequence may be dictated by the experimental necessity for short acquisition time (for instance in dynamic experiments involving contrast agents with rapid kinetics) or higher measurement precision.

The Modified Look-Locker Inversion Recovery (MOLLI) sequence is an alternative when small animal renal T_1 mapping is performed using a clinical MR system. One rationale for choosing a clinical platform for preclinical studies is the similarity between MR protocol played out on small animals and human kidneys. MOLLI was initially designed for myocardial T_1 mapping at 1.5 T [27]. A typical MOLLI sequence can be performed by acquiring single shot True FISP images at different inversion times after a single inversion pulse. MOLLI is routinely used clinically for T_1 mapping and is usually available on clinical MR systems equipped with a cardiac package. The original MOLLI sequence provided by the manufacturers' library is a good starting point for MOLLI optimization in the rodent kidney. However, translating the MOLLI technique for scanning rodent models on a clinical MR scanner requires a specific implementation. In human, MOLLI is usually acquired in breath hold. In rodent, a physiological monitoring system to track the respiration and synchronize the sequence is needed (*see* Fig. 1).

3.2.2 Types of Readouts, and Corresponding Specific Points of Attention

In recovery-type sequences, several options are possible for the imaging shots that are performed to sample the recovery period.

Fast low angle shots, where magnetization is spoiled before subsequent RF pulses, can be used. They have the advantage of a short TR (~3 ms) that is compatible with low flip angles (<10°) [9]. As such, they perturb the longitudinal regrowth of the magnetization only to a small extent.

Balanced readouts such as steady-state free precession (SSFP) can also be used, as they tend to yield higher signal to noise due to the conservation of magnetization from preceding shots [28]. The SSFP condition links the TE and TR. Because FISP involves radiofrequency phase coherence between shots, acquisition can be true-FISP, fid mode or echo mode. It acquires innermost the phase encoding (in-segments), then slices, then phase encoding (segments), then (optionally) averaging. SSFP is especially sensitive to careful shimming of the B_0. The segmenting can be performed either sequentially or by interleaving phase encode steps. The interleaved mode is recommended for inversion recovery experiments. The T_1 recovery sampling must then be setup by adjusting the time between the inversion pulse and the first imaging shot. This delay is incompressible due to the need for stabilizing the steady state condition of the magnetization. This is either done with a half flip angle pulse or with a starter (dummy) sequence, at the cost of a longer delay. Unfortunately for these reasons, the implementation of respiratory or cardiac triggering is challenging, and it is recommended to proceed by gating on the saturation or inversion pulse.

Finally, echoplanar imaging (EPI) readouts have also been proposed in that context [6, 7, 16, 29, 30]. Although they are quite advantageous due to their speed (in single shot EPI, a full k-space image may be acquired after a single excitation pulse), EPI sequences for kidney T_1 mapping are vulnerable to problems associated with EPI in general, particularly if both kidneys are to be assessed. In particular, the EPI train is sensitive to B_0 inhomogeneity, which can become problematic at higher magnetic field strengths and in large bore systems. This effect is more important for long echo train EPIs such as single shot EPI. In this situation there is also a long effective echo time to accommodate the train length required by the single shot mode. This can be detrimental because it can increase the point spread function diameter ("smearing"), thus reducing the effective spatial resolution [30]. The long echo time of single shot EPI also comes at a disadvantage in kidneys with short T_2^* such as kidneys after injection of high concentrations of contrast agents. EPI is also associated with signal dropouts and geometric distortions at regions of strong magnetic susceptibility gradients, which sometimes occur at the kidney edges [30].

These disadvantages can be mitigated by performing segmented EPI acquisitions. In segmented EPI, full k-space acquisition is subdivided over several recovery periods, thereby enabling for decreased echo times. Segmentation will, however, increase the acquisition time, since full k-space coverage will be performed over a greater number of recovery periods. Finally, EPI image quality is also adversely affected by the presence of fat, which may be abundant in some kidney disease models such as obesity-related disease models. This can be remedied by applying fat saturation pulses [7].

3.2.3 Duration of Imaging Readouts

The duration of the imaging readouts should be short relatively to the duration of the recovery. This enables to interrogate precise inversion recovery delays rather than long intervals during which the longitudinal magnetization does vary substantially. Furthermore, short imaging readout durations are also advantageous because more imaging shots can be positioned during longitudinal regrowth. The increased number of data points yields better numerical stability during the subsequent fitting procedure.

3.2.4 Number of Imaging Readouts

The total number of imaging readouts that can be fit in a single regrowth is limited by several factors. First, the imaging sequence (excitation and readout) itself takes an incompressible minimum amount of time. Second, there is a requirement to acquire full images at each of the recovery delays. Hence, if only a single k-space line is acquired at each recovery delay, this also means that to acquire the appropriate number of k-space lines for image reconstruction (e.g., 128), an equal number of saturation or inversion recovery periods will be necessary. Since full relaxation needs to be reached (typically 10 s or more) before the next inversion RF pulse can be applied, this implies very long acquisition times (20 min or more). Hence it is important to consider acceleration schemes such as echoplanar imaging, where partial k-spaces are acquired during the regrowth rather than single k-space lines. Finally, the image acquisition readouts perturb the growing longitudinal magnetization: the application of the imaging RF pulses slightly saturates the signal, which makes the signal regrow with a biased apparent T_1 (sometimes denoted T_1*) that is different than the true tissue T_1. This effect can be mitigated by using smaller flip angles and longer RF pulse repetition intervals. Postprocessing strategies are also available to correct for that effect (cf. the chapter by Garteiser P et al. "Analysis Protocols for MRI Mapping of Renal T_1").

3.2.5 Repetition Time

In saturation or inversion recovery type sequences, it is important to distinguish the time between RF inversion pulses and the time between imaging RF pulses. The time between saturation or inversion must take into account the T_1 of the kidney at the considered field strength. A sufficiently long recovery period must be taken into account to prevent to saturate the magnetization. Typically inversion pulses are separated by 10 s [16, 28], 18 s [6, 7] or even 20 s [30].

The repetition time between imaging segments represents the precision with which the inversion recovery will be sampled. If a high accuracy is required for the T_1, only short imaging segments with a few to a single k-space line can be adopted. This will ensure that there is only little confounding factor arising from the longitudinal regrowth occurring during each imaging segment. Conversely if a lower T_1 recovery sampling is acceptable, then imaging can be noticeably accelerated by k-space segmenting.

3.2.6 Inversion Pulses

Adiabatic passage pulses can be advantageous to ensure saturation (adiabatic half passage) or inversion (adiabatic full passage). These pulses maintain their rotation properties invariant to the B_1^+ field, provided that the pulse B_1 exceeds an adiabaticity threshold. This is of importance in the field of kidney imaging, where the presence of intraabdominal fat can be challenging for B_1 homogeneity. Hence adiabatic RF pulses such as the hyperbolic secant RF pulse, are often used in T_1-mapping protocols, as half passage for saturation recovery experiments [23, 31] or as full passage for inversion recovery experiments [16, 30]. However, these RF pulses tend to require long duration and RF power levels, which may not be compatible with all RF coils, and unless provided by the manufacturer, their frequency and phase modulation shapes may require careful design.

Generally non selective inversion RF pulses are used. Indeed, slice selective inversion RF pulses are exposed to inflow artifacts. Indeed, when a slice selective RF pulse is applied, the spins entering the imaging slice via perfusion effects, have not been resonantly exposed to the RF pulse. Hence their presence in the imaging slice will contribute to increase on average the magnetization. This effect will be higher if perfusion is elevated, and is in fact the basis for FLAIR sequences. Whenever the true tissue T_1 is the parameter of interest, perfusion becomes a confounding factor, and inflow artifacts should be minimized. This can be achieved either by selecting an inversion slice that is significantly larger than the imaging slice to minimize the inflow artifact by creating a large region adjacent to the imaging slice that the noninverted spins need to cross before entering the imaged slice. Alternately, a nonselective saturation pulse may be adopted. In this case, even the spins that enter the imaging slice by perfusion during the imaging train are inverted, and hence they will not modify the apparent tissue T_1. Some authors recommend offsetting the position of the kidney within the radiofrequency coil to ensure that the heart is present within the effective region of the coil, to ensure maximally inverted spins throughout the entire body of the animal [16].

Recommended acquisition parameters are given in section 4 below.

3.3 Variable Flip Angle Techniques

Variable flip angle (VFA) sequences vary the flip angle of the rf excitation pulse but keep TR constant. Data can be acquired in 3D volume, so such sequences are ideal when the entire kidney must be sampled, for example in the case of heterogeneous or focal pathology (Fig. 4). However, data acquisition takes longer than for 2D sequences, and they are not robust in the presence of B_1^+ inhomogeneity.

Variable flip angle sequences are usually based on spoiled gradient echo sequences (fast low angle shot) [12, 32, 33], but the same principles can be applied with UTE sequences [34]. By virtue of their 3D nature, they are well suited for analyzing entire kidney volumes. However, the acquisition scheme where a single angle is acquired at a time also limits the number of different flip angle acquisitions that can be achieved within reasonable scanning durations. A linearization of the VFA signal provides T_1 estimates based on as little as two flip angles, although this technique is prone to noise bias. In a study at clinical field strength of 3.0 T using a wrist coil, flip angles of 5° and 26° were proposed for a rat model of acute kidney injury [12]. The use of VFA-based protocols for kidney mapping is not yet widespread at higher magnetic field strengths, but this type of sequence is applicable in other organs [34] or in tumor models [32, 33]. VFA schemes are also prone to B_1^+ field heterogeneity. Indeed, the effectively achieved flip angle at a specific location in the kidney is function of not only pulse amplitude, but also the shape and electromagnetic properties of the animal, the radiofrequency pulse design and (to a lesser extent when volume RF coils are used for RF transmission) RF coil coverage homogeneity. Thus, the B_1 field may require to be mapped first. For instance a reference T_1 map using a recovery-based sequence can be obtained and then injected into the signal equation to extract the effective flip angle [35]. Another acquisition strategy consists of measuring the B_1^+ field directly with dual angle spin echo sequence

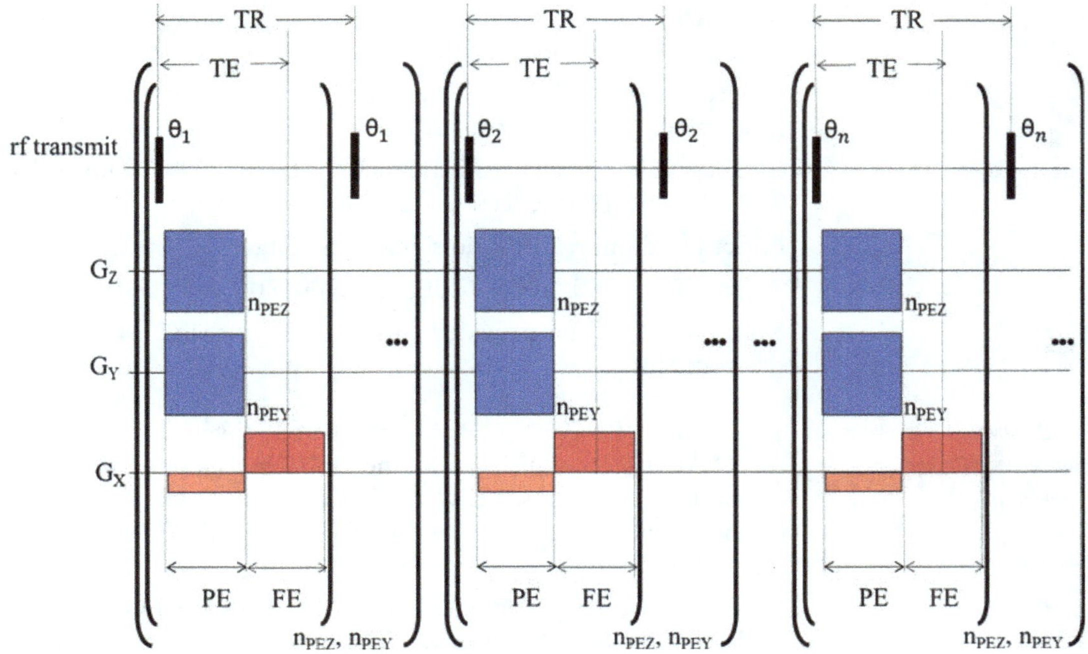

Fig. 4 3D variable flip angle protocol. *TR* repetition time (maintained constant for the duration of the acquisition), *TE* echo time, θ flip angle (flip angle is varied during the protocol), n_{PEY}, n_{PEZ} number of prescribed phase encoding lines in the *Y* and *Z* dimensions, *PE* phase encoding, *FE* frequency encoding. While the TR is maintained and constant during acquisition, the flip angle is varied several times until a complete dataset has been fully acquired for each prescribed flip angle. Accessory gradient lobes are not shown for clarity. Often, investigators need to suppress the signal from fat, in which case the hard pulse would be replaced by a spectrally selective "soft" pulse to excite ^1H_2O but not C^1H_2 or C^1H_3. During the phase-encoding (PE) step, spatial location is encoded by incrementing *X* and *Y* gradients i_X and G_Y multiple times n_{PEX} and n_{PEY}, typically 64 or 128. During this period magnetization is prephased using the *Z* gradient G_Z, so that a gradient echo may be formed by inverting the polarity of the gradient, yielding a return to phase at TE at the mid-point of the gradient echo. TE is set as short as possible, typically ~2–3 ms, in order to avoid T_2^* weighting, and to minimize total acquisition time. Practically, this is limited by the specification and performance of the gradient coils and amplifiers available to the investigator. TR is also set as short as possible, ~5 ms, in order to minimize the overall acquisition time

[36, 37]. Recommended acquisition parameters are given in section 4 below.

4 Methods

4.1 MR Protocol Setup

4.1.1 2D RARE VTR in Bruker ParaVision 6

1. Use the ParaVision RARE T1 saturation-recovery METHOD "T1map_RARE protocol" (Rat/Head/Relaxometry, or Mouse/Head/Relaxometry).
2. Set the geometry to coronal, 58 × 58 mm FOV (rat) or 40 × 30 mm FOC (mouse). These may need adjustment in studies on large (e.g., obese) animals.

3. Set the matrix size to 128 × 128; if acquisition length is too large, you may decrease the phase encoding resolution.
4. Use a single 90° 1.16 mm slice selection (optionally, apply spectrally selective fat suppression).
5. Select an180° train RARE factor 8, matching pulse bandwidths of 90° and 180°, effective TE 30 ms, echo spacing 7.5 ms.
6. Set five dummy scans; no signal averaging.
7. Set TR = 5500, 2000, 1200, 750, 500, 300, 200, and 100 ms.
8. A manufacturer-provided macro is available for data processing.

4.1.2 Inversion Recovery Sequence in Bruker ParaVision 6

1. Use the ParaVision Fluid-Attenuated Inversion Recovery (FLAIR) method using only the global inversion mode (Fair-Mode set to Nonselective), using Flow-sensitive Alternating Inversion Recovery FAIR-RARE or FAIR-EPI Bruker methods.
2. Set the geometry to axial or coronal, 58 × 58 mm FOV (rat) or 40 × 30 mm FOV (mouse). These may need adjustment on large (e.g., obese) animals.
3. Use a single 1 mm slice selection.
4. Set the matrix size to 128 × 128 matrix; if acquisition is too long, you may diminish the spatial resolution and adopt partial Fourier acceleration.
5. Set an TE of 36 ms (FAIR-RARE) or longer (FAIR-EPI).
6. Set the inversion pulse properties to calculated, as this provides a full passage adiabatic pulse with appropriately good flip angle homogeneity.
7. Use 21 inversion times starting at 30 ms with increments of 200 ms (to be adapted to the particular study at hand).
8. Select a recovery time of 10 s or greater.
9. Adjust the number of averages based on the available scan time.
10. In case of EPI usage, a careful shimming of B0 is paramount. The manufacturer-recommended method is MapShim using an ellipsoidal shim volume, in which a B_0 map is measured (accessible in the adjustments platform) and used to correct the B_0 with the shims coils available on the system.
11. A manufacturer-provided macro is provided for data processing.

1. Install rat in a wrist coil with conventional pressure pad to monitor breath rate. Figure 1 illustrates a dedicated small animal SA Instruments system connected to a Siemens clinical MR system.

4.1.3 Modified Look-Locker Inversion Recovery (MOLLI) [27] Sequence for Rats on a Siemens Clinical Scanner

2. Load the MOLLI sequence provided by the MRI system. The original MOLLI 3(3)3(3)5 scheme can be applied for kidney imaging. In this sampling scheme, multiple images are acquired at 11 time points on the recovery curve, with three inversions with slightly shifted inversion times, enabling a pixel-based T_1 quantification.
3. Start TI at 117 ms with TI increments (ΔTI) between inversion of 80 ms.
4. The slice thickness and in-plane resolution are particularly important to avoid partial volume effects. Use a slice with the lowest thickness and the highest in-plane resolution allowed by the MR system typically resulting voxel size around $0.7 \times 1.1 \times 3.5$ mm at 3 T.
5. Set TR/TE around 711/1.09 ms.
6. Set flip angle from 28° to 35° (default flip angle of 35°) T1 map relies on kidney being aligned between all TI images. As a consequence it is important to provide an additional motion correction method to mitigate residual respiratory motion. It is recommended to perform at least a rigid registration algorithm between images from various inversion times before the pixel-wise analysis of the relaxation curve (cf. the chapter by Garteiser P et al. "Analysis Protocols for MRI Mapping of Renal T_1"). Some vendors proposed on line motion correction algorithm, such as MOCCO from Siemens, during the reconstruction process.

4.2 Calibrated Phantom Acquisitions

1. Construct or procure a set of filled nickel/agarose phantoms without air bubbles. Each phantom should use a vial appropriate for the size of the animal abdomen (e.g., 25 mm diameter × 40 mm high for a mouse or 50 mm diameter × 80 mm high for a rat). Use 2% agarose, and a different concentration of nickel chloride in each phantom. Suitable nickel concentrations are 0 mM, 0.5 M, 1 mM, 2 mM, and 4 mM: 8 mM, and 16 mM can be added if very short T_1 values are expected (e.g., in DCEMRI). Add a preservative, such as 0.05% sodium azide, and seal.
2. Measure T_1 for each phantom using the method of Subheading 4.3 and the chapter by Garteiser P et al. "Analysis Protocols for MRI Mapping of Renal T_1." Repeat the measurements on a different day. Temperature should be controlled carefully, for instance by isolating the T_1 phantom in an ice–water mixture, or by inserting the phantom in a larger structure with high thermal inertia and preequilibrated at the target temperature.
3. In consultation with a professional statistician, calculate the repeatability and ensure the sample size is adequate to test the

hypothesis of interest. From an ethical perspective, this is mandatory before living animals are entered into the procedures.

4. Repeat **steps 2** and **3** in a group of living animals. The group size should be determined in consultation with a professional statistician: group sizes of between 6 and 15 are common.

4.3 Animal Experiments (Dedicated Small Animal MR Systems)

1. Use a volume RF coil of suitable diameter. In dedicated preclinical MRI, volume RF coils with an inner diameter of 38 mm for mice or 72 mm for rats could be used.
2. Anesthetize the animal with isoflurane as described in the chapter by Kaucsar T et al. "Preparation and Monitoring of Small Animals in Renal MRI" and transfer it to the scanner.
3. Set up the temperature monitoring (rectal probe) and respiratory monitoring (balloon on chest) unit.
4. Perform anatomical imaging as described in the chapter by Pohlmann A et al. "Essential Practical Steps for MRI of the Kidney in Experimental Research."
5. Perform localized shimming on the kidney imaging as described in the chapter by Pohlmann A et al. "Essential Practical Steps for MRI of the Kidney in Experimental Research." Wherever possible, appropriate tuning and matching of the used RF coil should be done.
6. Make sure the respiratory gating is setup properly, and that the anesthesia is stable.
7. Ensure that B_1^+ is correct, that is, that the relationship between the RF power and the desired flip angle is known in the region of space occupied by the kidneys. In *ParaVision* this is performed as part of the initial sequence adjustments when the reference pulse power is calibrated.

Acknowledgments

We thank Dr. Sascha Koehler (Bruker Biospin, Ettlingen, Germany) for helpful discussions.

This chapter is based upon work from COST Action PARENCHIMA, supported by European Cooperation in Science and Technology (COST). COST (www.cost.eu) is a funding agency for research and innovation networks. COST Actions help connect research initiatives across Europe and enable scientists to enrich their ideas by sharing them with their peers. This boosts their research, career, and innovation.

PARENCHIMA (renalmri.org) is a community-driven Action in the COST program of the European Union, which unites more than 200 experts in renal MRI from 30 countries with the aim to improve the reproducibility and standardization of renal MRI biomarkers.

References

1. Friedli I, Crowe LA, Berchtold L, Moll S, Hadaya K, de Perrot T et al (2016) New magnetic resonance imaging index for renal fibrosis assessment: a comparison between diffusion-weighted imaging and T1 mapping with histological validation. Sci Rep 6:30088
2. Waterton JC, Hines CDG, Hockings PD, Laitinen I, Ziemian S, Campbell S et al (2019) Repeatability, and reproducibility of longitudinal relaxation rate in 12 small-animal MRI systems. Magn Reson Imaging 59:121–129
3. Dekkers IA, Lamb HJ (2018) Clinical application and technical considerations of T1 & T2 (*) mapping in cardiac, liver, and renal imaging. Br J Radiol 91(1092):20170825
4. Waterton JC (2013) Translational magnetic resonance imaging and spectroscopy: opportunities and challenges. In: Garrido L, Beckmann N (eds) New applications of NMR in drug discovery and development. Royal Society of Chemistry, London, pp 333–360
5. O'Connor JP, Aboagye EO, Adams JE, Aerts HJ, Barrington SF, Beer AJ et al (2017) Imaging biomarker roadmap for cancer studies. Nat Rev Clin Oncol 14(3):169–186
6. Hueper K, Peperhove M, Rong S, Gerstenberg J, Mengel M, Meier M et al (2014) T1-mapping for assessment of ischemia-induced acute kidney injury and prediction of chronic kidney disease in mice. Eur Radiol 24(9):2252–2260
7. Tewes S, Gueler F, Chen R, Gutberlet M, Jang MS, Meier M et al (2017) Functional MRI for characterization of renal perfusion impairment and edema formation due to acute kidney injury in different mouse strains. PLoS One 12(3):e0173248
8. Hueper K, Hensen B, Gutberlet M, Chen R, Hartung D, Barrmeyer A et al (2016) Kidney transplantation: multiparametric functional magnetic resonance imaging for assessment of renal allograft pathophysiology in mice. Investig Radiol 51(1):58–65
9. Kierulf-Lassen C, Nielsen PM, Qi H, Damgaard M, Laustsen C, Pedersen M et al (2017) Unilateral nephrectomy diminishes ischemic acute kidney injury through enhanced perfusion and reduced pro-inflammatory and pro-fibrotic responses. PLoS One 12(12): e0190009
10. Wang JJ, Hendrich KS, Jackson EK, Ildstad ST, Williams DS, Ho C (1998) Perfusion quantitation in transplanted rat kidney by MRI with arterial spin labeling. Kidney Int 53 (6):1783–1791
11. Ogbron MR, Sareen S, Prychitko J, Buist R, Peeling J (1997) Altered organic anion and osmolyte content and excretion in rat polycystic kidney disease: an NMR study. Am J Phys 272(1 Pt 2):F63–F69
12. Ko SF, Yip HK, Zhen YY, Lee CC, Lee CC, Huang SJ et al (2017) Severe bilateral ischemic-reperfusion renal injury: hyperacute and acute changes in apparent diffusion coefficient, T1, and T2 mapping with immunohistochemical correlations. Sci Rep 7(1):1725
13. Keenan KE, Ainslie M, Barker AJ, Boss MA, Cecil KM, Charles C et al (2018) Quantitative magnetic resonance imaging phantoms: a review and the need for a system phantom. Magn Reson Med 79(1):48–61
14. Captur G, Gatehouse P, Keenan KE, Heslinga FG, Bruehl R, Prothmann M et al (2016) A medical device-grade T1 and ECV phantom for global T1 mapping quality assurance-the T1 mapping and ECV standardization in cardiovascular magnetic resonance (T1MES) program. J Cardiovasc Magn Reson 18(1):58
15. Lerski RA, McRobbie DW, Straughan K, Walker PM, de Certaines JD, Bernard AM (1988) Multi-center trial with protocols and prototype test objects for the assessment of MRI equipment. EEC Concerted Research Project. Magn Reson Imaging 6(2):201–214
16. Rajendran R, Lew SK, Yong CX, Tan J, Wang DJ, Chuang KH (2013) Quantitative mouse renal perfusion using arterial spin labeling. NMR Biomed 26(10):1225–1232
17. Christoffersson JO, Olsson LE, Sjoberg S (1991) Nickel-doped agarose gel phantoms in MR imaging. Acta Radiol 32(5):426–431
18. Kraft KA, Fatouros PP, Clarke GD, Kishore PR (1987) An MRI phantom material for quantitative relaxometry. Magn Reson Med 5 (6):555–562
19. Howe FA (1988) Relaxation times in paramagnetically doped agarose gels as a function of temperature and ion concentration. Magn Reson Imaging 6(3):263–270
20. Finney JS, Bach PH, Bushell MC, Gregg NM, Taylor DG (1990) The application of proton nuclear magnetic resonance imaging for the in vivo characterisation of chemically induced renal lesions in rats over a prolonged time study. Magn Reson Imaging 8(6):713–721
21. Jiang K, Tang H, Mishra PK, Macura SI, Lerman LO (2018) A rapid T1 mapping method for assessment of murine kidney viability using

dynamic manganese-enhanced magnetic resonance imaging. Magn Reson Med 80 (1):190–199

22. Korb JP, Bryant RG (2002) Magnetic field dependence of proton spin-lattice relaxation times. Magn Reson Med 48(1):21–26
23. Zhang J, Chamberlain R, Etheridge M, Idiyatullin D, Corum C, Bischof J et al (2014) Quantifying iron-oxide nanoparticles at high concentration based on longitudinal relaxation using a three-dimensional SWIFT Look-Locker sequence. Magn Reson Med 71 (6):1982–1988
24. Chow K, Flewitt JA, Green JD, Pagano JJ, Friedrich MG, Thompson RB (2014) Saturation recovery single-shot acquisition (SASHA) for myocardial T(1) mapping. Magn Reson Med 71(6):2082–2095
25. Stikov N, Boudreau M, Levesque IR, Tardif CL, Barral JK, Pike GB (2015) On the accuracy of T1 mapping: searching for common ground. Magn Reson Med 73(2):514–522
26. Akcakaya M, Weingartner S, Roujol S, Nezafat R (2015) On the selection of sampling points for myocardial T1 mapping. Magn Reson Med 73(5):1741–1753
27. Messroghli DR, Radjenovic A, Kozerke S, Higgins DM, Sivananthan MU, Ridgway JP (2004) Modified Look-Locker inversion recovery (MOLLI) for high-resolution T1 mapping of the heart. Magn Reson Med 52(1):141–146
28. Little RA, Jamin Y, Boult JKR, Naish JH, Watson Y, Cheung S et al (2018) Mapping hypoxia in renal carcinoma with oxygen-enhanced MRI: comparison with intrinsic susceptibility MRI and pathology. Radiology 288 (3):739–747
29. Hueper K, Gutberlet M, Rong S, Hartung D, Mengel M, Lu X et al (2014) Acute kidney injury: arterial spin labeling to monitor renal perfusion impairment in mice-comparison with histopathologic results and renal function. Radiology 270(1):117–124
30. Pastor G, Jimenez-Gonzalez M, Plaza-Garcia S, Beraza M, Reese T (2017) Fast T1 and T2 mapping methods: the zoomed U-FLARE sequence compared with EPI and snapshot-FLASH for abdominal imaging at 11.7 Tesla. MAGMA 30(3):299–307
31. Zhang J, Ring HL, Hurley KR, Shao Q, Carlson CS, Idiyatullin D et al (2017) Quantification and biodistribution of iron oxide nanoparticles in the primary clearance organs of mice using T1 contrast for heating. Magn Reson Med 78(2):702–712
32. Subashi E, Choudhury KR, Johnson GA (2014) An analysis of the uncertainty and bias in DCE-MRI measurements using the spoiled gradient-recalled echo pulse sequence. Med Phys 41(3):032301
33. Vautier J, Heilmann M, Walczak C, Mispelter J, Volk A (2010) 2D and 3D radial multi-gradient-echo DCE MRI in murine tumor models with dynamic R*2-corrected R1 mapping. Magn Reson Med 64(1):313–318
34. Alamidi DF, Smailagic A, Bidar AW, Parker NS, Olsson M, Hockings PD et al (2018) Variable flip angle 3D ultrashort echo time (UTE) T1 mapping of mouse lung: a repeatability assessment. J Magn Reson Imaging. https://doi.org/10.1002/jmri.25999
35. Marques JP, Kober T, Krueger G, van der Zwaag W, Van de Moortele PF, Gruetter R (2010) MP2RAGE, a self bias-field corrected sequence for improved segmentation and T1-mapping at high field. NeuroImage 49 (2):1271–1281
36. Yoon JH, Lee JM, Kim E, Okuaki T, Han JK (2017) Quantitative liver function analysis: volumetric T1 mapping with fast multisection B1 inhomogeneity correction in hepatocyte-specific contrast-enhanced liver MR imaging. Radiology 282(2):408–417
37. Stollberger R, Wach P (1996) Imaging of the active B1 field in vivo. Magn Reson Med 35 (2):246–251

12

Renal MRI Diffusion: Experimental Protocol

João S. Periquito, Martin Meier, Thoralf Niendorf, Andreas Pohlmann, and Neil Peter Jerome

Abstract

Renal diffusion-weighted imaging (DWI) can be used to obtain information on the microstructure of kidney tissue, and has the potential to provide MR-biomarkers for functional renal imaging. Here we describe in a step-by-step experimental protocol the MRI method for measuring renal diffusion coefficients in rodents using ADC or IVIM models. Both methods provide quantification of renal diffusion coefficients; however, IVIM, a more complex model, allows for the calculation of the pseudodiffusion and fraction introduced by tissue vascular and tubular components. DWI provides information of renal microstructure contributing to the understanding of the physiology and the underlying processes that precede the beginning of pathologies.

This chapter is based upon work from the COST Action PARENCHIMA, a community-driven network funded by the European Cooperation in Science and Technology (COST) program of the European Union, which aims to improve the reproducibility and standardization of renal MRI biomarkers. This experimental protocol chapter is complemented by two separate chapters describing the basic concept and data analysis.

Key words Magnetic resonance imaging (MRI), Kidney, Mice, Rats, Diffusion, ADC, IVIM

1 Introduction

Diffusion weighting imaging (DWI) is an MR imaging technique sensitive to the motion of water molecules within a voxel of tissue. The random movement, also known as Brownian motion, of fluid molecules makes them spread out until a boundary stops them. In general, extracellular water molecules will have a larger net displacement over time than intracellular molecules. Intracellular molecules have more chances to collide with cell walls, organelles, and macromolecules. Diseases and pathologies that influence tissue properties and structure may either increase or decrease the diffusion behavior of water in tissues, which can be quantified using DWI [1, 2].

In DWI, the image contrast is based on the displacement of water molecules. Voxels where molecules present a larger

Andreas Pohlmann and Thoralf Niendorf (eds.), *Preclinical MRI of the Kidney: Methods and Protocols*, Methods in Molecular Biology, vol. 2216, https://doi.org/10.1007/978-1-0716-0978-1_24,

displacement during the diffusion-sensitization preparation will appear darker on the resulting image.

Sensitization to diffusion can be achieved by using an extra pair of magnetic field gradients during the pulse sequence, generating images with diffusion-weighting determined by the magnitude, duration, and separation of the gradients, which can be quantified by the acquisition parameter *b*-value [3].

The DWI signal decay across a series of images with different diffusion-weightings can then be analyzed, using more or less complex mathematical models, to quantify the diffusion parameters. Ideally, the acquisition should be designed considering the signal model one wishes to use. The simplest model considers only the apparent diffusion coefficient (ADC), an empirical parameter reflecting the overall water molecule motion in the tissue averaged over one or more directions using a small number of *b*-values. ADC can be estimated by fitting a monoexponential curve to the DWI signal as a function of b-value, and fitting signal curves on a pixel-by-pixel basis allows construction of diffusion parameter maps [4].

Perfusion in tissue introduces a pseudodiffusion component to the DWI signal, which cannot be quantified using the ADC model (but it will influence the calculated ADC if low b-values are included). A more complex model is needed to take separate out this effect. Intravoxel incoherent motion (IVIM) intends to model flow processes, which manifest as pseudodiffusion with a larger coefficient, by assuming the DWI signal as a function of the *b*-value is not monoexponential but biexponential. This method requires the acquisition of several *b*-values before the pseudodiffusion decays away, especially between *b*-values of 0 and 200 s/mm^2 [5].

This experimental protocol chapter is complemented by two separate chapters describing the basic concept and data analysis, which are part of this book.

This chapter is part of the book Pohlmann A, Niendorf T (eds) (2020) Preclinical MRI of the Kidney—Methods and Protocols. Springer, New York.

2 Materials

2.1 Animals

This experimental protocol is tailored for mice (variants of C57BL/6) with a body mass of 15–35 g. Advice for adaptation to rats is given as *Notes* where necessary.

2.2 Lab Equipment and Chemicals

1. Anesthesia: typically, 0.5–1.5% isoflurane is used for anesthesia administered to the mice using an anesthetic gas vaporizer (Leica Biosystems, Maryland, USA). For nonrecovery experiments, urethane solution (Sigma-Aldrich, Steinheim,

Germany; 20% in distilled water) can provide anesthesia for several hours with comparatively fewer side effects on renal physiology, which is an important issue. For nonrecovery experiments urethane solution (Sigma-Aldrich, Steinheim, Germany; 20% in distilled water) can provide anesthesia for several hours with comparatively fewer side effects on renal physiology, which is an important issue. For an in-depth description and discussion of the anesthesia please refer to the chapter by Kaucsar T et al. "Preparation and Monitoring of Small Animals in Renal MRI."

2. Gases: O_2, N_2, and compressed air, as well as a gas-mixing system (FMI Föhr Medical Instruments GmbH, Seeheim-Ober Beerbach, Germany) or general inhalation anesthesia equipment, including an anesthetic vaporizer, a flow meter, and an induction chamber.

2.3 MRI Hardware

The general hardware requirements for renal ^{1}H MRI on mice and rats are described in the chapter by Ramos Delgado P et al. "Hardware Considerations for Preclinical Magnetic Resonance of the Kidney." The technique described in this chapter has been tailored for MR preclinical systems at magnetic fields higher than 3 T but advice for adaptation to other field strengths is given where necessary. No special or additional hardware is required, except for the following:

A physiological monitoring system that can track the respiration and which is connected to the MR system such that it can be used to trigger the MRI scanner with respiration. Typically, we use the MR-compatible rodent monitoring and gating system (Small Animal Instruments, New York, USA) equipped with an air-pillow to monitor breathing rate.

2.4 MRI Techniques

The diffusion MRI pulse sequence includes a diffusion preparation responsible for the diffusion sensitization. Specifically, sensitisation to diffusion and/or other motion of water molecules is achieved by inclusion of an extra pair of magnetic field gradients during the acquisition, generating images with varying degrees of diffusion-weighting. The degree of diffusion weighting depends on the area of each of the diffusion gradients (amplitude G and duration δ) as well as the time spacing between the pair (Δ); the resulting weighting is commonly specified by the compound parameter *b*-value (Fig. 1). The diffusion module is followed by fast image readout such as echo planar imaging (EPI). Other readouts are available for DWI (*see* **Note 1**), but DW-EPI is the standard since it provides the higher SNR in acceptable acquisition times, and so will be used in this chapter.

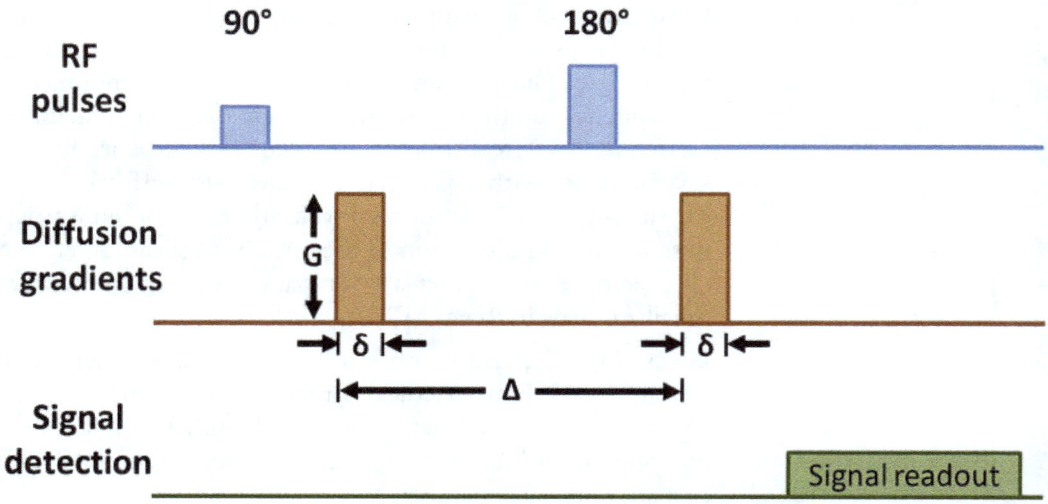

Fig. 1 Diffusion preparation ("Diffusion gradients"). The degree of diffusion weighting (measured by the "*b*-value" [mm/s^2]) depends on the area of the extra pair of gradients (amplitude *G* and duration δ) as well as the time spacing between them (Δ): $b = \gamma^2 G^2 \delta^2 \left(\Delta - \frac{\delta}{3}\right)$

3 Methods

3.1 MR Protocol Setup

All the mentioned MR parameters are adjustable; the provided suggestions are based on experience, but the end protocol is likely to be adjusted from these values. For more details on what goes toward making these decisions please refer to the chapter by Jerome NP et al. "Renal Diffusion-Weighted Imaging (DWI) for Apparent Diffusion Coefficient (ADC), Intravoxel Incoherent Motion (IVIM), and Diffusion Tensor Imaging (DTI): Basic Concepts"of this book.

3.1.1 DW-EPI for ADC

1. Load the DW-EPI sequence.
2. Sequence type: 2D Echo Planar Imaging sequence with diffusion preparation module that has a defined Δ and δ and a G which can be incremented within a single scan. This is a standard sequence on Bruker MRI systems, called "DW-EPI."
3. The diffusion parameters are then adjusted to allow detection of incoherent movement of molecules. The range of displacements measured with DWI is typically in the order of 1–20 μm, allowing for quantitative measurements that reflect micromorphological and physiological changes in tissues. As a recommendation a $\delta = 3.5$ ms and a $\Delta = 8.5$ ms should be used (*see* **Note 2**).
4. Set up your *b*-values to the following values: 0, 200, 600 s/mm^2 over three orthogonal directions *x*: (1,0,0), *y*: (0,1,0) and *z*: (0,0,1).

5. Repetition time (TR): choose ~500 ms for good signal stability and signal-to-noise per time (SNR/t) efficiency. TR will be limited by the length of the excitation pulse, length of echo train and the number of slices you acquire.
6. Echo time (TE): use the shortest TE. Acquisition bandwidth should be considered to shorten the inter-echo-time.
7. Segments: as low as possible to reduce scan time, however 1 segment (single-shot) might create unacceptable distortions on phase encoding. A high number of segments will increase scan time and makes the acquisition more prone to motion artifacts. As a recommendation two segments should be used (multishot DW-EPI) with a matrix size of 172 × 172 with an FOV of 30 × 30 mm.
8. Acquisition bandwidth (BW): ~ 350.000 Hz, one wants to acquire as many lines of k-space as possible to minimize motion distortions of the images. For that reason, it is advantageous to have a low inter-echo-time. Larger inter-echo-times are not advisable because the SNR in the kidney will be so low that these images must be excluded.
9. Enable fat saturation. On ultrahigh field systems this works well to avoid fat signal overlaying the kidney due to chemical shift. At lower field strengths it might work less efficient.
10. Enable the respiration trigger (per slice). This is essential to reduce motion artefacts, reduce motion blurring and unwanted intensities variations among the images acquired with different *b*-values (*see* **Note 3**).
11. Choose as phase-encoding direction the L-R direction and adapt the geometry so that the FOV in this direction includes the entire animal.
12. Use frequency encoding in head-feet (rostral-caudal) direction to avoid severe aliasing. Adjust the FOV to your needs keeping in mind that in this direction the FOV can be smaller than the animal and a smaller FOV permits a smaller acquisition matrix, and in turn a shorter echo-spacing.
13. Increase the number of averages to improve signal-to-noise ratio by a factor of $\sqrt{}$averages, especially important for higher *b*-values (use nine averages as a recommendation).
14. To reach a steady-state magnetization is advisable to use dummy scans, two as a recommendation.
15. For an example of a specific parameter set please *see* **Notes 4** and **5**.
16. For adaptation of the geometry to rats (*see* **Note 6**).

3.1.2 DW-EPI for IVIM

1. Load the DW-EPI sequence.
2. Use the same parameters as DWI-EPI for ADC (TE, TR, matrix size, dummy scans, averages, bandwidth, segments).
3. Keep the same diffusion parameters as for the ADC but increase the number of *b*-values from 3 to at least 7 (e.g., 0, 50, 100, 200, 400, 600, and 740 s/mm^2) to probe fast diffusion from blood perfusion.

3.2 In Vivo DWI

3.2.1 Animal Preparation

1. Anesthetize the animal and transfer it to scanner. For an in-depth description and discussion of the anesthesia please refer to the chapter by Kaucsar T et al. "Preparation and Monitoring of Small Animals in Renal MRI."
2. Start the temperature monitoring system, apply some surgical lubricant to the temperature probe and place it in the rectum of the animal.
3. Attach the respiration sensor (e.g., balloon) to the chest of the animal using adhesive tape. Start and set up the respiratory monitoring system. If necessary, adjust the position of the respiration sensor until the amplitude of the respiration trace is sufficiently large for the system to reliably detect the trigger points at the beginning of expiration (*see* **Note 3**).

3.2.2 Scanner Adjustments and Anatomical Imaging

1. Acquire a fast pilot scan to obtain images in three orthogonal planes *x*, *y*, and *z*.
2. Acquire anatomical images in several oblique orientations to facilitate planning a coronal slice orientation with regard to the long axis of the kidney, as described in the chapter by Pohlmann A et al. "Essential Practical Steps for MRI of the Kidney in Experimental Research" (open-access).
3. Perform localized shimming on the kidney as described in the chapter by Pohlmann A et al. "Essential Practical Steps for MRI of the Kidney in Experimental Research" (open-access). NB: shimming is crucial for DW-EPI (*see* **Note 7**), because a poor shim can lead to large distortions and add errors in the measured diffusion coefficients.
4. Acquire a 3D B_0 field-map without adaptation of the geometry (optional; *see* **Notes 8** and **9**).

3.2.3 Baseline Condition

1. Load the 2D multishot EPI sequence, adapt the slice orientation to provide a coronal or axial view with respect to the kidney (in scanner coordinates this is double-oblique).
2. In the monitoring unit set the trigger delay so that the trigger starts at the beginning of the expiratory plateau (no chest or diaphragm motion) and the duration such that it covers the

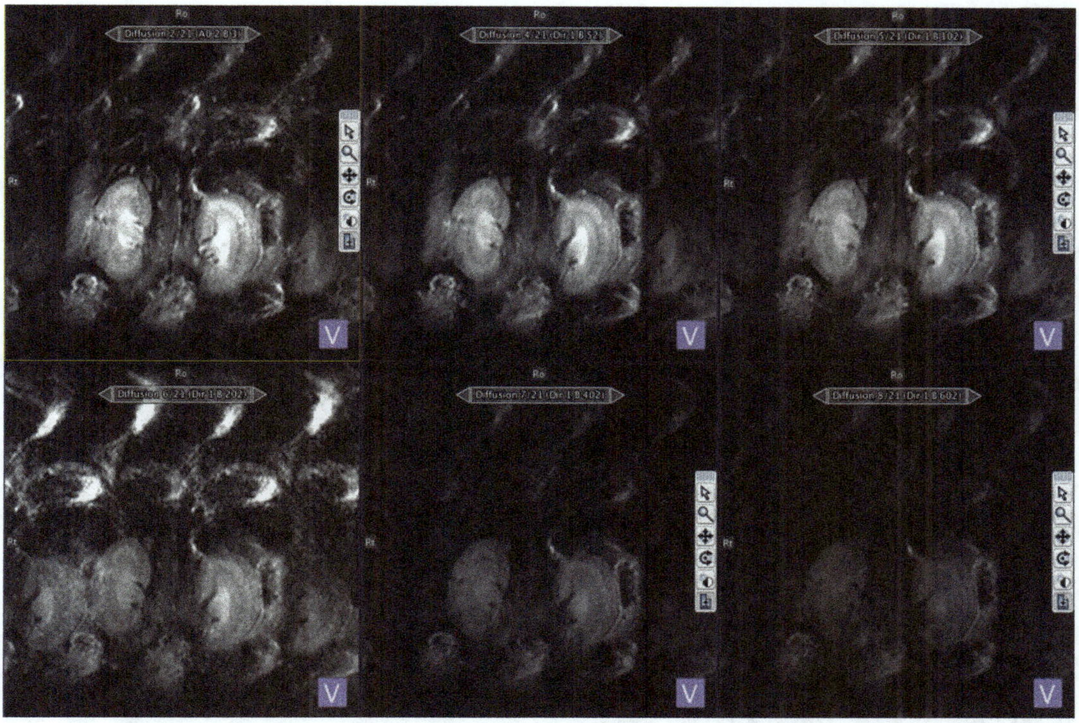

Fig. 2 Series of six diffusion-weighted images of a healthy mouse kidney acquired with DW-EPI sequence at 7.0 T. Images correspond to *b*-values: 0, 50, 100, 200, 400, and 600 mm/s^2. EPI readouts are prone to magnetic susceptibility artifacts, low-phase encoding bandwidth leads to ΔB_0 induced frequency dispersions which causes image distortion. When using a segmented EPI readout a phase deviation occurs between the different segments in k-space leading to ghosting artefacts visible in the above images [7]

entire expiratory phase, that is, until just before inhalation starts (1/2–2/3 of breath-to-breath interval) (*see* **Note 3**).

3. In the monitoring unit set the trigger delay so that the trigger starts at the beginning of the expiratory plateau (no chest or diaphragm motion) and the duration to a short value, such as 10 ms (*see* **Note 3**).
4. Run the EPI scan. Example images are shown in Fig. 2.

4 Notes

1. Other readouts apart from EPI can be use in DWI such as rapid acquisition with relaxation enhancement (RARE) (Fig. 3) which is less prone to suffering from geometric distortion specially at ultrahigh magnetic fields [6].
2. Gradients systems might differ from MR scanner to MR scanner even for the same magnetic field. If the gradient system cannot reach *b*-value of 600, consider to adjust $\delta = 3.5$ ms and

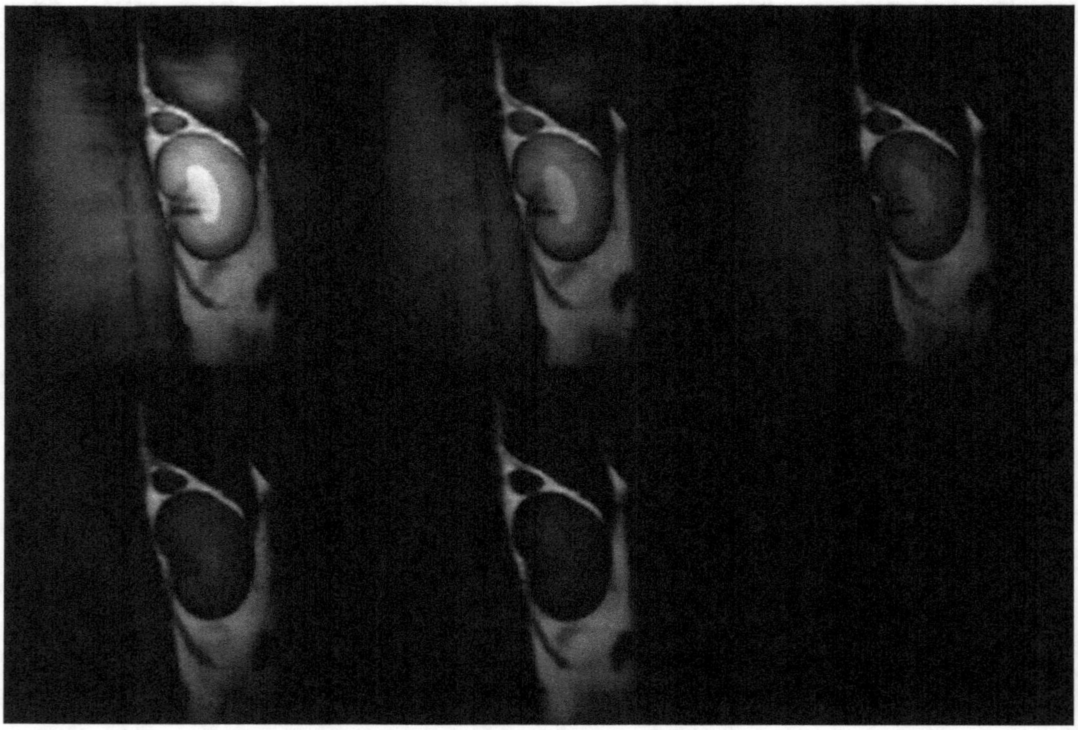

Fig. 3 Series of five diffusion-weighted images of a healthy mouse kidney acquired with single-shot DW-RARE sequence at 9.4 T. Images correspond to *b*-values: 0, 200, 300, 400, and 600 mm/s^2. A RARE readout can be used to minimize the magnetic susceptibility artifacts which cause geometric distortions on DW-EPI. DW-RARE is not commercially available, pulse programming skills are needed to implement it [6]

a $\Delta = 8.5$ to higher values. Record and report all diffusion parameters used.

3. You must monitor the respiration continuously throughout the entire experiment.
4. *Example for ADC of a 30 g mouse at 7 T (Bruker small animal system)*: TR = 500 ms; 3 *b*-values: 0, 200, 600 s/mm^2, diffusion directions: 3 (orthogonal), effective TE = 56.87 ms; Segments = 2; averages = 9; slice thickness = 1.2 mm; slice orientation = axial; frequency encoding = head-feet; FOV = 30 × 30 mm; matrix size = 172 × 172; Bandwidth = 350.000 Hz; fat suppression = on; scan time ≈ 80 s.
5. *Example for ADC of a 270 g rat at 9.4 T (Bruker small animal system)*: TR = 500 ms; 3 *b*-values: 0, 200, 600 s/mm^2, diffusion directions: 3 (orthogonal), effective TE = 56.87 ms; Segments = 2; averages = 9; slice thickness = 1.2 mm; slice orientation = axial; frequency encoding = head-feet; FOV = 45 × 45 mm; matrix size = 172 × 172; Bandwidth = 350.000 Hz; fat suppression = on;, scan time ≈ 80 s.

6. For rats increase the FOV to the body width and keep the matrix size the same or similar. The relative resolution is then identical and the SNR should also be similar, because the larger rat RF coil provides worse SNR (e.g., eight-channel rat body phase array receive coil vs eight-channel mouse body phase array receive coil).
7. Shimming is particularly important, since macroscopic magnetic field inhomogeneities affect EPI readout and might create severe geometric distortions. Shimming should be performed on a voxel enclosing the kidney using either the default iterative shimming method or the Mapshim technique (recommended).
8. *Example parameters for field mapping of a 30 g mice at 9.4 T (Bruker small animal system)*: use the vendors default protocol *AnyObject > AnyRegion > Adjustments > ADJ_B0MAP.* TR = 20 ms; flip angle = 30°; first echo = 1.60 ms; echo spacing = 3.57 ms; fat/water in-phase = on; slice orientation = main orientations (no angles) and offset = 0; FOC = (58 × 58 × 58) mm; matrix size =64 × 64 × 64; resolution = (0.904 × 0.904 × 0.904) mm; respiration trigger = off; acquisition time = 1–2 min.
9. This serves to keep a record of the B_0 influence on the measured DW-EPI images. It allows explanation of unusually distortions due to an imperfect shim.

Acknowledgments

This work was funded, in part (Thoralf Niendorf, Andreas Pohlmann, and Joao Periquito), by the German Research Foundation (Gefoerdert durch die Deutsche Forschungsgemeinschaft (DFG), Projektnummer 394046635, SFB 1365, RENOPROTECTION. Funded by the Deutsche Forschungsgemeinschaft (DFG, German Research Foundation), Project number 394046635, SFB 1365, RENOPROTECTION).

This chapter is based upon work from COST Action PARENCHIMA, supported by European Cooperation in Science and Technology (COST). COST (www.cost.eu) is a funding agency for research and innovation networks. COST Actions help connect research initiatives across Europe and enable scientists to enrich their ideas by sharing them with their peers. This boosts their research, career, and innovation.

PARENCHIMA (renalmri.org) is a community-driven Action in the COST program of the European Union, which unites more than 200 experts in renal MRI from 30 countries with the aim to improve the reproducibility and standardization of renal MRI biomarkers.

References

1. Hahn EL (1950) Spin echoes. Phys Rev 80:580–594
2. Carr HY, Purcell EM (1954) Effects of diffusion on free precessions in nuclear magnetic resonance experiments. Phys Rev 94:630–635
3. Stejskal EO, Tanner JE (1965) Spin diffusion measurements: spin echoes in the presence of a time-dependent field gradient. J Chem Phys 42:288–292. https://doi.org/10.1063/1.1695690
4. Le Bihan D et al (1950) Imagerie de diffusion in-vivo par resonance magnetique. CR Acad Sci 15:1109–1112
5. Le Bihan D et al (1988) Separation of diffusion and perfusion in intravoxel incoherent motion MR imaging. Radiology 168(2):497–505
6. Periquito J et al (2020) Diffusion-weighted renal MRI at 9.4 Tesla using RARE to improve anatomical integrity. *Scientific Reports* 9(1):1–12
7. Paul K et al (2015) Diffusion-sensitized ophthalmic magnetic resonance imaging free of geometric distortion at 3.0 and 7.0 T: a feasibility study in healthy subjects and patients with intraocular masses. Investig Radiol 50:309–321

13

Renal Blood Flow Using Arterial Spin Labeling (ASL) MRI: Experimental Protocol and Principles

Kai-Hsiang Chuang, Martin Meier, María A. Fernández-Seara, Frank Kober, and Min-Chi Ku

Abstract

A noninvasive, robust, and reproducible method to measure renal perfusion is important to understand the physiology of kidney. Arterial spin labeling (ASL) MRI technique labels the endogenous blood water as freely diffusible tracers to measure perfusion quantitatively without relying on exogenous contrast agent. Therefore, it alleviates the safety concern involving gadolinium chelates. To obtain quantitative tissue perfusion information is particularly relevant for multisite and longitudinal imaging of living subjects.

This chapter is based upon work from the PARENCHIMA COST Action, a community-driven network funded by the European Cooperation in Science and Technology (COST) program of the European Union, which aims to improve the reproducibility and standardization of renal MRI biomarkers. This experimental protocol chapter is complemented by two separate chapters describing the basic concept and data analysis.

Key words Magnetic resonance imaging (MRI), Kidney, Mice, Arterial spin labeling (ASL)

1 Introduction

Arterial spin labeling (ASL) is a magnetic resonance imaging (MRI) method for measuring tissue perfusion [1, 2]. The term perfusion refers to the delivery of blood to capillary beds, and is quantified by the amount of blood delivered to the tissue per unit time, per unit volume or mass of tissue. The quantification of renal tissue perfusion is essential because it determines the rate of nutrients (e.g., oxygenation and glucose) to the renal tissue, and the rate of clearance of waste products.

The principle of ASL-MRI is to label the arterial blood as an endogenous diffusible tracer. Before the blood flows into the target tissue, the blood proton spins are "labeled" (tagged) by inverting the longitudinal magnetization using radiofrequency (RF) pulses. The labeled blood then flows into the kidney tissue, resembling direct exogenous contrast more than MRI contrast agents that act

Andreas Pohlmann and Thoralf Niendorf (eds.), *Preclinical MRI of the Kidney: Methods and Protocols*, Methods in Molecular Biology, vol. 2216, https://doi.org/10.1007/978-1-0716-0978-1_26,

on relaxation times. The labeled blood, however, loses its contrast on its way to kidney tissue within a few seconds due to the T_1 relaxation of blood. This makes ASL only suitable for probing renal perfusion, but not later processes in the kidney such as glomerular filtration. On the other hand, the intrinsic signals from the static kidney tissue have to be eliminated. For this, a control image without labeling arterial blood is acquired, and subtraction of the two images with and without labeling would result in an image enhanced with only the labeled arterial blood.

The most frequently used ASL technique for kidney imaging is flow-sensitive alternating inversion recovery (FAIR) which uses an inversion pulse for spin labeling [3]. Its principle is illustrated in the chapter by Ku M-C et al. "Noninvasive Renal Perfusion Measurement Using Arterial Spin Labeling (ASL) MRI: Basic Concept." In this technique, two acquisitions with different inversions are alternatingly applied: one acquisition with selective inversion of a slab that is slightly larger than the imaging slice (no labeling of in-flowing blood) and a second acquisition with global inversion of all blood within the RF coil (nonselective inversion). Subtraction of the image with global inversion from the image with spatially selective inversion results in a perfusion-weighted image, as the difference between the two images is caused by the noninverted blood spins moving from outside the selective inversion slab into the imaging plane.

Here we describe ASL-MRI using FAIR method for monitoring of the renal blood flow in the kidney of rodents in a step-by-step experimental protocol. The rationale for the chosen acquisition parameters is given in generic terms, together with specific parameter examples.

This experimental protocol chapter is complemented by two separate chapters describing the basic concept and data analysis, which are part of this book.

This chapter is part of the book Pohlmann A, Niendorf T (eds) (2020) Preclinical MRI of the Kidney—Methods and Protocols. Springer, New York.

2 Materials

2.1 Animals

This experimental protocol is tailored to mice (e.g., wild type C57BL/6 or disease model in immune-deficient nude mice) with a body mass of 20–40 g. Some advice for adaptation to other rodents such as rats is given as *Notes* when necessary.

2.2 Lab Equipment

1. Anesthesia: For an in-depth description and discussion of anesthesia please refer to the chapter by Kaucsar T et al. "Preparation and Monitoring of Small Animals in Renal MRI." Typically 0.5–1.5% isoflurane is used for anesthesia administered to the mice using an anesthetic gas vaporizer (Dräger Vapor® FMI Föhr Medical Instruments GmbH, Seeheim-Ober Beerbach, Germany).

2. Gases: O_2, N_2 and compressed air, as well as a gas-mixing system or general inhalation anesthesia equipment, including an anesthetic vaporizer, a flow meter and an induction chamber.

2.3 MRI Hardware

The general hardware requirements for renal ^{1}H MRI on mice and rats are described in the chapter by Ramos Delgado P et al. "Hardware Considerations for Preclinical Magnetic Resonance of the Kidney." The technique described in this chapter was tailored for a 7 T MR system (Biospec 70/20, Bruker Biospin, Ettlingen, Germany) but advice for adaptation to other field strengths is given where necessary. No special or additional hardware is required, except for:

1. A physiological monitoring system that can track the respiration, and is connected to the MR system such that it can be used to trigger the image acquisition. Typically, the MR-compatible rodent monitoring and gating system (Small Animal Instruments, New York, USA) equipped with an air-pillow to monitor breath rate can be used.
2. Mouse cradle and RF-antenna (*see* **Note 1**): The 2 × 2 cardiac coil array (Bruker), originally designed for mouse heart is integrated into corresponding animal cradle tips. The combination of receive-only coil array and a circularly polarized volume transmitter coil (Bruker) will improve signal to noise ratio (SNR). Alternatively, a single-loop surface coil could be used for receiving provided that a volume coil is used for transmit in any case.

2.4 MRI Sequences

1. *Sequence type*: For the choice of type of sequence to use for renal ASL in rodents please refer to the chapter by Ku M-C et al. "Noninvasive Renal Perfusion Measurement Using Arterial Spin Labeling (ASL) MRI: Basic Concept." A 2D sequence composed by FAIR for labeling and EPI for image acquisition is described in this chapter. This is a standard sequence on Bruker MRI systems, where it is called "FAIR-EPI." To minimize the susceptibility artifact and geometric distortion in the abdomen, spin-echo EPI or RARE acquisition is desirable as alternative ("FAIR-RARE").
2. *Echo time (TE)*: To preserve signal from T_2/T_2^* decay, a minimum TE should always be used (~10 ms) to maximize SNR.

   Avoid crusher gradients: Although they reduce flow-related artifacts, they require prolongation of the minimum TE. They would reduce SNR and introduce more T_2 (T_2^*) contrast into the ASL image. Crusher gradients also remove potentially important information, such as the presence of delayed or collateral flow.

3. *Repetition time (TR)*: There are two considerations on choosing appropriate TR. First, to allow substantial relaxation of labeled spins between acquisitions, TR should be long enough (~10,000 ms). Since T_1 time is field dependent, TR as well. The long TR (~10,000 ms) is recommended for a 7 T system. For other field strength this value need to be justified. Second, if respiratory induced artifact is severe and the respiratory trigger is needed, a long TR that is at least five times greater than the tissue T_1 (e.g., 10 s) can be used to minimize the variable T_1-weighting due to irregular respiration rate. If the respiratory trigger is not needed, a shorter TR that has good signal-to-noise per time (SNR/t) efficiency could be used. TR will be limited by the maximum inversion time (TI) and the number of acquired slices.
4. *TR mode*: TR must allow tag washout and refreshing, TE should be short to minimize T2 contamination.
5. *Repetition spacing*: Choose "Const_Rep" to use the same TR.
6. *FAIR Experiment Mode*: Choose "Interleaved (TI loop outside)" to measure control-label pairs, followed by different TI.
7. *Inversion mode (TI Setting)*: Set for "User" TIR.
8. *Inversion time* (TI): TI should be long enough to permit tagging to leave tagging region and ensure tag exchange with tissue water (i.e., the arterial arrival time), but short enough to reduce loss of tag. TI should be increased whenever slow arterial flows (i.e., long arterial arrival time) are expected. For example, in the case of poor cardiac output. Shorter TI values are recommended in case of more rapid circulation times (this depends on the anesthesia level). Unless the arterial arrival time is known, measurement with multiple TI is recommended, e.g., from 25, 50, 100, 150, 200, 300, 500, 1000, 1500, 2000, to 5000 ms. The arrival time increases with the selective inversion slab thickness. For single slice FAIR, the arrival time is typically very short (*see* **Note 2**).
9. *Inversion pulse*: For inversion, an adiabatic full passage frequency-selective inversion pulse (e.g., hyperbolic secant-shaped pulse) should be used with a high bandwidth of 5190 Hz. A calculated adiabatic pulse can be used as well.
10. *Inversion slab thickness*: This depends on the imaging slice thickness. Usually at least 2.5 times of slice package thickness. For example, the slice package margin should be at least 1.5 mm resulting in a 5 mm inversion slice when you use 2 mm slice thickness.
11. *Acquisition bandwidth (BW)*: Use a high BW (e.g., 200 kHz) for EPI readout to shorten TE. Keep an eye on the SNR while modifying BW. SNR decreases with increasing BW. Low SNR

may be balanced out with more averages or repetitions. For scanning with a short TE, an SNR of at least 60 is recommended (*see* **Note 3**).

12. *Fat saturation*: Turn on. Important to avoid fat signal overlaying the kidney due to chemical shift.
13. *Geometry*: this is a tricky part. To cover the whole kidney in one slice, an oblique coronal slice will be needed. It is important to avoid the selective inversion slab crossing the feeding arteries (aorta) as this will reduce the labeled arterial blood spins. Use a rectangular field of view (FOV) and use a frequency encoding in H-F direction to avoid aliasing (*see* **Note 4**).
14. *Respiration trigger*: Turn on (per repetition). This is essential when respiration is very irregular or motion artifact is induced in multishot imaging such as RARE.
15. *Number of slice and thickness*: Slice thickness is typically no less than 1 mm in mice or rats due to the low SNR of ASL. The number of slices and thickness determines the selective inversion slab thickness. It should be noted that ASL using FAIR is not suitable for multislice imaging per se, because the labeled blood magnetization decreases with increasing inversion slab thickness. This is due to relaxation during transit, but also to the excitation pulses related to imaging readout in the various slices. Therefore, usually no more than three slices are recommended. Besides, ASL has generally low SNR due to a relatively small fractional magnetization of available labeled arterial blood (1–5%). Therefore, rather thick imaging slices ($\geq$1 mm) are needed to reduce noise.
16. *T_1 map*: A T_1 map is useful to improve the quantification accuracy as it provides a measured tissue T_1 (which is different in medulla and cortex) and inversion efficiency. It can be adapted from the ASL sequence by selecting the "nonselective inversion" mode in "FAIR Experiment." Set up at least six TI in logarithmic order (e.g., 10, 50, 200, 1000, 2000, 5000, 9000 ms) with long constant TR (e.g., 10 s). A few (e.g., 3) data averaging will be needed to increase SNR.

3 Methods

3.1 Animal Preparations and Initial Setups for Imaging

1. Anesthetize the animal with isoflurane in an induction box (approximately 3–3.5% isoflurane for induction with air and oxygen mixed at a 3:1 ratio) and then transfer the animal to the scanner (*see* **Note 5**).
2. Set up the temperature monitoring (rectal probe) and respiratory monitoring (balloon on chest) unit. Ophthalmic ointment should be applied to the eyes of the animal.

3. If isoflurane is used, adjust anesthesia level (e.g., 1.5–2%) to maintain regular respiration rate around 90 breaths per minute (bpm) in mouse or 60 bpm in rat during the scan. The level of isoflurane may need to be adjusted regularly to maintain a rather constant respiration rate (*see* **Note 6**).
4. Carefully position the RF-antenna to be near the kidney and place it to the magnet isocenter based on the initial anatomical imaging.
5. Perform coil tuning/matching and *global* shimming (*see* **Note 7**).
6. Acquire kidney anatomical imaging (i.e., routine respiratory triggered T_2-weighted turbo spin echo sequences in axial and coronal planes) as described in the chapter by Pohlmann A et al. "Essential Practical Steps for MRI of the Kidney in Experimental Research" (*see* **Note 8**).
7. In the case of use a sequence with FAIR for labeling and EPI for image readout (FAIR-EPI), please perform the trajectory adjustment (*see* **Note 9**).

3.2 Renal Perfusion Imaging

3.2.1 Baseline Condition (Healthy Animal)

1. Load the ASL (FAIR-EPI) sequence (*see* **Note 10**), adapt the slice orientation to provide either a coronal or axial view with respect to the kidney (in scanner coordinates this is double-oblique). Adjust the geometry of a flow saturation slice onto aorta and perpendicular to the ASL imaging slices (Fig. 1) (*see* **Note 11**).
2. Acquire a pilot scan to evaluate slice location and image quality by setting repetition and average to 1. Fine tune the slice position based on the pilot scan to maximize the coverage of

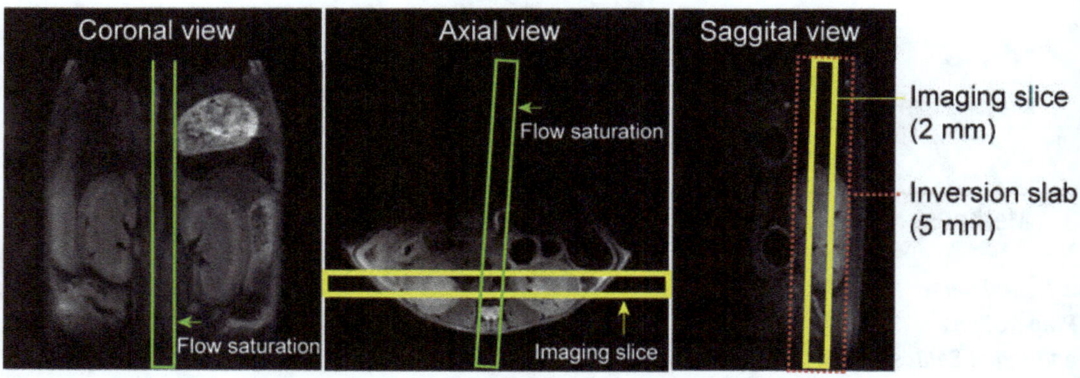

Fig. 1 Anatomical images with 3 planes (coronal, axial and sagittal views of mouse kidneys). Imaging is performed in a central coronal plane, adjusted to the long axis of the kidneys. The green box outlines slice position for a saturation slice. The yellow box outlines the imaging slice for a coronal view. The red dotted box outlines the inversion slab. Please note that the inversion slab has to be thicker than the imaging slice

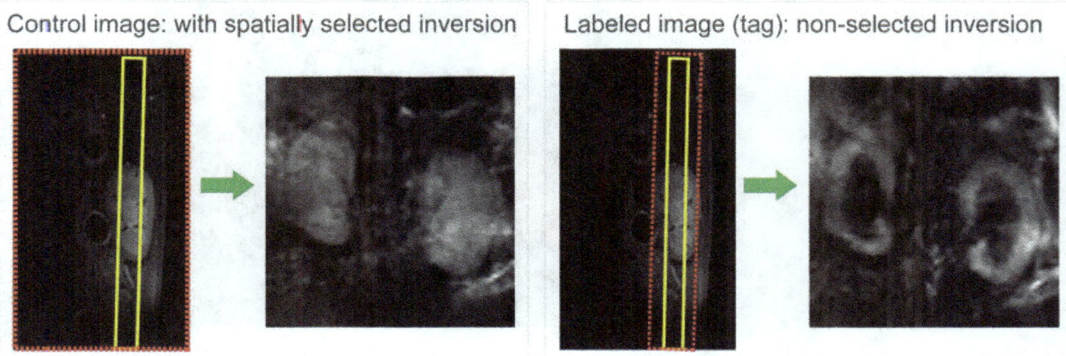

Fig. 2 Left: A resulted ASL image with coronal view from nonselective inversion pulse. Right: A resulted ASL image with coronal view from selective inversion

kidney while avoiding the selective inversion slab (imaging slab) to cross the feeding arteries (Fig. 2).

3. Perform subtraction between label and control images to evaluate the level of perfusion signal.
4. Acquire ASL scans with multiple repetitions. Increase repetition if SNR is not optimal (*see* **Note 12**).
5. Inspect the acquired image time series. If motion artifacts are severe, use respiratory trigger and then repeat scans (*see* **Note 13**).
6. When use respiration triggering: in the monitoring unit set the trigger delay so that the trigger starts at the beginning of the expiratory plateau (no chest motion) and the duration such that it covers the entire expiratory phase, that is, until just before the next inhalation starts.
7. Clone (duplicate) the ASL scan and set all the optimized parameters. Run the sequence for ASL scanning.
8. Load the T_1-mapping (IR-EPI) scan using the same slice geometry and resolution.

3.2.2 Hypoxia/Hyperoxia/Hypercapnia for Benchmarking (Optional)

1. Duplicate the ASL (FAIR-EPI) scan.
2. Start of hypoxia: Change the gas flowing through the respiratory mask to 10% O_2/90% N_2.
3. Exactly 5 min after the start of hypoxia run the ASL and T_1-mapping scans.
4. End of Hypoxia: Change the gas flowing through the respiratory mask back to air (21% O_2).
5. Similarly, hyperoxia and hypercapnia conditions could be assessed by switching to 100% O_2 and 5% CO_2 in air, respectively.

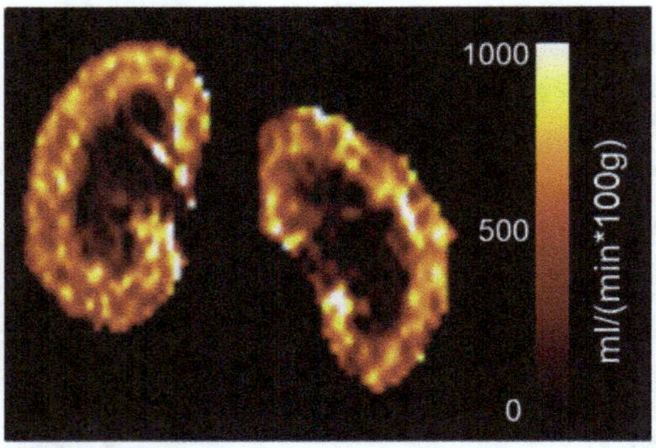

Fig. 3 A noninvasive, robust, and reproducible functional MRI method to characterize the physiology of kidney: An example of resulted renal perfusion maps in C57BL/6 mouse

3.2.3 Perfusion Map

1. The demonstration of a perfusion map that can be expected in physiological condition is shown in Fig. 3. Please note that the detailed protocol for the image analysis is given in the chapter by Chuang K-H et al. "Quantitative Analysis of Renal Perfusion by Arterial Spin Labeling." Briefly, the perfusion-weighted signals at different TIs, $\Delta M(\mathrm{TI})$, can be fitted to a kinetic function by a nonlinear least square routine in Matlab (Mathworks, MA, USA) [4–6]:

$$\Delta M(\mathrm{TI}) = 2M_0\alpha f/\lambda\left[\frac{\exp\left(-\mathrm{TI}/T_{1\mathrm{app}}\right) - \exp\left(-\mathrm{TI}/T_{1a}\right)}{\left(1/T_{1a} - 1/T_{1\mathrm{app}}\right)}\right],$$

   where $1/T_{1\mathrm{app}} = 1/T_1 + f/\lambda$, f is the perfusion (when lambda is in ml/100 g and T_1 in minutes), T_{1a} is the arterial blood T_1, and λ is the blood/tissue partition coefficient. In this equation, three parameters can be derived from the additional T_1 mapping: M_0 represents the equilibrium magnetization, T_1 the tissue longitudinal relaxation time, and α the inversion efficiency. They can be calculated by three-parameter curve fitting of the inversion recovery T_1 mapping data. Please note that the above equation assumes minimal and negligible arterial transit time.

2. In the Macro manager, choose Calculate Global T_1 Map. Note that if there is a bug, you need to select each map twice in the macro.
3. Step through the macro by first loading the ASL experiment.
4. Before selecting Compute Perfusion Map, check the T_1 of blood [7] (Fig. 3).

4 Notes

1. The ASL technique is SNR limited. Multichannel array coils or cryoprobes are a better choice. Particularly, as FAIR requires a global inversion, a volume transmit coil is necessary. Using surface transmit/receive coil would lead to underestimation of perfusion. Parallel acceleration should be avoided due to its SNR penalty. For mice reduce the FOV to the body width and keep the matrix size the same as that used in rats. The relative resolution in resolving kidney is then comparable to that in rats. The SNR would also be similar because the smaller mouse RF coil gives better SNR, that is, mouse heart four-element surface coil vs rat heart four-element surface coil.
2. For using CASL or pCASL instead of FAIR, depending on the field strength and expected flow velocities, the labeling duration and postlabeling delay should be adapted. Labeling durations of $\geq$1600 ms for (p)CASL with *postlabeling delay* $< =$500 ms are suitable.
3. As the labeling effect of ASL on image contrast is weak, SNR considerations mandate acquisition of images that are of lower spatial resolution. For ASL in plane matrices are in the range of 64×64 to 128×128. To maintain acceptable SNR at reasonable imaging times (2–6 min), multiple signal averages/repetitions are required ($N > =3$).
4. In CASL or pCASL but not for FAIR, the labeling plane should be perpendicular to the feeding artery. As the labeling plane in CASL is typically designed to be in parallel to the imaging plane, that would limit the images to be acquired in transverse planes so that labeling can be perpendicular to the aorta.
5. The renal oxygen (O_2) demand is associated primarily with renal tubular O_2 consumption necessary for solute reabsorption. Increasing O_2 delivery such as giving pure oxygen to the animals makes animal hyperoxia and leads to vasoconstriction which changes the basal physiology.
6. The respiration rate must be monitored continuously throughout the entire experiment and if necessary adapt the TR accordingly to ensure full relaxation (~5 times of T_1).
7. Shimming is particularly important for nonselective (global) inversion, since adiabatic condition depends on B0 field homogeneity. If localized or high-order shim is used, the global field uniformity required for nonselective inversion (which is for labeling arterial spins) will be compromised and leads to inferior inversion (and spin labeling). Shimming should be performed on a global level to optimize uniformity over the whole

body. Neither the default iterative shimming method nor the Mapshim technique is recommended.

8. Example for a 25 g mouse at 7 T: Anatomical images can be acquired with routine respiratory-triggered T_2-weighted turbo spin echo (RARE) sequences in axial and coronal planes. Additionally, bSSFP is a fast imaging that could be used for acquiring anatomical image with minimal motion artefact, with parameters such as TR = 3 ms, TE = 1.07 ms, flip angle of 70°, matrix = 128 × 128 and 16 averages (TA = 6.2 s for one slice without trigger).
9. EPI sequence is highly depending on the gradient system therefore a good trajectory measurement is recommended.
10. Example for a 25 g mouse at 7 T [4, 5, 8, 9]: a respiratory triggered, FAIR sequence with an EPI readout: TR = 16,000 ms; TE = 16.6 ms; TIR = 30, 100, 200, 300, 500, 700, 1000, 1200, 1500, 2000, 3000, 5000, 8000 ms; calculated inversion pulse; effective bandwidth 350 kHz; pulse bandwidth = 2000 Hz; FOV = 3.5 × 3.5 mm^2, slice thickness = 2 mm, inversion slab = 5 mm, IR-spoiler duration = 10 ms, IR-Spoiler amplitude = 40%. As kidney has very high perfusion, the perfusion signal is expected to be high even with just a single pair of ASL scan. If perfusion signal is weak, the nonselective inversion may not be effective. Try increasing the bandwidth of the inversion pulse (i.e., from 2000 to 5000 Hz or higher). This will increase the RF power demand so be mindful about the safe limit of the RF coil and the amplifier.
11. Optional: The flow saturation slice shown in Fig. 1 is a spatially selective saturation band applied to suppress unwanted flow artifacts from vessels entering a slice. This is not the most optimal way of suppressing when using FAIR, but it reduces flow artifacts significantly.
12. Use repetition instead of averaging as repetition allows image registration in post-processing before averaging to minimize residual motion artefacts, whereas direct averaging on the scanner may lead to a blurred image in the presence of motion.
13. If SE-EPI readout causes severe distortion, consider using RARE acquisition instead.

Acknowledgments

This chapter is based upon work from COST Action PARENCH IMA, supported by European Cooperation in Science and Technology (COST). COST (www.cost.eu) is a funding agency for research and innovation networks. COST Actions help connect research initiatives across Europe and enable scientists to enrich their ideas by sharing them with their peers. This boosts their research, career, and innovation.

PARENCHIMA (renalmri.org) is a community-driven Action in the COST program of the European Union, which unites more than 200 experts in renal MRI from 30 countries with the aim to improve the reproducibility and standardization of renal MRI biomarkers.

References

1. Williams DS, Detre JA, Leigh JS, Koretsky AP (1992) Magnetic resonance imaging of perfusion using spin inversion of arterial water. Proc Natl Acad Sci U S A 89:212–216
2. Kwong KK, Belliveau JW, Chesler DA, Goldberg IE, Weisskoff RM, Poncelet BP, Kennedy DN, Hoppel BE, Cohen MS, Turner R et al (1992) Dynamic magnetic resonance imaging of human brain activity during primary sensory stimulation. Proc Natl Acad Sci U S A 89:5675–5679
3. Kim SG (1995) Quantification of relative cerebral blood flow change by flow-sensitive alternating inversion recovery (FAIR) technique: application to functional mapping. Magn Reson Med 34:293–301
4. Hueper K, Gutberlet M, Rong S, Hartung D, Mengel M, Lu X, Haller H, Wacker F, Meier M, Gueler F (2014) Acute kidney injury: arterial spin labeling to monitor renal perfusion impairment in mice-comparison with histopathologic results and renal function. Radiology 270:117–124
5. Rajendran R, Lew SK, Yong CX, Tan J, Wang DJ, Chuang KH (2013) Quantitative mouse renal perfusion using arterial spin labeling. NMR Biomed 26:1225–1232
6. Pell GS, Thomas DL, Lythgoe MF, Calamante F, Howseman AM, Gadian DG, Ordidge RJ (1999) Implementation of quantitative FAIR perfusion imaging with a short repetition time in time-course studies. Magn Reson Med 41:829–840
7. Rane SD, Gore JC (2013) Measurement of T1 of human arterial and venous blood at 7T. Magn Reson Imaging 31:477–479
8. Hueper K, Schmidbauer M, Thorenz A, Brasen JH, Gutberlet M, Mengel M, Hartung D, Chen R, Meier M, Haller H, Wacker F, Rong S, Gueler F (2017) Longitudinal evaluation of perfusion changes in acute and chronic renal allograft rejection using arterial spin labeling in translational mouse models. J Magn Reson Imaging 46:1664–1672
9. Tewes S, Gueler F, Chen R, Gutberlet M, Jang MS, Meier M, Mengel M, Hartung D, Wacker F, Rong S, Hueper K (2017) Functional MRI for characterization of renal perfusion impairment and edema formation due to acute kidney injury in different mouse strains. PLoS One 12: e0173248

14

Sodium (^{23}Na) MRI of the Kidney: Experimental Protocol

James T. Grist, Esben Søvsø Hansen, Frank G. Zöllner, and Christoffer Laustsen

Abstract

Sodium handling is a key physiological hallmark of renal function. Alterations are generally considered a pathophysiologic event associated with kidney injury, with disturbances in the corticomedullary sodium gradient being indicative of a number of conditions. This experimental protocol review describes the individual steps needed to perform ^{23}Na MRI; allowing accurate monitoring of the renal sodium distribution in a step-by-step experimental protocol for rodents.

This chapter is based upon work from the PARENCHIMA COST Action, a community-driven network funded by the European Cooperation in Science and Technology (COST) program of the European Union, which aims to improve the reproducibility and standardization of renal MRI biomarkers. This experimental protocol chapter is complemented by two separate chapters describing the basic concept and data analysis.

Key words Magnetic resonance imaging (MRI), Kidney, Mice, Rats, ^{23}Na, Sodium

1 Introduction

Sodium is an essential body fluid electrolyte, with serum concentration tightly controlled by the renal proximal and distal tubules, the loop of Henle, and the collecting duct through a complex process of active reabsorption via transport proteins [1]. Electrolyte reabsorption requires large quantities of adenosine triphosphate (ATP), to move ions against the concentration gradient, produced via the mitochondrial tricarboxylic acid (TCA) cycle [1–3]. To fuel TCA activity, oxygen is delivered via a network of arterial vessels to the renal system. However, should the renal system undergo injury, for example in acute kidney injury or chronic renal disease, the delivery of oxygen to local tissues may be disrupted, and subsequently the gradient of sodium from the cortex to the medulla impaired [4].

In this chapter we describe the process of undertaking sodium MRI for assessing alterations of the corticomedullary sodium

Andreas Pohlmann and Thoralf Niendorf (eds.), *Preclinical MRI of the Kidney: Methods and Protocols*, Methods in Molecular Biology, vol. 2216, https://doi.org/10.1007/978-1-0716-0978-1_28,

gradient in the kidney of rodents in a step-by-step experimental protocol. We also describe the rationale for acquisition parameter selection, with generic terms, with specific examples for rodent imaging on a small-bore animal MR system (Bruker Biospin, Ettlingen, Germany), and porcine imaging on whole body human MR scanner (General Electric, Waukesha, USA). Finally, we discuss the effects of acute diuretics such as furosemide to demonstrate alterations in renal sodium handling.

This experimental protocol chapter is complemented by two separate chapters describing the basic concept and data analysis, which are part of this book.

This chapter is part of the book Pohlmann A, Niendorf T (eds) (2020) Preclinical MRI of the Kidney—Methods and Protocols. Springer, New York.

2 Materials

2.1 Calibration Phantom Preparation: Rodent

2.1.1 Lab Equipment and Components

1. 5 mL Eppendorf tubes.
2. Agarose.
3. 5 g Sodium chloride.
4. Microwave oven.
5. Beaker (microwave safe).
6. Deionized water.

2.1.2 Process to Make 4% Agarose Phantoms (Example 60 and 150 mmol/L Phantoms)

1. Weigh 350 mg sodium chloride.
2. Weight 25 g agarose.
3. Add both to a beaker with 100 mL of deionized water and stir until dissolved.
4. Heat solution in a microwave oven in 30 s intervals, until thickened.
5. Pipette 5 mL of solution in to Eppendorf tubes.
6. Repeat for 150 mmol/L phantom, weighing 875 mg sodium chloride for an equivalent volume of water.
7. Leave Eppendorf tubes to cool for 24 h and seal with Parafilm.

2.2 Animals

This experimental protocol is tailored for rats (Wistar, Sprague-Dawley or Lewis) with a body mass of 300–350 g or pigs 20–40 kg.

2.3 Lab Equipment

1. Anesthesia: please refer to the chapter by Kaucsar T et al. “Preparation and Monitoring of Small Animals in Renal MRI” for an in-depth description and discussion of the anesthesia. For nonrecovery experiments urethane solution (Sigma-Aldrich, Steinheim, Germany; 20% in distilled water) can provide anesthesia for several hours with comparatively fewer side effects on renal physiology, which is an important issue.

2. Gases: O_2, N_2, and compressed air, as well as a gas-mixing system (FMI Föhr Medical Instruments GmbH, Seeheim-Ober Beerbach, Germany) to achieve required changes in the oxygen fraction of inspired gas mixture (FiO_2).
3. Device for FiO_2 monitoring in gas mixtures: for example, Capnomac AGM-103 (Datex GE, Chalfont St Gils, UK).
4. A physiological monitoring system that can track the respiration, and which is connected to the MR system such that it can be used to trigger the image acquisition.

2.4 MRI Hardware

The general hardware requirements for renal ^1H MRI on mice and rats are described in the chapter by Ramos Delgado P et al. "Hardware Considerations for Preclinical Magnetic Resonance of the Kidney." The technique described in this chapter has been tailored for a 7 and 3 T MR system (Biospec 94/20, Bruker Biospin, Ettlingen, Germany and MR750, General Electric, Milwaukee, USA), but advice for adaptation to other field strengths is given where necessary. An additional dual or single tuned $^1H/^{23}Na$ surface or volume coil is required, as well as multinuclear capabilities of the MR system.

3 Methods

3.1 MR Protocol Setup

3.1.1 Total Sodium Imaging (BRUKER)

1. Sequence type: 3D gradient echo sequence. This is a standard sequence on Bruker MRI systems. *See* **Notes 1–3** for details.
2. Repetition time (TR): Choose 2.5× greater than the T_1 of sodium in free fluid (T_1 approx. 70 ms at 7 T).
3. Flip angle (FA): 90°.
4. Echo time (TE): The minimum TE achievable on the system is used to acquire the rapidly decaying signal.
5. Acquisition bandwidth (BW): Use the highest acquisition bandwidth possible to shorten the echo time; however, this will lead to a decrease in SNR. Low SNR may be countered by signal averaging.
6. Respiration trigger: on (per excitation).
7. Geometry: adapt so that animal fits into FOV in L-R direction.
8. Spatial resolution: adapt to the physiological resolution aimed for in the study at hand. Recommend 1 mm × 1 mm in rats.
9. Crushing: Ensure signal is crushed at the end of each readout, to ensure spoiling of latent T_2^* signal.

3.1.2 Total Sodium Imaging (General Electric)

1. Sequence type: Fidall. This is a research pulse sequence from GE. *See* **Notes 4–6** for sequence details.
2. Calibration can be performed using the inbuilt Bloch–Siegert calibration sequence.

3. Readout type: 3D cones. Waveforms can be generated using code available online (http://www-mrsrl.stanford.edu/~ptgurney/cones.php).
4. Repetition time (TR): Choose 2.5× greater than the T_1 of sodium in free fluid (T_1 approx. 50 ms at 3 T).
5. Flip angle (FA): Ernst-angle (typically 70–90°).
6. Echo time (TE): The minimum TE achievable on the system is used to acquire the rapidly decaying signal.
7. Acquisition bandwidth (BW): Use the highest acquisition bandwidth possible to shorten TE, however this will lead to a decrease in SNR. Low SNR may be countered by signal averaging.
8. Respiration trigger: on (minimum 6 per excitation).
9. Geometry: adapt so that animal fits into FOV in L-R direction.
10. Crushing: Ensure signal is crushed at the end of each readout, to ensure spoiling of latent T_2^* signal using crusher gradients.

3.1.3 T_2^* Mapping (BRUKER)

1. Sequence type: 3D gradient echo sequence. This is a standard sequence on Bruker MRI systems, where it is called "3D gradient echo" (*see* **Note 1** for sequence details).
2. Repetition time (TR): Choose 2.5× greater than the T_1 of sodium in free fluid (T_1 approx. 70 ms at 7 T).
3. Flip angle (FA): 90°.
4. Echo time (TE): The minimum TE achievable on the system is used to acquire the rapidly decaying signal.
5. Acquisition bandwidth (BW): Use the highest acquisition bandwidth possible to shorten TE, however this will lead to a decrease in SNR. Low SNR may be countered by signal averaging.
6. Geometry: adapt so that animal fits into FOV in L-R direction.
7. Spatial resolution: adapt to the physiological resolution aimed for in the study at hand. Recommend 1 mm × 1 mm in rats.
8. Crushing: Ensure signal is crushed at the end of each readout to ensure spoiling of latent T_2^* signal using crusher gradients.
9. Repeat acquisition using same prescan parameters with incremented TE, ensuring at least five echo times are collected. We recommended eight echo times: 0.5, 1, 2, 4, 5, 10, 15, and 20 ms.

3.1.4 Total Sodium Imaging Agilent)

1. Sequence type: 2D or 3D chemical shift imaging sequence. This is a standard sequence on preclinical MRI and clinical MRI systems. *See* **Notes 7** and **8** for sequence details.

2. Repetition time (TR): Choose 2.5× greater than the T_1 of sodium in free fluid (T_1 approx. 70 ms at 7 T).
3. Echo time (TE): choose the shortest possible for good signal-to-noise.
4. Flip angle (FA): 90° or according to the Ernst angle.
5. Acquisition bandwidth (BW): Choose BW and NP to ensure sufficient resolution and acquisition time of approximately $2.5 \times T_2^*$.

3.1.5 Calibration Scans

1. Perform a reference scan with above given parameters using a homogeneous phantom to acquire the receive sensitivity of the RF coils and gradient trajectory (*see* **Note 8**).
2. Coregistration of reference and the scans of Subheading 3.1.1–3.1.4.
3. Obtain sensitivity corrected images by the quotient image of both coregistered images concentration.
4. For B_1 mapping (double angle method) perform a measurement using a homogeneous phantom and scan parameters reported in Subheading 3.1.1 and flip angles of $\alpha_1 = 40°$, $\alpha_2 = 80°$.

3.2 In Vivo Sodium Imaging

3.2.1 Preparations

1. Anesthetize the animal, obtained venous access (tail vein for rat and ear vein for pig) and transfer it to scanner.
2. Set up the temperature monitoring (rectal probe) and respiratory monitoring (balloon on chest) unit.
3. Fixate the sodium phantoms to the animal near the imaging area.
4. Perform anatomical imaging as described in the chapter by Pohlmann A et al. "Essential Practical Steps for MRI of the Kidney in Experimental Research."

3.2.2 Baseline Condition

1. Load the 3D GRE sequence, altering the slice orientation to the desired acquisition plane.
2. Triggering: in the monitoring unit set the trigger delay so that the trigger starts at the beginning of the expiratory plateau (no chest motion) and the duration such that it covers the entire expiratory phase, that is, until just before inhalation starts.
3. Run the sodium scan. Example images are shown in Fig. 1.

3.2.3 Imaging Furosemide Action

1. Duplicate the sodium scan.
2. Introduction of furosemide: Inject 10 mg/kg furosemide via tail vein catheter and begin image acquisition.

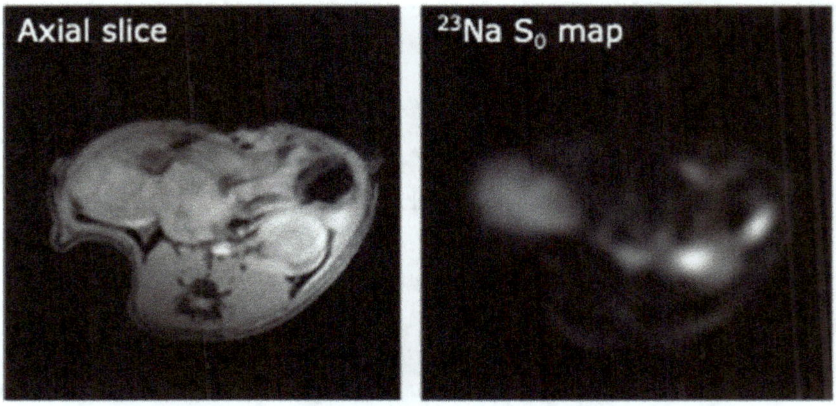

Fig. 1 Example ^{1}H (left) and ^{23}Na (right) rodent renal imaging acquired at 9.4 T, acquisition time = 3.5 min

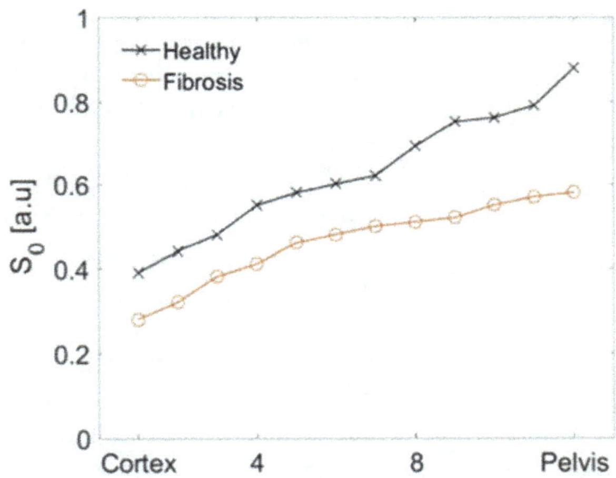

Fig. 2 Example corticomedullary sodium gradient, healthy (black) and impaired rodent kidney (orange)

3. Continue to acquire sodium imaging for up to one hour post the introduction of furosemide.
4. A demonstration of the sodium changes that can be expected in pathophysiological scenarios is given in Fig. 2.

3.2.4 T_2^* Mapping

1. Load the 3D GRE multiecho sequence, altering the slice orientation to the desired acquisition plane.
2. Triggering: in the monitoring unit set the trigger delay so that the trigger starts at the beginning of the expiratory plateau (no chest motion) and the duration such that it covers the entire expiratory phase, that is, until just before inhalation starts.
3. Run the sodium scan.

4 Notes

1. *Example 3D gradient echo sequence parameters at 4.7 T*: 90° sine/cosine adiabatic pulse, echo-time/repetition-time (TE/TR) of 1.7/60 ms, FOV 12 × 12 × 5–8 cm^3, and a matrix of 128 × 128 × 16 with ten scans (20 min scan time).
2. *Example 3D gradient echo sequence parameters at 7 T*: 90° sine/cosine adiabatic pulse, echo-time/repetition-time (TE/TR) of 1.7/180 ms, FOV 12 × 12 × 5–8 cm^3, and a matrix of 128 × 128 × 16 with ten scans (60 min scan time).
3. *Example dynamic imaging protocol at 4.7 T*: 90° sine/cosine adiabatic pulse, echo-time/repetition-time (TE/TR) of 1.7/60 ms, FOV 12 × 12 × 5–8 cm^3, and a matrix of 128 × 128 × 16 with two scans (4 min scan time).
4. *3D cones sequence parameters at 3 T*: TR = 48 ms; TE = 0.5 ms, flip angle = 90°; pulse length 500 μs; receiver bandwidth = 250 kHz; readout length = 30 ms, averages = 10; slice orientation = coronal oblique; FOV = (240 × 240 × 240) mm; matrix size = 60 × 60 × 60 zero-filled to 120 × 120 × 120 (10 min scan time).
5. *Example dynamic imaging protocol at 3 T*: TR = 48 ms; TE = 0.5 ms, flip angle = 90°; pulse length 500 μs; receiver bandwidth = 250 kHz; readout length = 30 ms, averages = 5; slice orientation = coronal oblique; FOV = (240 × 240 × 240) mm; matrix size = 60 × 60 × 60 zero-filled to 120 × 120 × 120 (5 min scan time).
6. *Example 3D radial UTE protocol at 9.4 T*: TR = 150 ms; TE = 185 μs; 90° block pulse length of 350 μs; each radial projection was recorded in 6.4 ms of read out time (Tro) using a low acquisition bandwidth of 5 kHz; undersampling factor of 3; number of projections to 4206, nominal anisotropic resolution of (1 × 1 × 4) mm^3, and FOV = 64 mm × 64 mm × 64 mm; TR = 50 ms.
7. *2D CSI sequence parameters at 9.4 T*: Example for a 300 g rat at 9.4 T: TR = 65 ms; TE = 0.65 ms, flip angle = 90°; pulse length 500 μs; receiver bandwidth = 8 kHz; number of points = 256 complex points, averages = 8; slice orientation = axial oblique; FOV = (60 × 60) mm; matrix size = 32 × 32 zero-filled to 64 × 64; 1 slice with 1–2 cm thickness; TA = 67 s (without triggering).
8. Rapid MR-imaging sequences using non-Cartesian sampling are known to be sensitive to gradient hardware imperfections and eddy-current effects that can superimpose acquired data. This is a common problem on preclinical MRI systems which compared with human MRI systems are equipped with

approximately 20-fold stronger (740 mT/m maximal gradient amplitude) and 30-fold faster gradient systems (6900 T/m/s gradient slew rate). To overcome this a calibration by measuring the readout trajectory on a phantom should be performed. For further details please *see* [5].

Acknowledgments

This chapter is based upon work from COST Action PARENCHIMA, supported by European Cooperation in Science and Technology (COST). COST (www.cost.eu) is a funding agency for research and innovation networks. COST Actions help connect research initiatives across Europe and enable scientists to enrich their ideas by sharing them with their peers. This boosts their research, career, and innovation.

PARENCHIMA (renalmri.org) is a community-driven Action in the COST program of the European Union, which unites more than 200 experts in renal MRI from 30 countries with the aim to improve the reproducibility and standardization of renal MRI biomarkers.

References

1. Kiil F (1977) Renal energy metabolism and regulation of sodium reabsorption. Kidney Int 11:153–160
2. Klahr S, Hamm LL, Hammerman MR, Mandel LJ (2011) Renal metabolism: integrated responses. Compr Physiol. https://doi.org/10.1002/cphy.cp080249
3. Deng A, Miracle CM, Suarez JM et al (2005) Oxygen consumption in the kidney: effects of nitric oxide synthase isoforms and angiotensin II. Kidney Int 68:723–730
4. Hansell P, Welch WJ, Blantz RC, Palm F (2013) Determinants of kidney oxygen consumption and their relationship to tissue oxygen tension in diabetes and hypertension. Clin Exp Pharmacol Physiol 40:123–137
5. Zhang Y, Hetherington HP, Stokely EM et al (1998) A novel k-space trajectory measurement technique. Magn Reson Med 39:999–1004

15

Hyperpolarized Carbon (^{13}C) MRI of the Kidneys: Basic Concept

Cornelius von Morze, Galen D. Reed, Zhen J. Wang, Michael A. Ohliger, and Christoffer Laustsen

Abstract

Existing clinical markers for renal disease are limited. Hyperpolarized (HP) ^{13}C MRI is based on the technology of dissolution dynamic nuclear polarization (DNP) and provides new avenues for imaging kidney structure, function, and most notably, renal metabolism, addressing some of these prior limitations. Changes in kidney structure and function associated with kidney disease can be evaluated using [^{13}C]urea, a metabolically inert tracer. Metabolic changes can be assessed using [1-^{13}C]pyruvate and a range of other rapidly metabolized small molecules, which mainly probe central carbon metabolism. Results from numerous preclinical studies using a variety of these probes demonstrated that this approach holds great potential for monitoring renal disease, although more work is needed to bridge intelligently into clinical studies. Here we introduce the general concept of HP ^{13}C MRI and review the most relevant probes and applications to renal disease, including kidney cancer, diabetic nephropathy and ischemic kidney injury.

This chapter is based upon work from the PARENCHIMA COST Action, a community-driven network funded by the European Cooperation in Science and Technology (COST) program of the European Union, which aims to improve the reproducibility and standardization of renal MRI biomarkers. This introduction chapter is complemented by two separate chapters describing the experimental procedure and data analysis.

Key words Dynamic nuclear polarization, Kidney, Preclinical models, Carbon-13

1 Introduction

While renal MRI has traditionally been limited largely to morphologic depiction of vascular disease and neoplasia, hyperpolarized (HP) ^{13}C MRI supplies new metabolic and/or functional insight that could be valuable for a range of kidney diseases. The high renal delivery of intravenously injected small molecules, which provides extraordinary sensitivity for renal imaging of HP ^{13}C MRI probes, suggests great potential for application of this nascent medical imaging modality to kidney disease.

Andreas Pohlmann and Thoralf Niendorf (eds.), *Preclinical MRI of the Kidney: Methods and Protocols*, Methods in Molecular Biology, vol. 2216, https://doi.org/10.1007/978-1-0716-0978-1_16,

Commonly used clinical markers for kidney disease have significant limitations, especially in the context of early disease. Serum creatinine is frequently utilized as a functional marker, but has a wide reference interval, and the mathematical corrections applied for the estimation of glomerular filtration rate (GFR) are inexact. For example, GFR is unpredictably overestimated in glomerulopathic patients as a result of increased creatinine secretion [1]. Even accurately measured GFR, such as by the "gold standard" inulin clearance, is insensitive to early disease [2]. Blood urea nitrogen (BUN) fluctuates due to factors unrelated to kidney function, such as hydration status and diet. Proteinuria at baseline is a significant risk factor for renal disease, but has poor negative predictive value [3]. In general, clinical markers do not exhibit definitive changes until a significant fraction of kidney function is already lost.

Medical imaging has clear potential to address these limitations by providing localized functional data, but this has yet to be translated on a large scale. Nuclear medicine plays a significant role, with (mercaptoacetyltriglycine) MAG_3 scintigraphy estimated to account for >400,000 renograms per year [4], commonly for evaluation of renal function (often pre- or post-transplant), split function, collecting duct/urinary tract obstruction, renovascular hypertension, and renal artery stenosis. However, nuclear scans typically have relatively poor spatial resolution and lack the rich tissue contrast of MRI. Furthermore, these studies carry the risks of exposure to ionizing radiation. Ultrasound is also commonly used for assessing kidney disease [5], but is generally limited to evaluating advanced damage reflected in alterations in kidney size and shape, and to some extent blood flow. For patients with impaired renal function, iodinated Computer Tomography (CT) contrast media carry an increased risks of acute kidney injury [6]. Gadolinium based MRI contrast media are associated with nephrogenic systemic fibrosis [7].

HP ^{13}C MRI has unique potential for improved, safer clinical imaging studies of renal structure and function, and perhaps most notably offers an unprecedented avenue toward assessing renal metabolism in vivo. Indeed, results of numerous preclinical studies conducted to date, as summarized below, show the clear potential of this new approach to fill pressing unmet clinical needs for improved markers of various diseases affecting the kidneys, both malignant and nonmalignant. More preclinical work with realistic renal disease models is, however, needed in order to bridge effectively into clinical studies.

This introduction chapter is complemented by two separate chapters describing the experimental procedure and data analysis, which are part of this book.

This chapter is part of the book Pohlmann A, Niendorf T (eds) (2020) Preclinical MRI of the Kidney—Methods and Protocols. Springer, New York.

2 Measurement Concept

2.1 Basic Concept of HP ^{13}C MRI

HP ^{13}C MRI is based on a transient enhancement of the nuclear magnetism of ^{13}C-enriched liquids, by up to five orders of magnitude over states readily attainable in a clinical MRI magnet, thereby offsetting the limitation of poor sensitivity that previously hampered in vivo ^{13}C MRI. Although multiple alternate approaches exist for producing HP material, the method of dissolution dynamic nuclear polarization (DNP) [8] provides an especially robust avenue for hyperpolarizing a wide variety of ^{13}C-labeled substrates, using commercially available instruments. In this approach, the ^{13}C substrate is first prepolarized in a separate magnet at low temperature (*see* **Note 1**), primarily through microwave irradiation applied near the electron paramagnetic resonance (EPR) frequency in the presence of a stable organic free radical (aka electron paramagnetic agent or EPA, usually a trityl radical) (*see* **Note 2**). Following a period of polarization buildup, the solid sample is rapidly dissolved into a liquid state where it temporarily maintains its hyperpolarization, and is quickly transferred to the MRI scanner for intravenous injection and imaging (*see* **Note 3**). The overall process is illustrated in Fig. 1. The transient hyperpolarized state persists for a period of time determined by the substrate's T_1 relaxation time, an exponential time constant governing the rate of decay of polarization (*see* **Note 4**). Inverse scaling of T_1 with molecular size limits the scope of applicable probes to small molecules, with labels preferably located distal to bonded hydrogen atoms, which can destroy the ^{13}C magnetization via ^{13}C-^{1}H dipolar coupling (*see* **Note 5**). During the decay period, ^{13}C MRI data is collected, capitalizing on the sensitivity enhancement afforded by hyperpolarization. Specific methods for data acquisition and processing of HP ^{13}C MRI data are described in the relevant sections to follow.

2.2 Renal Functional and Metabolic Investigations Using HP ^{13}C MRI

HP ^{13}C MRI offers many new possibilities for renal functional and metabolic investigations. Dynamic images of the real-time delivery of metabolically inert tracers such as ^{13}C urea from arterial vasculature to the kidneys can be used to quantify renal function. Real-time in vivo processing of metabolically active HP probes by the kidneys can be tracked by spectroscopic imaging, which yields separate images of injected tracer(s) and their downstream metabolic product(s) based on chemical shift differences. Notably, multiple probes can also be simultaneously copolarized to yield multiparametric data sets [9], for example spanning both renal functional and metabolic parameters. In this section, we review the most promising HP ^{13}C MRI probes of renal function/metabolism proposed to date, and the relevant associated principles. These probes and their metabolic pathways are illustrated in Fig. 2.

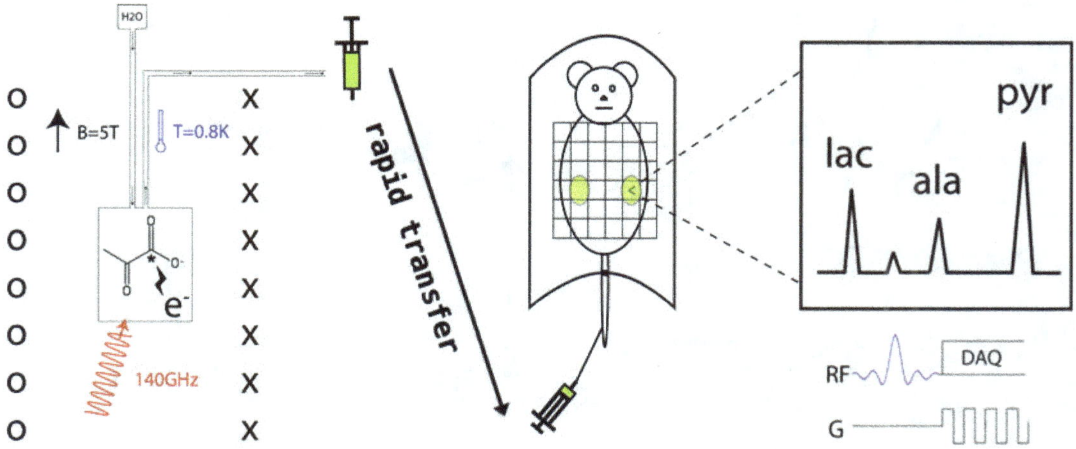

Fig. 1 Illustration of the process of HP ^{13}C MRI via dissolution dynamic nuclear polarization. The agent (e.g., [1-^{13}C]pyruvate) is mixed with the EPA and cooled to 0.8 K in a magnetic field of 5 T, then irradiated at 140GHz to transfer polarization from unpaired electrons in the EPA to the ^{13}C nuclei. The sample is then rapidly dissolved and transferred to the MRI scanner for intravenous injection and MR imaging

2.2.1 [^{13}C]Urea

The key osmolyte and metabolic end product urea was one of the first ^{13}C-labeled molecules to be hyperpolarized ($T_1 = 45$ s at 3 T) [8] and imaged in vivo [10], and high quality dynamic images of the kidneys and the feeding arterial vasculature can readily be generated [11–13]. Quantitative estimates of renal function require dynamic measurements from both the renal parenchyma and arterial vasculature [11, 14]. Urea is largely reabsorbed by urea transporters (UTs) expressed at the inner medullary collecting ducts (IMCD), and accordingly renal imaging shows distinct modulation by hydration state [13, 15], based on differential action of vasopressin. Despite this significant reabsorption, it has been suggested that urea can also be used to estimate glomerular filtration rate (GFR) [14], based on the first-order transfer coefficient between arterial vasculature and renal parenchyma. Secondary labeling of [^{13}C]urea with $^{15}N_2$ is helpful in terms of prolonging both T_1 (at low magnetic fields only) [16] and T_2 relaxation times [12] of urea, with the latter factor allowing imaging rat kidneys at spatial resolutions approaching 1 mm isotropic (using refocused image acquisition) [13]. Furthermore, relaxation mapping shows great promise for improved contrast between the individual kidney compartments and various functional states [12, 13, 17]. Urea is distinguished by an exceptionally good safety profile among medical imaging contrast agents, even in patients with reduced kidney function, and therefore has potential for clinical translation for imaging patients with kidney diseases.

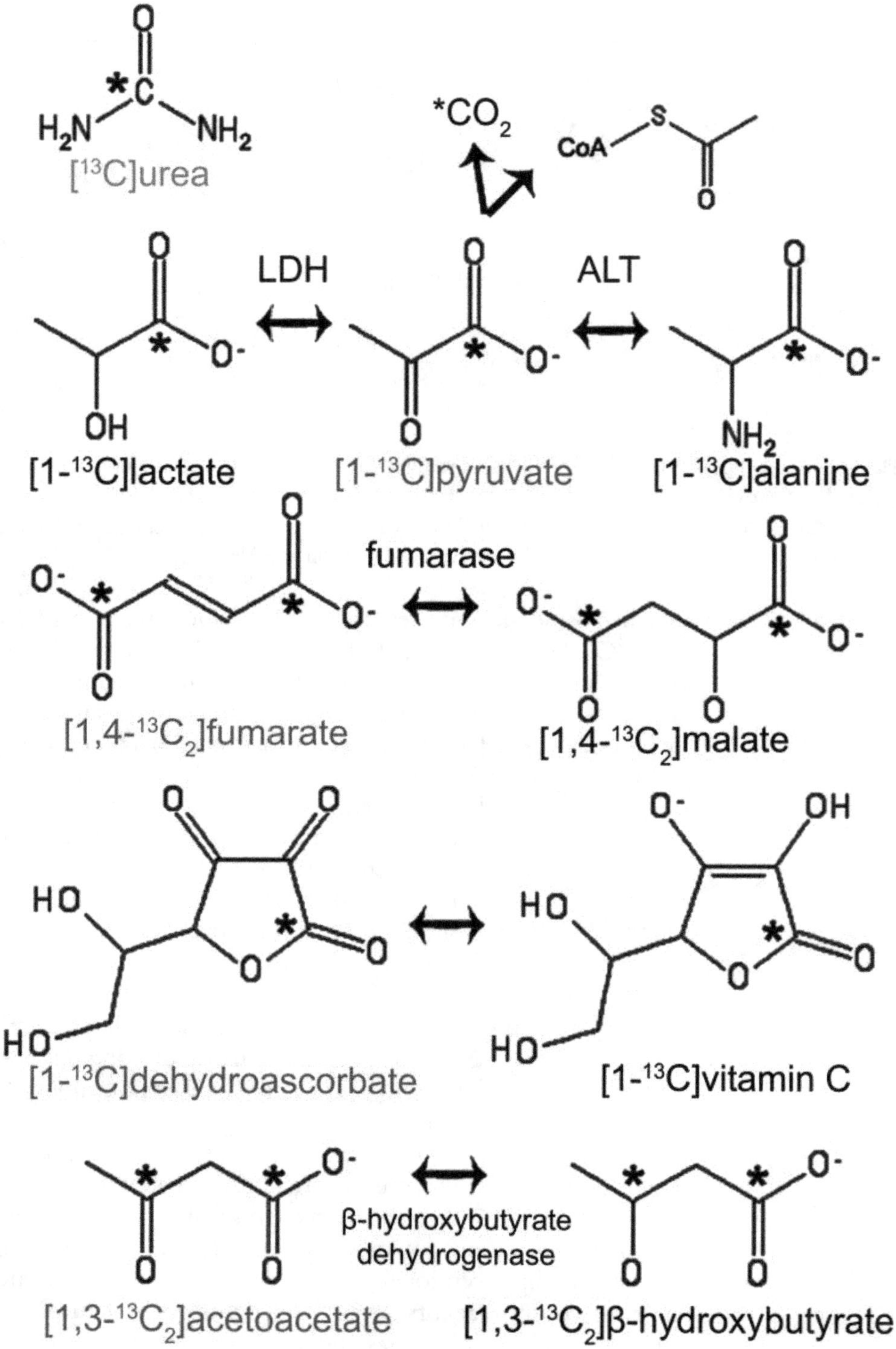

Fig. 2 HP ^{13}C MRI probes of interest for monitoring renal disease, and the associated metabolic conversions (if any). Positions of the ^{13}C labels are indicated by stars

2.2.2 [1-^{13}C]Pyruvate

Pyruvate, the end product of glycolysis and key metabolic intermediate, is the most widely studied ^{13}C probe, in C_1-labeled form ($T_1 = 60$s at 3 T) [18]. In the kidneys, its interconversions with lactate (via lactate dehydrogenase, LDH) and alanine (via alanine transaminase, ALT), as well as its decarboxylation yielding [^{13}C] bicarbonate (via pyruvate dehydrogenase or PDH) can readily be tracked by spectroscopic imaging. The extent of metabolic conversion observed reflects a complex series of biophysical processes, including vascular delivery, cellular uptake (via monocarboxylate transporters), and finally enzymatic conversion, which in turn may be influenced by multiple factors. For the conversion via LDH, the lactate pool size is especially important [19, 20]. For quantitative comparison among subjects, all of these factors are usually grouped into simple parameters such as metabolite area-under-the-curve (AUC) ratios or related apparent first-order conversion rates (e.g., $k_{pyruvate\text{-}to\text{-}lactate}$ or k_{pl}) [21, 22], derived from a series of dynamic spectroscopic imaging data. From a metabolic perspective, while the conversion to bicarbonate is clearly a net flux, the conversions to lactate and alanine via the respective bidirectional, highly active enzymes appear to represent largely isotopic exchange fluxes into the respective product metabolite pools [19, 20, 23]. Because of the high bidirectional activity of LDH (which is restricted to cytoplasm), the ratio of lactate to pyruvate has frequently been interpreted as a marker for the cytosolic free NADH/NAD$^+$ ratio [24]. This suggests that the conversion of HP pyruvate to lactate is driven by this NAD(H) redox state, a parameter that is fundamentally inter-connected with numerous related biochemical reactions.

2.2.3 [1,4-$^{13}C_2$]Fumarate

Cellular uptake of injected fumarate, a tricarboxylic acid (TCA) cycle intermediate, is ordinarily highly restricted on the timescale of HP experiments, due to its dicarboxylate structure. Compromise of the cellular membrane (e.g., due to necrosis) allows access of injected HP [1,4-$^{13}C_2$]fumarate (a singlet due to molecular symmetry, with $T_1 = 58$ s at 3 T) [25] to cellular fumarase, and consequently detectable conversion of product HP [1,4-$^{13}C_2$] malate. Thus, HP fumarate has been investigated as a specific marker of cellular necrosis with potentially significant applicability to detection of renal tubular necrosis [26].

2.2.4 [1-^{13}C] Dehydroascorbate

HP [1-^{13}C]dehydroascorbate ($T_1 = 56$ s at 3 T) [27, 28] can be used to probe oxidative stress in a direct manner. Vitamin C, a key physiologic antioxidant, exists in a NADP(H)-mediated equilibrium with its oxidized form, dehydroascorbate (DHA). Conversion of injected HP [1-^{13}C]DHA, which is rapidly taken up by glucose transporters, to [1-^{13}C]vitamin C is detectable in vivo. The observed extent of conversion of HP DHA to vitamin C, a reaction whose reducing power is likely mostly derived from reduced glutathione (GSH), is attenuated by oxidative stress.

2.2.5 [^{13}C]Acetoacetate

The ketone body acetoacetate, a universal oxidative fuel, rapidly interconverts with its reduced form, beta-hydroxybutyrate, in mitochondria via beta-hydroxybutyrate dehydrogenase. In analogy with lactate/pyruvate, the BOHB–AcAc ratio has frequently been interpreted as a marker of the free mitochondrial NADH–NAD$^+$ ratio, suggesting an analogous interpretation of conversion of HP acetoacetate [29, 30] as being driven by the mitochondrial NAD (H) redox state. Metabolic conversion of injected [1,3-$^{13}C_2$]acetoacetate (58 s at 3 T, C_1 position) can be detected in rat kidney in vivo (via the C_1 label) [29], suggesting applicability of this new probe to interrogate mitochondrial-driven kidney disease.

3 Overview of Applications

3.1 Kidney Cancer

Multiple studies have reported elevated conversion of HP [1-^{13}C] pyruvate to [1-^{13}C]lactate and rapid export of [1-^{13}C]lactate in renal cell carcinoma (RCC), in both RCC cells ex vivo [31–33] and in vivo in mice orthotopically implanted with human RCC cells [34]. These findings suggest that HP [1-^{13}C]pyruvate MRI could have clinical value for improved characterization of kidney cancer in patients. Moreover, a recent study showed that HP [1-^{13}C]pyruvate MRI could be used to predict RCC treatment response to mTOR inhibition, which varies greatly among individual patients, thus potentially informing treatment decisions [35].

3.2 Diabetic Nephropathy

Diabetes results in profound shifts in central carbon metabolism, directly shifting several pathways accessible to HP ^{13}C MRI. Although diabetes is detectable using relatively simple testing, sustained hyperglycemia over time leads to serious end-organ complications including diabetic nephropathy, a significant source of morbidity, the detection/prediction of which is a difficult clinical problem where HP ^{13}C MRI could be valuable. Though cancer has been the main focus of the HP ^{13}C MRI community, several recent studies have reported differences in renal HP ^{13}C signals detected in type 1 and type 2 diabetes models as compared to normal controls, based on multiple HP probes including [1-^{13}C]pyruvate [23, 36, 37], [^{13}C]urea [38, 39], and [1-^{13}C]DHA [40]. Not surprisingly, standard antidiabetic agents including insulin and metformin have been found to induce large renal HP signal changes as well [29, 41, 42]. Renal HP lactate levels are attenuated with hyperbaric [43] and antioxidant treatment [44] in diabetic rats. HP [^{13}C]acetate has so far failed to show any significant metabolic change associated with the diabetic kidney [45]. Further work is needed in animal models of frank diabetic nephropathy, which may display changes additive to the fundamental metabolic shifts observed in diabetes, to address this important clinical problem.

3.3 Ischemic Kidney Injury

Effective detection of acute kidney injury (AKI) is an unresolved clinical problem especially affecting hospitalized patients. Rapid treatment of AKI is critical but is impeded by existing clinical indicators which are poor in diagnosing early AKI. Several studies of models of ischemia reperfusion injury (i.e., unilateral renal artery clamp) have shown clear effects of AKI on renal HP ^{13}C MRI using [^{13}C]urea [46, 47], pyruvate [48], and [1-^{13}C]pyruvate–[1-^{13}C] DHA combination [49], and fumarate [50]. However, these relatively simple models likely do not reflect the etiology of ischemic injuries more frequently encountered in patients, such as those resulting from atherosclerotic disease. Further work using more realistic models of ischemic kidney injury is needed to answer, for example, the important question of predicting treatment response in renal artery stenosis. Finally, HP [1,4-$^{13}C_2$]fumarate has also been investigated as a probe of tissue necrosis in a toxic folic acid model of acute tubular necrosis (ATN) [26]. A nonzero urinary fumarase activity could potentially be used as a clinical indicator for a hyperpolarized fumarate examination to investigate the extent and the origin of the renal damage [50].

4 Notes

1. The state-of-the-art GE SPINLab polarizer operates at 5 T and a temperature of 0.8 K. Microwave irradiation is applied near the EPR frequency corresponding to this magnetic field (~140 GHz), with a typical power of ~20 mW. A buildup time of ~3 h is typically required.
2. Urea and many other agents including fumarate and acetoacetate require the addition of a glassing agent such as glycerol or DMSO to prevent crystallization upon freezing, which impedes the polarization process.
3. The ^{13}C concentration is made as high as possible in the starting material (in the molar range), facilitating efficient polarization, but the concentration typically drops >10-fold on dissolution. In contrast, the concentration of the radical is only ~15 mM in the starting material.
4. The T_1 exponential decay constant of HP ^{13}C probe is directly proportional to its "half-life," by a factor of ln 2 (i.e., $t_{1/2} = 0.69 \times T_1$).
5. T_1 values of 30–60 s are typical for the most useful probes, and T_1 values are magnetic field- and temperature-dependent.

Acknowledgments

Grant support from National Institutes of Health (NIH) K01DK099451 is gratefully acknowledged.

This chapter is based upon work from COST Action PARENCHIMA, supported by European Cooperation in Science and Technology (COST). COST (www.cost.eu) is a funding agency for research and innovation networks. COST Actions help connect research initiatives across Europe and enable scientists to enrich their ideas by sharing them with their peers. This boosts their research, career, and innovation.

PARENCHIMA (renalmri.org) is a community-driven Action in the COST program of the European Union, which unites more than 200 experts in renal MRI from 30 countries with the aim to improve the reproducibility and standardization of renal MRI biomarkers.

References

1. Shemesh O, Golbetz H, Kriss JP, Myers BD (1985) Limitations of creatinine as a filtration marker in glomerulopathic patients. Kidney Int 28:830–838
2. Metcalfe W (2007) How does early chronic kidney disease progress? A background paper prepared for the UK Consensus Conference on early chronic kidney disease. Nephrol Dial Transplant 22(Suppl 9):ix26–ix30. https://doi.org/10.1093/ndt/gfm446
3. Ishani A, Grandits GA, Grimm RH, Svendsen KH, Collins AJ, Prineas RJ, Neaton JD (2006) Association of single measurements of dipstick proteinuria, estimated glomerular filtration rate, and hematocrit with 25-year incidence of end-stage renal disease in the multiple risk factor intervention trial. J Am Soc Nephrol 17:1444–1452. https://doi.org/10.1681/ASN.2005091012
4. Esteves FP, Taylor A, Manatunga A, Folks RD, Krishnan M, Garcia EV (2006) 99mTc-MAG3 renography: normal values for MAG3 clearance and curve parameters, excretory parameters, and residual urine volume. AJR Am J Roentgenol 187:W610–W617. https://doi.org/10.2214/AJR.05.1550
5. O'Neill WC (2014) Renal relevant radiology: use of ultrasound in kidney disease and nephrology procedures. Clin J Am Soc Nephrol 9:373–381. https://doi.org/10.2215/CJN.03170313
6. PA MC, Stacul F, Becker CR, Adam A, Lameire N, Tumlin JA, Davidson CJ, CIN Consensus Working Panel (2006) Contrast-induced nephropathy (CIN) consensus working panel: executive summary. Rev Cardiovasc Med 7:177–197
7. Kuo PH, Kanal E, Abu-Alfa AK, Cowper SE (2007) Gadolinium-based MR contrast agents and nephrogenic systemic fibrosis. Radiology 242:647–649. https://doi.org/10.1148/radiol.2423061640
8. Ardenkjaer-Larsen JH, Fridlund B, Gram A, Hansson G, Hansson L, Lerche MH, Servin R, Thaning M, Golman K (2003) Increase in signal-to-noise ratio of > 10,000 times in liquid-state NMR. Proc Natl Acad Sci U S A 100:10158–10163. https://doi.org/10.1073/pnas.1733835100
9. Wilson DM, Keshari KR, Larson PEZ, Chen AP, Hu S, Van Criekinge M, Bok R, Nelson SJ, Macdonald JM, Vigneron DB, Kurhanewicz J (2010) Multi-compound polarization by DNP allows simultaneous assessment of multiple enzymatic activities in vivo. J Magn Reson 205:141–147. https://doi.org/10.1016/j.jmr.2010.04.012
10. Golman K, Ardenkjaer-Larsen JH, Petersson JS, Månsson S, Leunbach I (2003) Molecular imaging with endogenous substances. Proc Natl Acad Sci U S A 100:10435–10439. https://doi.org/10.1073/pnas.1733836100
11. von Morze C, Larson PEZ, Hu S, Keshari K, Wilson DM, Ardenkjaer-Larsen JH, Goga A, Bok R, Kurhanewicz J, Vigneron DB (2011) Imaging of blood flow using hyperpolarized [C-13] urea in preclinical cancer models. J

Magn Reson Imaging 33:692–697. https://doi.org/10.1002/jmri.22484

12. Reed GD, von Morze C, Bok R, Koelsch BL, Van Criekinge M, Smith KJ, Shang H, Larson PEZ, Kurhanewicz J, Vigneron DB (2014) High resolution (13)C MRI with hyperpolarized urea: in vivo T(2) mapping and (15)N labeling effects. IEEE Trans Med Imaging 33:362–371. https://doi.org/10.1109/TMI.2013.2285120
13. Reed GD, von Morze C, Verkman AS, Koelsch BL, Chaumeil MM, Lustig M, Ronen SM, Bok RA, Sands JM, Larson PEZ, Wang ZJ, Larsen JHA, Kurhanewicz J, Vigneron DB (2016) Imaging renal urea handling in rats at millimeter resolution using hyperpolarized magnetic resonance relaxometry. Tomography 2:125–135. https://doi.org/10.18383/j.tom.2016.00127
14. Østergaard Mariager C, Nielsen PM, Qi H, Schroeder M, Bertelsen LB, Laustsen C (2017) Can hyperpolarized 13C-urea be used to assess glomerular filtration rate? A retrospective study. Tomography 3:146–152. https://doi.org/10.18383/j.tom.2017.00010
15. von Morze C, Bok RA, Sands JM, Kurhanewicz J, Vigneron DB (2012) Monitoring urea transport in rat kidney in vivo using hyperpolarized C-13 magnetic resonance imaging. Am J Physiol Renal Physiol 302: F1658–F1662. https://doi.org/10.1152/ajprenal.00640.2011
16. Chiavazza E, Kubala E, Gringeri CV, Düwel S, Durst M, Schulte RF, Menzel MI (2013) Earth's magnetic field enabled scalar coupling relaxation of 13C nuclei bound to fast-relaxing quadrupolar 14N in amide groups. J Magn Reson 227:35–38. https://doi.org/10.1016/j.jmr.2012.11.016
17. Laustsen C, Stokholm Nørlinger T, Christoffer Hansen D, Qi H, Mose Nielsen P, Bonde Bertelsen L, Henrik Ardenkjaer-Larsen J, Stødkilde Jørgensen H (2016) Hyperpolarized 13C urea relaxation mechanism reveals renal changes in diabetic nephropathy. Magn Reson Med 75:515–518. https://doi.org/10.1002/mrm.26036
18. Golman K, in 't Zandt R, Thaning M (2006) Real-time metabolic imaging. Proc Natl Acad Sci U S A 103:11270–11275. https://doi.org/10.1073/pnas.0601319103
19. Day SE, Kettunen MI, Gallagher FA, Hu D-E, Lerche M, Wolber J, Golman K, Ardenkjaer-Larsen JH, Brindle KM (2007) Detecting tumor response to treatment using hyperpolarized 13C magnetic resonance imaging and spectroscopy. Nat Med 13:1382–1387. https://doi.org/10.1038/nm1650
20. Hurd RE, Spielman D, Josan S, Yen Y-F, Pfefferbaum A, Mayer D (2013) Exchange-linked dissolution agents in dissolution-DNP (13)C metabolic imaging. Magn Reson Med 70:936–942. https://doi.org/10.1002/mrm.24544
21. Hill DK, Orton MR, Mariotti E, Boult JKR, Panek R, Jafar M, Parkes HG, Jamin Y, Miniotis MF, Al-Saffar NMS, Beloueche-Babari M, Robinson SP, Leach MO, Chung Y-L, Eykyn TR (2013) Model free approach to kinetic analysis of real-time hyperpolarized 13C magnetic resonance spectroscopy data. PLoS One 8:e71996. https://doi.org/10.1371/journal.pone.0071996
22. Daniels CJ, McLean MA, Schulte RF, Robb FJ, Gill AB, McGlashan N, Graves MJ, Schwaiger M, Lomas DJ, Brindle KM, Gallagher FA (2016) A comparison of quantitative methods for clinical imaging with hyperpolarized (13)C-pyruvate. NMR Biomed 29:387–399. https://doi.org/10.1002/nbm.3468
23. von Morze C, Allu PKR, Chang GY, Marco-Rius I, Milshteyn E, Wang ZJ, Ohliger MA, Gleason CE, Kurhanewicz J, Vigneron DB, Pearce D (2018) Non-invasive detection of divergent metabolic signals in insulin deficiency vs. insulin resistance in vivo. Sci Rep 8:2088. https://doi.org/10.1038/s41598-018-20264-w
24. Williamson D, Lund P, Krebs H (1967) Redox state of free nicotinamide-adenine dinucleotide in cytoplasm and mitochondria of rat liver. Biochem J 103:514–527
25. Gallagher FA, Kettunen MI, Hu D-E, Jensen PR, I' nt Zandt R, Karlsson M, Gisselsson A, Nelson SK, Witney TH, Bohndiek SE, Hansson G, Peitersen T, Lerche MH, Brindle KM (2009) Production of hyperpolarized [1,4-13C2]malate from [1,4-13C2]fumarate is a marker of cell necrosis and treatment response in tumors. Proc Natl Acad Sci U S A 106:19801–19806. https://doi.org/10.1073/pnas.0911447106
26. Clatworthy MR, Kettunen MI, Hu D-E, Mathews RJ, Witney TH, Kennedy BWC, Bohndiek SE, Gallagher FA, Jarvis LB, Smith KGC, Brindle KM (2012) Magnetic resonance imaging with hyperpolarized [1,4-(13)C2]fumarate allows detection of early renal acute tubular necrosis. Proc Natl Acad Sci U S A 109:13374–13379. https://doi.org/10.1073/pnas.1205539109
27. Keshari KR, Kurhanewicz J, Bok R, Larson PEZ, Vigneron DB, Wilson DM (2011) Hyperpolarized 13C dehydroascorbate as an endogenous redox sensor for in vivo metabolic

imaging. Proc Natl Acad Sci U S A 108:18606–18611. https://doi.org/10.1073/pnas.1106920108

28. Bohndiek SE, Kettunen MI, Hu D-E, Kennedy BWC, Boren J, Gallagher FA, Brindle KM (2011) Hyperpolarized [1-13C]-ascorbic and dehydroascorbic acid: vitamin C as a probe for imaging redox status in vivo. J Am Chem Soc 133:11795–11801. https://doi.org/10.1021/ja2045925
29. von Morze C, Ohliger MA, Marco-Rius I, Wilson DM, Flavell RR, Pearce D, Vigneron DB, Kurhanewicz J, Wang ZJ (2018) Direct assessment of renal mitochondrial redox state using hyperpolarized 13 C-acetoacetate. Magn Reson Med 79(4):1862–1869. https://doi.org/10.1002/mrm.27054
30. Miller JJ, Ball DR, Lau AZ, Tyler DJ (2018) Hyperpolarized ketone body metabolism in the rat heart. NMR Biomed 31:e3912. https://doi.org/10.1002/nbm.3912
31. Keshari KR, Sriram R, Koelsch BL, Van Criekinge M, Wilson DM, Kurhanewicz J, Wang ZJ (2013) Hyperpolarized 13C-pyruvate magnetic resonance reveals rapid lactate export in metastatic renal cell carcinomas. Cancer Res 73:529–538. https://doi.org/10.1158/0008-5472.CAN-12-3461
32. Sriram R, Van Criekinge M, Hansen A, Wang ZJ, Vigneron DB, Wilson DM, Keshari KR, Kurhanewicz J (2015) Real-time measurement of hyperpolarized lactate production and efflux as a biomarker of tumor aggressiveness in an MR compatible 3D cell culture bioreactor. NMR Biomed 28:1141–1149. https://doi.org/10.1002/nbm.3354
33. Sriram R, Van Criekinge M, Delos Santos J, Keshari KR, Wilson DM, Peehl D, Kurhanewicz J, Wang ZJ (2016) Non-invasive differentiation of benign renal tumors from clear cell renal cell carcinomas using clinically translatable hyperpolarized 13C pyruvate magnetic resonance. Tomography 2:35–42. https://doi.org/10.18383/j.tom.2016.00106
34. Sriram R, Gordon J, Baligand C, Ahamed F, Delos Santos J, Qin H, Bok RA, Vigneron DB, Kurhanewicz J, Larson PEZ, Wang ZJ (2018) Non-invasive assessment of lactate production and compartmentalization in renal cell carcinomas using hyperpolarized 13C pyruvate MRI. Cancers (Basel) 10:313. https://doi.org/10.3390/cancers10090313
35. Dong Y, Eskandari R, Ray C, Granlund KL, Dos Santos-Cunha L, Miloushev VZ, Tee SS, Jeong S, Aras O, Chen Y-B, Cheng EH, Hsieh JJ, Keshari KR (2019) Hyperpolarized MRI visualizes Warburg effects and predicts treatment response to mTOR inhibitors in patient-derived ccRCC xenograft models. Cancer Res 79(1):242–250. https://doi.org/10.1158/0008-5472.CAN-18-2231
36. Laustsen C, Østergaard JA, Lauritzen MH, Nørregaard R, Bowen S, Søgaard LV, Flyvbjerg A, Pedersen M, Ardenkjaer-Larsen JH (2013) Assessment of early diabetic renal changes with hyperpolarized [1-13C]pyruvate. Diabetes Metab Res Rev 29:125–129. https://doi.org/10.1002/dmrr.2370
37. von Morze C, Chang GY, Larson PE, Shang H, Allu PK, Bok RA, Crane JC, Olson MP, Tan CT, Marco-Rius I, Nelson SJ, Kurhanewicz J, Pearce D, Vigneron DB (2017) Detection of localized changes in the metabolism of hyperpolarized gluconeogenic precursors 13C-lactate and 13C-pyruvate in the kidneys and liver. Magn Reson Med 77(4):1429–1437
38. Qi H, Nørlinger TS, Nielsen PM, Bertelsen LB, Mikkelsen E, Xu Y, Stødkilde Jørgensen H, Laustsen C (2016) Early diabetic kidney maintains the corticomedullary urea and sodium gradient. Physiol Rep 4:e12714. https://doi.org/10.14814/phy2.12714
39. Bertelsen LB, Nielsen PM, Qi H, Nørlinger TS, Zhang X, Stødkilde Jørgensen H, Laustsen C (2017) Diabetes induced renal urea transport alterations assessed with 3D hyperpolarized 13 C,15 N-urea. Magn Reson Med 77:1650–1655. https://doi.org/10.1002/mrm.26256
40. Keshari KR, Wilson DM, Sai V, Bok R, Jen K-Y, Larson P, Van Criekinge M, Kurhanewicz J, Wang ZJ (2015) Noninvasive in vivo imaging of diabetes-induced renal oxidative stress and response to therapy using hyperpolarized 13C dehydroascorbate magnetic resonance. Diabetes 64:344–352. https://doi.org/10.2337/db13-1829
41. Laustsen C, Lipsø K, Østergaard JA, Nørregaard R, Flyvbjerg A, Pedersen M, Palm F, Ardenkjaer-Larsen JH (2014) Insufficient insulin administration to diabetic rats increases substrate utilization and maintains lactate production in the kidney. Physiol Rep 2:e12233. https://doi.org/10.14814/phy2.12233
42. Qi H, Nielsen PM, Schroeder M, Bertelsen LB, Palm F, Laustsen C (2018) Acute renal metabolic effect of metformin assessed with hyperpolarised MRI in rats. Diabetologia 61:445–454. https://doi.org/10.1007/s00125-017-4445-6
43. Nørlinger TS, Nielsen PM, Qi H, Mikkelsen E, Hansen K, Schmidt NH, Pedersen M, Agger P, Palm F, Laustsen C (2017) Hyperbaric oxygen therapy reduces renal lactate production.

Physiol Rep 5:e13217. https://doi.org/10.14814/phy2.13217

44. Laustsen C, Nielsen PM, Nørlinger TS, Qi H, Pedersen UK, Bertelsen LB, Østergaard JA, Flyvbjerg A, Ardenkjaer-Larsen JH, Palm F, Stødkilde Jørgensen H (2017) Antioxidant treatment attenuates lactate production in diabetic nephropathy. Am J Physiol Renal Physiol 312:F192–F199. https://doi.org/10.1152/ajprenal.00148.2016
45. Koellisch U, Laustsen C, Nørlinger TS, Østergaard JA, Flyvbjerg A, Gringeri CV, Menzel MI, Schulte RF, Haase A, Stødkilde Jørgensen H (2015) Investigation of metabolic changes in STZ-induced diabetic rats with hyperpolarized [1-13C]acetate. Physiol Rep 3:e12474. https://doi.org/10.14814/phy2.12474
46. Nielsen PM, Szocska Hansen ES, Nørlinger TS, Nørregaard R, Bonde Bertelsen L, Stødkilde Jørgensen H, Laustsen C (2016) Renal ischemia and reperfusion assessment with three-dimensional hyperpolarized 13 C,15 N2-urea. Magn Reson Med 76:1524–1530. https://doi.org/10.1002/mrm.26377
47. Mariager CØ, Nielsen PM, Qi H, Ringgaard S, Laustsen C (2018) Hyperpolarized 13 C,15 N2 -urea T2 relaxation changes in acute kidney injury. Magn Reson Med 80:696–702. https://doi.org/10.1002/mrm.27050
48. Nielsen PM, Laustsen C, Bertelsen LB, Qi H, Mikkelsen E, Kristensen MLV, Nørregaard R, Stødkilde Jørgensen H (2017) In situ lactate dehydrogenase activity: a novel renal cortical imaging biomarker of tubular injury? Am J Physiol Renal Physiol 312:F465–F473. https://doi.org/10.1152/ajprenal.00561.2015
49. Baligand C, Qin H, True-Yasaki A, Gordon JW, von Morze C, Delos Santos J, Wilson DM, Raffai R, Cowley PM, Baker AJ, Kurhanewicz J, Lovett DH, Wang ZJ (2017) Hyperpolarized C-13 magnetic resonance evaluation of renal ischemia reperfusion injury in a murine model. NMR Biomed 30(10). https://doi.org/10.1002/nbm.3765
50. Nielsen PM, Eldirdiri A, Bertelsen LB, Jørgensen HS, Ardenkjaer-Larsen JH, Laustsen C (2017) Fumarase activity: an in vivo and in vitro biomarker for acute kidney injury. Sci Rep 7:40812. https://doi.org/10.1038/srep40812

16

Experimental Protocol for MRI Mapping of the Blood Oxygenation-Sensitive Parameters T_2* and T_2 in the Kidney

Andreas Pohlmann, Kaixuan Zhao, Sean B. Fain, Pottumarthi V. Prasad, and Thoralf Niendorf

Abstract

Renal hypoxia is generally accepted as a key pathophysiologic event in acute kidney injury of various origins, and has also been suggested to play a role in the development of chronic kidney disease. Here we describe a step-by-step experimental protocol for indirect monitoring of renal blood oxygenation in rodents via the deoxyhemoglobin sensitive MR parameters T_2* and T_2—a contrast mechanism known as the blood oxygenation level dependent (BOLD) effect. Since an absolute quantification of renal oxygenation from T_2*/T_2 remains challenging, the effects of controlled and standardized variations in the fraction of inspired oxygen are used for bench marking. This MRI method may be useful for investigating renal blood oxygenation of small rodents in vivo under various experimental (patho)physiological conditions.

This chapter is based upon work from the COST Action PARENCHIMA, a community-driven network funded by the European Cooperation in Science and Technology (COST) program of the European Union, which aims to improve the reproducibility and standardization of renal MRI biomarkers. This experimental protocol chapter is complemented by two separate chapters describing the basic concept and data analysis.

Key words Magnetic resonance imaging (MRI), Kidney, Mice, Rats, T_2, T_2*, BOLD

1 Introduction

Renal tissue oxygenation relies on a delicate balance between delivery of O_2, as determined by renal blood flow and arterial O_2 content, and consumption of O_2, which is predominantly determined by energy-dependent tubular reabsorption. Even under physiological conditions, tissue partial pressure of O_2 is low in the medulla. Hence renal tissue hypoxia may result from even a small detrimental imbalance between O_2 delivery and consumption. Based largely upon studies on animal models, intrarenal hypoxia is generally accepted as a key pathophysiologic event in acute kidney injury of various origins, and has also been suggested to promote its progression to chronic kidney disease CKD.

Andreas Pohlmann and Thoralf Niendorf (eds.), *Preclinical MRI of the Kidney: Methods and Protocols*, Methods in Molecular Biology, vol. 2216, https://doi.org/10.1007/978-1-0716-0978-1_23,

The parametric mapping of the transverse relaxation times T_2* and T_2 (or relaxation rates $R_2* = 1/T_2*$ and $R_2 = 1/T_2$) has the potential to allow inferences about renal oxygenation, because both parameters are sensitive to blood oxygenation. The underlying mechanism is the inherent difference in the magnetic properties of oxygenated hemoglobin (diamagnetic) vs. deoxygenated hemoglobin (paramagnetic). The presence of deoxyhemoglobin in a voxel decreases both relaxation times, T_2* and T_2. Additional factors that influence this relationship between renal venous blood oxygenation and renal T_2* include the blood volume fraction, the hematocrit and the oxygen binding curve.

Here we describe quantitative mapping of the blood oxygenation sensitive parameter T_2* in the kidney of small rodents in a step-by-step experimental protocol. The rationale for the chosen acquisition parameters is given in generic terms, together with specific parameter examples.

Mapping of renal T_2 is described as an optional component of the experiment. This may serve two purposes. Firstly, T_2* includes the dynamic (irreversible) dephasing effects described by T_2 plus the additional effects that are due to static (reversible) dephasing effects described by T_2'. Hence, the additional measurement of T_2 permits calculation of $R_2' = R_2* - R_2 = 1/T_2* - 1/T_2$.

Secondly, blood oxygenation affects primarily T_2* (often referred to as blood oxygenation level dependent, BOLD) but also T_2 to a lesser extent. The T_2 effect is via water diffusion within the magnetic field gradient created by deoxyhemoglobin. This contrast mechanism results in T_2 being dominated by blood oxygenation effects in the microvasculature, which makes it a valuable complement to conventional T_2* measurements.

The effects of controlled and standardized variations in T_2* relaxation parameters in response to the fraction of inspired oxygen (hypoxia, hyperoxia) are used for benchmarking. This MRI method may be useful for investigating renal blood oxygenation of rodents in vivo under various experimental (patho)physiological conditions.

This experimental protocol chapter is complemented by two separate chapters describing the basic concept and data analysis, which are part of this book.

This chapter is part of the book Pohlmann A, Niendorf T (eds) (2020) Preclinical MRI of the Kidney—Methods and Protocols. Springer, New York.

2 Materials

2.1 Animals

These experimental protocols are tailored for rats (Wistar, Sprague-Dawley, or Lewis) with a body mass of 250–350 g. Advice for adaptation to mice is given in where necessary.

2.2 Lab Equipment

Anesthesia: For nonrecovery experiments urethane solution (Sigma-Aldrich, Steinheim, Germany; 20% in distilled water) can provide anesthesia for several hours with comparatively little side effects on renal physiology, which is an important issue. For an in-depth description and discussion of the anesthesia please refer to the chapter by Kaucsar T et al. "Preparation and Monitoring of Small Animals in Renal MRI."

Gases: O_2, N_2, and compressed air, as well as a gas-mixing system (FMI Föhr Medical Instruments GmbH, Seeheim-Ober Beerbach, Germany) to achieve required changes in the oxygen fraction of inspired gas mixture (FiO_2). Besides air, the following gas mixtures are required during the experiment: 10% O_2–90% N_2 for hypoxia and 100% O_2 for hyperoxia.

Device for FiO_2 monitoring in gas mixtures: for example Capnomac AGM-103 (Datex GE, Chalfont St Gils, UK).

2.3 MRI Hardware

The general hardware requirements for renal ^1H MRI on mice and rats are described in the chapter by Ramos Delgado P et al. "Hardware Considerations for Preclinical Magnetic Resonance of the Kidney." The technique described in this chapter was tailored for a 9.4 T MR system (Biospec 94/20, Bruker Biospin, Ettlingen, Germany) but advice for adaptation to other field strengths and systems (e.g., 3 T Siemens Skyra or GE MR 750 human MR scanner using a wrist coil for signal reception or transmit-receive knee RF coil is given where necessary. No special or additional hardware is required, except for the following:

1. A physiological monitoring system that can track the respiration, and which is connected to the MR system such that it can be used to trigger the image acquisition.

2.4 MRI Techniques

Repeated measurements with a gradient-echo or spin-echo method and variable echo times (TE) would provide the most accurate T_2^* and T_2 but require very long acquisition times. Here we describe fast multiecho MRI methods: multi-gradient-echo (MGE) for T_2^* measurement and multi–spin-echo (also called "MSME") for T_2 assessment. They provide relaxation times that underestimate T_2^* and overestimate T_2. With increasing echo number additional diffusion weighting is added due to the repeated magnetic field gradients (NB: this effect is much more pronounced in small animal systems because of the much stronger magnetic field gradients used compared to clinical systems). The superposition of stimulated echoes in multi–spin-echo imaging may lead to an overestimation of T_2. Although these biases depend on the acquisition parameters, they are fixed and reproducible for each protocol and hence acceptable in studies of relative differences/changes in T_2^* and T_2, where precision is far more important than accuracy. If needed, more accurate T_2 values can be obtained from multiecho data using sophisticated postprocessing [1].

1. 2D multi-gradient-echo sequence for T_2*-mapping. This is a standard sequence that should be available on all MRI systems. (Bruker "MGE," Siemens "gre"; HE Healthcare 2D ME SPGR or ME FGRE) (*see* **Note 1**).
2. 2D multi-spin-echo sequence for T_2-mapping (optional; Bruker "MSME," Siemens "se_mc"; GE Healthcare "T2 Map" within the 2D ME FGRE family of sequences).
3. 3D double gradient echo sequence for acquiring a quantitative map of the static magnetic field B_0 (optional; Bruker "Field-Map"). The reconstruction performs a phase difference calculation, phase unwrapping, and a conversion to a frequency map. A similar sequence exists with Siemens ("AdjGreSeq"), however there is no reconstruction applied to the data. Choosing Magnitude and Phase under Reconstruction will save both Magnitude and Phase information, but no processing is performed to correct for the B_0 map. Similarly, for GE Healthcare clinical MR systems "IDEAL-IQ" allows for return of fat, water, R_2*, in-phase and out-of-phase water/fat images, but research mode is required to obtain magnitude, phase, and B_0 images.

3 Methods

3.1 MR Protocol Setup

3.1.1 Multi-gradient-Echo Sequence for T_2*-Mapping

1. Load the 2D multi–gradient-echo sequence.
2. Set the shortest echo time (TE) and echo spacing (ΔTE) possible, under the condition that fat and water are in phase (*see* **Note 2**). The last TE should be close to the largest expected $T_2^{(*)}$ in the kidney multiplied by 1.5 (*see* **Note 3**). The aim is to acquire ten or more echo images. Fewer TEs or larger ΔTE are not advisable because during strong hypoxia the SNR in the kidney at high TEs can be so low that only a few data points above the noise level are available for the analysis. Consider increasing the acquisition bandwidth and using half Fourier acceleration to shorten the first TE and ΔTE (*see* **Note 4**).
3. Choose the shortest possible repetition time (TR) for good signal-to-noise per time (SNR/t) efficiency. TR will be limited by the length of the echo train and the number of slices you acquire.
4. Adapt the flip angle (FA) to the TR and T_1 in order to achieve the best possible SNR. Use the Ernst angle $\alpha_E = \arccos(\exp(-TR/T_1))$ as a good starting value. Then try a few smaller and larger FAs and determine the optimal FA experimentally by comparing the measured SNRs in a phantom with a T_1 comparable to that of the renal cortex (1–1.2 s at 3 T).

5. Set a high acquisition bandwidth (BW) to shorten ΔTE, while keeping an eye on the SNR, which decreases with the square root of BW. SNR may be increased with signal averaging. (*see* **Note 5**).
6. Enable fat saturation. On ultrahigh field systems this works well to avoid fat signal overlaying the kidney due to chemical shift. At lower clinical field strengths fat saturation is less efficient.
7. Enable the respiration trigger (per slice). This is essential to reduce motion artefacts, reduce motion blurring and unwanted intensity variations between the images acquired with different TEs.
8. Choose as phase-encoding direction the L-R direction and adapt the geometry so that the FOV in this direction includes the entire animal (approx. 40 mm).
9. Use frequency encoding in head-feet (rostral-caudal) direction to avoid severe aliasing. Adjust the FOV to your needs keeping in mind that in the frequency encoding direction the FOV can be smaller than the animal and a smaller FOV permits a smaller acquisition matrix, and in turn a shorter echo-spacing.
10. Use the lowest slice thickness the SNR allows, typically around 1.5 mm. The thinner the slices the better, as this reduces the unwanted T_2*-effects of macroscopic field inhomogeneities associated with the large voxel size in slice direction. For adaptation of the geometry to mice *see* **Note 6**.
11. Use highest in-plane resolution that the SNR allows, typically between 100 and 200 μm. The higher the resolution the better, as this reduces the unwanted T_2*-effects of macroscopic field inhomogeneities. Zero-filling in phase encoding direction can be helpful to speed up acquisition when monitoring of fast oxygenation changes is required. One may use half Fourier in the frequency encoding direction (asymmetric echo) to further shorten the first TE, if very short T_2* (<5 ms) can occur. Reducing the excitation pulse length to below 1 ms would then also help to shorten TE. For adaptation to mice *see* **Note 7**.
12. For examples of a specific parameter set please *see* **Notes 8–10**.

3.1.2 Multi-spin-Echo Sequence for T_2-Mapping (Optional)

1. Load the 2D multi–spin-echo sequence.
2. Use the same FOV, matrix size and slice thickness as for the multi–gradient-echo sequence.
3. Adapt the repetition time (TR) to the respiration: The effective TR will be given by the respiration trigger and will be the respiration interval, that is, one excitation per breath. Choose TR to be a little shorter (about 100 ms) than the average

respiration interval that is displayed on the physiological monitoring unit (*see* **Note 11**).

4. Set the number of echoes to 12 (*see* **Note 12**.).
5. Set the echo spacing (ΔTE) as small as possible (more echoes are effectively more data points for the analysis and reduce the error; consider that with increasing number of echoes also the SAR increases) and that the last TE is close to the largest expected T_2 in the kidney multiplied by 1.5 (*see* **Note 3**).
6. Due to the artificial increase in signal intensity of fat with a multi–spin-echo sequence, enable fat saturation. Note that the spectral fat saturation does not usually suppress the fat signal completely with some of residual fat signal overlaying the kidney due to chemical shift (Fig. 2).
7. Enable the respiration trigger (per slice).
8. For an example of a specific parameter set please *see* **Notes 13–15**.

3.1.3 Field Map (Optional)

1. Load the field map sequence.
2. Store the field mapping scan protocol with the default parameters when using a small animal system (*see* **Note 16**) or those adapted for a clinical system (*see* **Notes 17** and **18**). Make sure the 3D B_0 field-map has isotropic resolution and a FOV that includes the entire MR-visible part of the animal.

3.2 In Vivo Blood Oxygenation Sensitive Imaging

3.2.1 Animal Preparation

1. Anesthetize the animal and transfer it to scanner. For more information on the choice and use of anesthesia please refer to the chapter by Kaucsar T et al. "Preparation and Monitoring of Small Animals in Renal MRI."
2. Start the temperature monitoring system, apply some surgical lubricant to the temperature probe and place it in the rectum of the animal.
3. Attach the respiration sensor (e.g., balloon) to the chest of the animal using adhesive tape. Start and setup the respiratory monitoring system. If necessary, adjust the position of the respiration sensor until the amplitude of the respiration trace is sufficiently large for the system to reliably detect the trigger points at the beginning of expiration.

3.2.2 Scanner Adjustments and Anatomical Imaging

1. Acquire a fast pilot scan to obtain images in the three orthogonal planes *x*, *y*, and *z*.
2. Acquire anatomical images in several oblique orientations to facilitate planning a coronal slice orientation with regard to the long axis of the kidney, as described in the chapter by Pohlmann A et al. "Essential Practical Steps for MRI of the Kidney in Experimental Research."

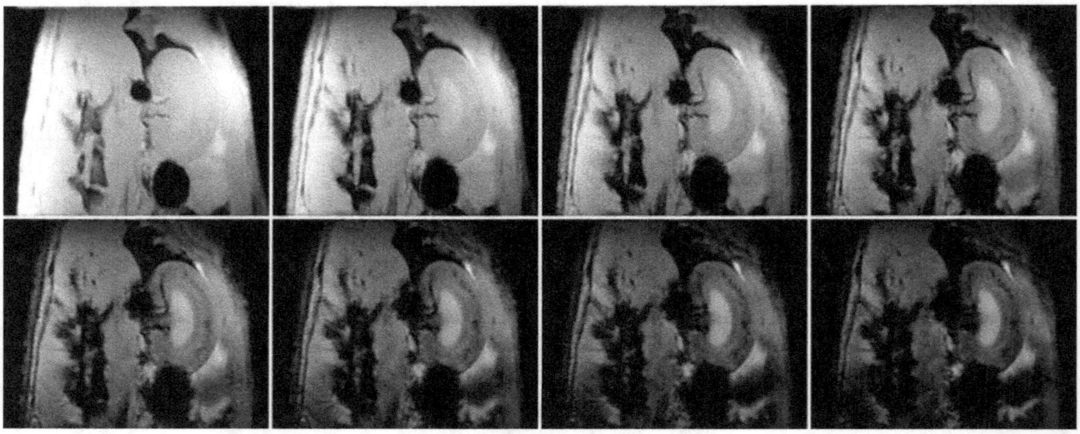

Fig. 1 Series of 8 T_2*-weighted images of a healthy rat kidney acquired with a multi–gradient-echo sequence at 9.4 T. Images correspond to TE = 1.43, 3.57, 5.71, 7.85 ms (top row), TE = 9.99, 12.13, 14.27, 16.41 ms (bottom row)

3. Perform localized shimming on the kidney as described in the chapter by Pohlmann A et al. "Essential Practical Steps for MRI of the Kidney in Experimental Research" (*see* **Note 19**).
4. Acquire a 3D B0 field-map without adaptation of the geometry (optional; *see* **Note 20**).

3.2.3 Baseline Condition

1. Load the T_2*-mapping sequence, adapt the slice orientation to provide a coronal or axial view with respect to the kidney (in scanner coordinates this is double-oblique).
2. In the monitoring unit set the trigger delay so that the trigger starts at the beginning of the expiratory plateau (no chest or diaphragm motion) and the duration such that it covers the entire expiratory phase, that is, until just before inhalation starts (1/2 to 2/3 of breath-to-breath interval) (*see* **Note 11**).
3. Run the T_2*-mapping scan. Example images are shown in Fig. 1.
4. Load the T_2-mapping sequence, adapt the slice orientation to provide a coronal or axial view with respect to the kidney (in scanner coordinates this is double-oblique).
5. Adapt TR to be a little shorter (about 100 ms) than the average respiration interval that is displayed on the physiological monitoring unit.
6. In the monitoring unit set the trigger delay so that the trigger starts at the beginning of the expiratory plateau (no chest or diaphragm motion) and the duration to a short value, such as 10 ms (**Note 11**).
7. Run the T_2-mapping scan. Example images are shown in Fig. 2.

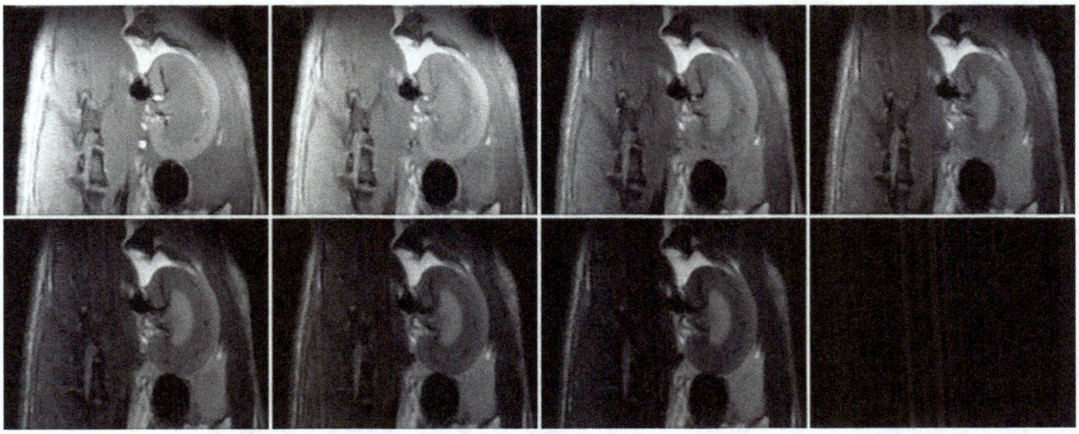

Fig. 2 Series of 7 T_2-weighted images of a healthy rat kidney acquired with a 2D multi-spin-echo sequence at 9.4 T. Images correspond to TE = 10, 20, 30, 40 ms (top row) and TE = 50, 60, 70 ms (bottom row)

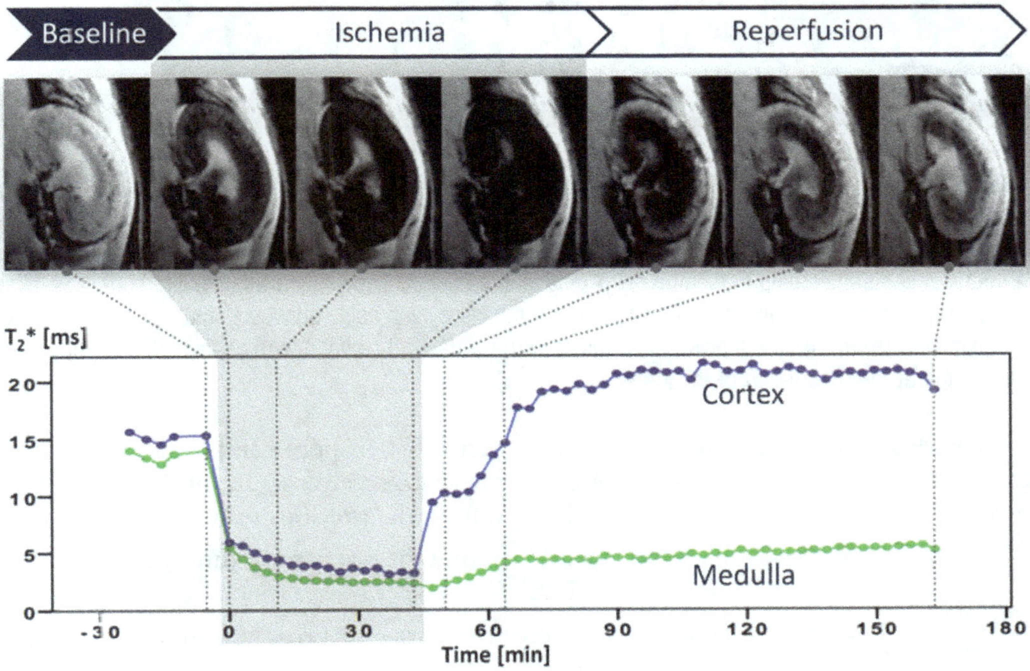

Fig. 3 Demonstration of the contrast changes that can be expected in pathophysiological scenarios. T_2*-weighted images (from a 2D multi–gradient-echo acquisition, TE = 3.57 ms) of rat kidneys throughout an ischemia–reperfusion experiment, together with a plot of T_2* in regions-of-interest in renal cortex and medulla

A demonstration of the contrast changes that can be expected in pathophysiological scenarios is given in Fig. 3. Example parametric maps of T_2* and T_2 are shown in Fig. 4.

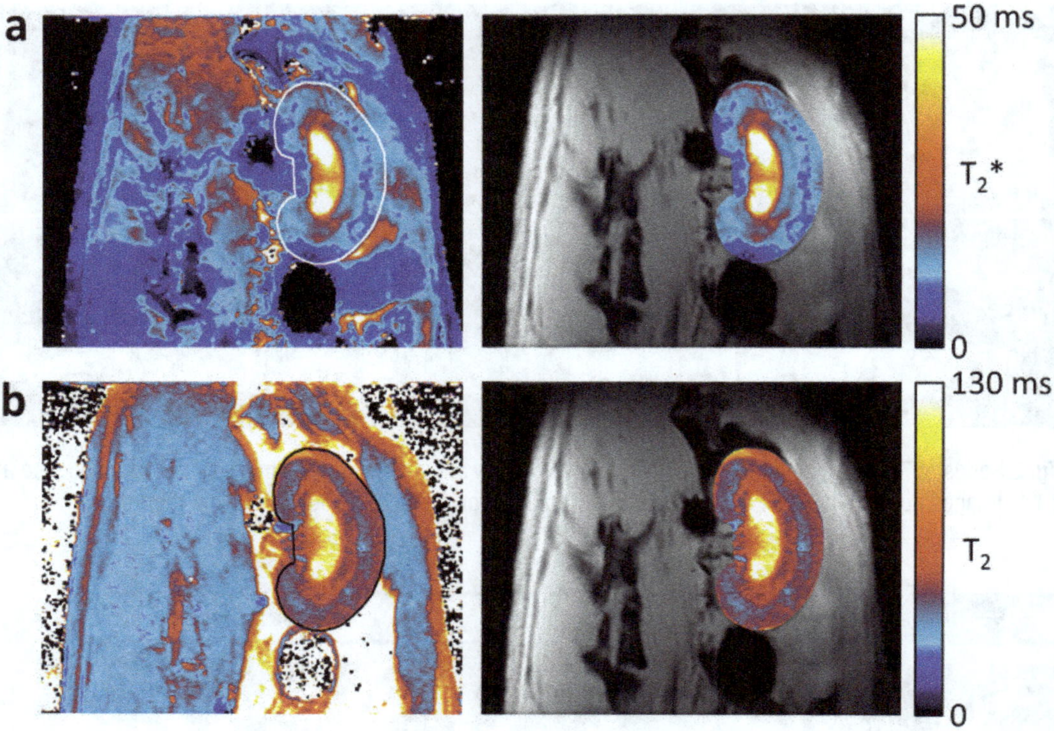

Fig. 4 Example parametric maps of T_2* (**a**) and T_2 (**b**) acquired in a rat at 9.4 T. Shown are the entire map with the kidney outlined (left) as well as an overlay of the map onto an anatomical MR image (right). While the overlays are preferable because they focus on the relevant part and do not distract the eye, looking at the entire map can sometimes help to identify extra-renal sources of susceptibility artefacts, like here the bowel gas below the kidney and an implanted device near the hilus, which cast "shadows" onto the renal cortex. Beware to exclude from the ROI analysis any regions with overlaid fat signal due to chemical shift, here seen as a thin stripe at the rostral end of the kidney

3.2.4 Hypoxia/Hyperoxia for Benchmarking (optional)

1. Duplicate the two scans (T_2*-mapping and T_2-mapping) and disable all adjustments (e.g., receiver gain, shimming) so that they are not changed from the previous scan.
2. Start hypoxia by changing the gas flowing through the respiratory mask to 10% O_2/90% N_2.
3. Three minutes after the start of hypoxia run the T_2*-mapping and T_2-mapping scans. Hypoxia should not exceed 5 min in order to avoid long lasting effects.
4. Immediately after the two scans end, change the gas flowing through the respiratory mask back to air (21% O_2).
5. Wait for a recovery time of at least 5 min.
6. Start hyperoxia by changing the gas flowing through the respiratory mask to 100% O_2.
7. Two minutes after the start of hyperoxia run the T_2*-mapping and T_2-mapping scans.

8. Immediately after the two scans end change the gas flowing through the respiratory mask back to air (21% O_2).
9. Wait for a recovery time of at least 5 min before conducting any further interventions.

3.2.5 Noise Scan

We highly recommend acquiring one scan with the T_2*-mapping protocol and T_2-mapping protocol that only contains noise. This is the best way to estimate the noise standard deviation, which is needed for correcting the noise bias during the data analysis (*see* **Note 21**). Alternatively it is possible to estimate the noise standard deviation from an ROI in the "background" of the study images, but it is often difficult to find a suitable region outside the subject that is large enough and artefact free.

1. Create a copy of the T_2*-mapping protocol.
2. Open the protocol and in the parameter setting set either the flip angle to 0° degrees or the reference power for the flip angle calibration to 0 W.
3. Run the T_2*-mapping scan.
4. Repeat **steps 1–3** for the T_2-mapping protocol.

4 Notes

1. A 3D version of this sequence is also available, which allows for thinner slices with better SNR, but tends to be too slow for most in vivo applications.
2. The fat signal has a slightly different Lamor frequency ($\Delta f = 220$ Hz/Tesla) than the water signal. The faster precession of the fat protons means that with increasing time the fat and water signal fractions within a voxel are sometimes in phase (signals add up) and sometimes out of phase (signals subtract). This can lead to an additional unwanted variation in the signal along the exponential decay curve. This is mostly relevant for diseased kidneys with increased fat content (e.g., diabetes), but we recommend to generally take this into account, that is, also for healthy kidneys. The TEs at which fat and water are in phase depend on the field strength: $\text{TE [ms]} = n \cdot (6.7069/B_0[T])$.
3. Larger TEs are needed to accurately calculate longer $T_2^{(*)}$ under normal or hyperoxic conditions. We recommend using the largest expected $T_2^{(*)}$ in the kidney multiplied by 1.5 as the largest TE. Since the largest $T_2^{(*)}$ is typically in the inner medulla—if this region is not relevant to your research then use the largest $T_2^{(*)}$ in the cortex/outer medulla. With increasing TE the signal intensity decreases and may reach the noise floor at large TEs. This can introduce a noise bias during data

analysis. To account for this we recommend performing a retrospective noise correction (preferred) or exclude images acquired at larger TEs from the analysis. Both approaches are described in the chapter by Periquito JS et al. "Analysis Protocols for MRI Mapping of the Blood Oxygenation–Sensitive Parameters T_2^* and T_2 in the Kidney."

4. Renal T_2* may be quite short at ultrahigh field strengths and in particular under hypoxia, which is what one wishes to detect. One needs to consider the shortest renal T_2* that could occur during experiment; under extreme conditions this could be only a few milliseconds, so several TEs around that value are needed.
5. When establishing the MR technique you need to define an SNR acceptance threshold for the image with the shortest TE. The aim is to have at least three (better five or more) number of echoes with an SNR > 5. This threshold will depend on the expected $T_2^{(*)}$ values, which in turn depends on parameters like the magnetic field strength, shim quality, and tissue properties (pathology). Example: for a rat imaged at 9.4 T using a 4-element rat heart array receive surface coil together with a volume resonator for excitation in combination with interventions leading to strong hypoxia, an SNR > 60 was needed.
6. For mice reduce the FOV to the body width and keep the matrix size the same. The relative resolution is then identical and the SNR should also be similar, because the smaller mouse RF coil gives better SNR, for example, mouse heart four-element surface coil vs rat heart four-element surface coil.
7. A good starting point is to use the same relative resolution as for rats. For this, reduce the FOV to the mouse body width and keep the matrix size the same.
8. *Example parameters for T_2* mapping of a 300 g rat at 9.4 T (Bruker small animal system)*: TR = 50 ms; flip angle = 16°; pulse length 1.0 ms; pulse bandwidth 5.4 kHz; receiver bandwidth = 109 kHz; number of echoes = 12; first echo = 2.14 ms; echo spacing 2.14 ms; TE = 2.14, 4.28, 6.42, 8.56, 10.7, 12.84, 14.98, 17.12, 19.26, 21.40, 23.54, 25.68 ms; averages = 4; slice orientation = coronal to kidney; frequency encoding = head-feet; FOV = (38.2 × 48.5) mm; matrix size = 169 × 115 zero-filled to 169 × 215; resolution = (0.226 × 0.421) mm; 1–3 slices with 1.4 mm thickness; fat suppression = on; respiration trigger = per slice; acquisition time = 40–60 s (with triggering under urethane anaesthesia).
9. *Example parameters for T_2* mapping of a 30 g mouse at 4.7 T (Agilent small animal system)*: TR = 350 ms; flip angle = 30°; receiver bandwidth = 100 kHz; number of echoes = 32; first

echo = 2.0 ms; echo spacing 2.4 ms; TE = 2.00, 4.40, 6.80, 9.20, 11.60, 14.00, 16.40, 18.80, 21.20, 23.60, 26.00, …, 76.40 ms; averages = 4; slice orientation = coronal to kidney; frequency encoding = head-feet; FOV = (30 × 30) mm; matrix size = 128 × 128; resolution = (0.230 × 0.230) mm; 1 slice with 1.0 mm thickness; fat suppression = on; respiration trigger = on; acquisition time = 3.5–9.0 min (with triggering under isoflurane anaesthesia).

10. *Example parameters for T_2* mapping of a 300 g rat at 3.0 T (Siemens Skyra^{fit}, a clinical system)*: Animal position: Right decubitus; Coil: Knee; TR = 69 ms; flip angle = 30°; receiver bandwidth = 320 Hz/pixel; number of echoes = 12; first echo = 3.56 ms; echo spacing 3.43 ms; TE = 3.56, 6.99, 10.42, 13.85, 17.28, 20.71, 24.14, 27.57, 31.00, 34.43, 37.86, 41.29 ms; averages = 20; slice orientation = axial; frequency encoding = anterior-posterior; FOV = (120 × 60) mm; matrix size = 256 × 128; resolution = (0.470 × 0.470) mm; 3 slices with 2.0 mm thickness; fat suppression = on; respiration trigger = off; acquisition time ~ 3 min. If one desires in-phase echoes, use first echo = 4.92 and echo spacing = 4.92 ms. If no specific animal holder is used, it is preferable to position the animals in left of right decubitus position to keep the bowels away from the kidneys to mitigate susceptibility artifacts.
11. You must monitor the respiration continuously throughout the entire experiment and if necessary adapt the TR accordingly.
12. Acquiring more echoes with smaller echo spacing will be beneficial because it improves the fitting, but keep in mind the SAR associated with sending many 180° RF pulses in a short time could heat up the tissue. This will usually not be detectable via a rectal temperature probe, but measurements with a temperature probe placed in the abdomen next to the kidney showed that significant temperature increases are possible with a multi–spin-echo sequence.
13. *Example parameters for T_2 mapping of a 300 g rat at 9.4 T (Bruker small animal system)*: TR = [respiration interval] − 100 ms; receiver bandwidth = 50 kHz; number of echoes = 12; first echo = 10.0 ms; echo spacing 10.0 ms; TE = 10, 20, 30, 40, 50, 60, 70, 80, 90, 100, 110, 120 ms; averages = 1; slice orientation = coronal to kidney; frequency encoding = head-feet; FOV = (38.2 × 48.5) mm; matrix size = 169 × 115 zero-filled to 169 × 215; resolution = (0.226 × 0.421) mm; 1 slice with 1.4 mm thickness; fat suppression = on; respiration trigger = per slice; acquisition time = 55–75 s (with triggering under urethane anaesthesia).

14. *Example parameters for T_2 mapping of a 30 g mouse at 4.7 T (Agilent small animal system)*: TR = [respiration interval] -100 ms; receiver bandwidth = 50 kHz; number of echoes = 12; first echo = 10.0 ms; echo spacing 10.0 ms; TE = 10, ..., 120 ms; averages = 1; slice orientation = coronal to kidney; frequency encoding = head-feet; FOV = (30 × 30) mm; matrix size = 128 × 128; resolution = (0.230 × 0.230) mm; 1 slice with 2.0 mm thickness; fat suppression = on; respiration trigger = on; acquisition time = 2–4 min (with triggering under isoflurane anaesthesia).
15. *Example parameters for T_2 mapping of a 300 g rat at 3.0 T (Siemens Skyra^{fit}, a clinical system)*: Animal position: Right decubitus; Coil: Knee; TR = [respiration interval] – 500 ms; receiver bandwidth = 399 Hz/pixel; number of echoes = 12; first echo = 10.0 ms; echo spacing 10.0 ms; TE = 10, ..., 120 ms; averages = 2; slice orientation = axial; frequency encoding = left-right; FOV = (120 × 60) mm; matrix size = 256 × 128; resolution = (0.470 × 0.470) mm; 1 slice with 2.0 mm thickness; fat suppression = on; respiration trigger = off; acquisition time ~2 min. If no specific animal holder is used, it is preferable to position the animals in left of right decubitus position to keep the bowels away from the kidneys to mitigate susceptibility artifacts.
16. *Example parameters for field mapping of a 300 g rat at 9.4 T (Bruker small animal system)*: use the vendors default protocol *AnyObject > AnyRegion > Adjustments > ADJ_B0MAP*. TR = 20 ms; flip angle = 30°; first echo = 1.60 ms; echo spacing = 3.57 ms; fat/water in-phase = on; slice orientation = main orientations (no angles) and offset = 0; FOV = (58 × 58 × 58) mm; matrix size = 64 × 64 × 64; resolution = (0.906 × 0.906 × 0.906) mm; respiration trigger = off; acquisition time = 1–2 min.
17. *Example parameters for field mapping of a 300 g rat at 3.0 T (Siemens Skyra^{fit}, a clinical system)*: The default setup uses the BODY Coil. TR = 20 ms; flip angle = 15°; in-phase echo times, first echo = 4.78 ms, and second echo = 7.17 ms; slice orientation = main orientations (no angles) and offset = 0; FOV = (350 × 350) mm; matrix size = 96 × 96; resolution = (3.6 × 3.6 × 8.0) mm; GRAPPA factor = 2; respiration trigger = off; acquisition time = 17 s.
18. *Example parameters for field mapping of a 300 g rat at 4.7 T (Agilent small animal system)*: TR = 34 ms; flip angle = 30°; number of echoes = 8; first echo = 4.23 ms; echo spacing 0.4 ms; averages = 8; slice orientation = coronal to kidney; frequency encoding = head-feet; FOV = (30 × 30) mm; matrix size = 128 × 128; resolution = (0.230 × 0.230) mm;

1 slice with 2.0 mm thickness; fat suppression = on; respiration trigger = on; acquisition time = 7.0–11.0 min (with triggering under isoflurane anaesthesia).

19. Shimming is particularly important, since macroscopic magnetic field inhomogeneities shorten T_2*, but provide no tissue specific information—rather they overshadow the microscopic T_2* effects of interest and hinder quantitative intra- and inter-subject comparisons. Shimming should be performed on a voxel enclosing only the kidney using either the default iterative shimming method or the Mapshim technique (recommended).
20. This serves to keep a record of the B_0 influence on the measured T_2*. It allows explanation of unusually small T_2* due to a bad shim. It may also be used later during the prost-processing for calculating a corrected T_2* by removing the influence B_0 inhomogeneities.
21. During the data analysis care must be taken to avoid noise biasing the mapping of T_2* and T_2. With increasing echo time the signal intensity in the images approaches more and more the noise floor, where the signal is so small that it is not detectable anymore. However, even though only noise is detected the signal is still above 0, because of the Ricean nature of the noise (negative values are "flipped" to the positive side). This means that the shape of the exponential curve will not fit well, as it expects the signal to decay toward 0. Adding an offset parameter to the fitted curve does not solve the problem because an offset will affect the signal intensities of all echoes, but the noise bias only affects those echoes where the true signal is very small. Instead a noise bias correction should be performed, which is described in the chapter by Periquito JS et al. "Analysis Protocols for MRI Mapping of the Blood Oxygenation–Sensitive Parameters T_2* and T_2 in the Kidney." Please note that you may not need to perform such a noise correction if all echo images are well above the noise floor.

Acknowledgments

This work was funded, in part (Thoralf Niendorf and Andreas Pohlmann), by the German Research Foundation (Gefoerdert durch die Deutsche Forschungsgemeinschaft (DFG), Projektnummer 394046635, SFB 1365, RENOPROTECTION. Funded by the Deutsche Forschungsgemeinschaft (DFG, German Research Foundation), Project number 394046635, SFB 1365, RENOPROTECTION).

This publication is based upon work from COST Action PARENCHIMA, supported by European Cooperation in Science and

Technology (COST). COST (www.cost.eu) is a funding agency for research and innovation networks. COST Actions help connect research initiatives across Europe and enable scientists to grow their ideas by sharing them with their peers. This boosts their research, career and innovation.

PARENCHIMA (renalmri.org) is a community-driven Action in the COST program of the European Union, which unites more than 200 experts in renal MRI from 30 countries with the aim to improve the reproducibility and standardization of renal MRI biomarkers.

Reference

1. Ben-Eliezer N, Sodickson DK, Block KT (2015) Rapid and accurate T2 mapping from multi-spin-echo data using bloch-simulation-based reconstruction. Magn Reson Med 73:809–817

Permissions

All chapters in this book were first published in PMRITKMP, by Springer; hereby published with permission under the Creative Commons Attribution License or equivalent. Every chapter published in this book has been scrutinized by our experts. Their significance has been extensively debated. The topics covered herein carry significant findings which will fuel the growth of the discipline. They may even be implemented as practical applications or may be referred to as a beginning point for another development.

The contributors of this book come from diverse backgrounds, making this book a truly international effort. This book will bring forth new frontiers with its revolutionizing research information and detailed analysis of the nascent developments around the world.

We would like to thank all the contributing authors for lending their expertise to make the book truly unique. They have played a crucial role in the development of this book. Without their invaluable contributions this book wouldn't have been possible. They have made vital efforts to compile up to date information on the varied aspects of this subject to make this book a valuable addition to the collection of many professionals and students.

This book was conceptualized with the vision of imparting up-to-date information and advanced data in this field. To ensure the same, a matchless editorial board was set up. Every individual on the board went through rigorous rounds of assessment to prove their worth. After which they invested a large part of their time researching and compiling the most relevant data for our readers.

The editorial board has been involved in producing this book since its inception. They have spent rigorous hours researching and exploring the diverse topics which have resulted in the successful publishing of this book. They have passed on their knowledge of decades through this book. To expedite this challenging task, the publisher supported the team at every step. A small team of assistant editors was also appointed to further simplify the editing procedure and attain best results for the readers.

Apart from the editorial board, the designing team has also invested a significant amount of their time in understanding the subject and creating the most relevant covers. They scrutinized every image to scout for the most suitable representation of the subject and create an appropriate cover for the book.

The publishing team has been an ardent support to the editorial, designing and production team. Their endless efforts to recruit the best for this project, has resulted in the accomplishment of this book. They are a veteran in the field of academics and their pool of knowledge is as vast as their experience in printing. Their expertise and guidance has proved useful at every step. Their uncompromising quality standards have made this book an exceptional effort. Their encouragement from time to time has been an inspiration for everyone.

The publisher and the editorial board hope that this book will prove to be a valuable piece of knowledge for researchers, students, practitioners and scholars across the globe.

List of Contributors

Min-Chi Ku, Adrian Schreiber, Paula Ramos Delgado, Philipp Boehm-Sturm, Ralph Kettritz and Sonia Waiczies

Christian Prinz, Ludger Starke, Jason M. Millward, Jens Rosenberg, Marc Nazaré and Helmar Waiczies

Andreas Pohlmann and Thoralf Niendorf

Cornelius von Morze and Galen D. Reed

Pietro Irrera, Lorena Consolino, Walter Dastrù, Michael Pedersen, Frank G. Zöllner and Dario Livio Longo

Suraj D. Serai and Meng Yin

Kowsalya Devi Pavuluri, Lorena Consolino, Phillip Zhe Sun and Michael T. McMahon

Kathleen Cantow, Mechthild Ladwig-Wiegard, Bert Flemming and Erdmann Seeliger

Andreas Müller

James T. Grist, Frank and Christoffer Laustsen

Philippe Garteiser, Octavia Bane, Sabrina Doblas, Iris Friedli, Stefanie Hectors, Gwenaë l Pagé, Bernard E. Van Beers and John C. Waterton

João S. Periquito and Neil Peter Jerome

Kai-Hsiang Chuang, Martin Meier, Marıà A. Fernández-Seara and Frank Kober

James T. Grist and Esben Søvsø Hansen

Cornelius von Morze, Galen D. Reed, Zhen J. Wang and Michael A. Ohliger

Kaixuan Zhao, Sean B. Fain and Pottumarthi V. Prasad

Index